Applying Metaverse Technologies to Human-Computer Interaction for Healthcare

The concept of the metaverse signifies the forthcoming stage of development of the Internet, wherein it will facilitate the creation of virtual worlds that are enduring, decentralized, and capable of providing immersive experiences in real time. The metaverse has vast potential for utilization in the domains of life sciences and healthcare, hence motivating investigations in contemporary trends, early adoption use cases, and the forthcoming opportunities it presents. The metaverse also possesses the capacity to fundamentally transform decentralized clinical trials through the elimination of physical and geographical constraints. This change in thinking entails the relocation of clinical trials from conventional settings to the comfort and convenience of patients' residences, resulting in improvements in health behavior, medication adherence, remote monitoring, and other associated factors.

Applying Metaverse Technologies to Human-Computer Interaction for Healthcare focuses on the current developments in the metaverse, investigates its applications in the life sciences and healthcare industry based on metaverse powered human—computer interactions (HCI), analyzes early adoption use cases that provide measurable commercial benefits, and anticipates prospects in this rapidly evolving domain.

The book examines the treatment, management, and prevention of illnesses with the use of immersive therapeutics that use augmented reality (AR), virtual reality (VR), and mixed reality (MR). It examines applications in cognitive therapy, support groups, psychiatric examinations, rehabilitation, and even physical therapy The book covers how healthcare practitioners have the capability to provide such services as diagnosis, treatment, monitoring, and care in remote settings, through the utilization of AR headsets and wearable devices. It concludes by discussing the continuous development of technology to facilitate the growth and maturation of the metaverse, hence enabling substantial business benefits for the life sciences and healthcare industries.

B. Sundaravadivazhagan, PhD, is a faculty member in the Department of Information Technology at the University of Technology, and Applied Science—AL Mussanah in Oman.

Balasubramaniam S, PhD, is an assistant professor in the School of Computer Science and Engineering, Kerala University of Digital Sciences, Innovation and Technology, Digital University Kerala, India.

Pethuru Raj, PhD, is a chief architect at the Edge AI division of Reliance Jio Platforms Ltd. (JPL) Bangalore, India.

K. Shantha Kumari, PhD, is with the Department of Data Science and Business Systems, SRM Institute of Science and Technology, Chengalpattu, Tamil Nadu, India.

Applying Metaverse Technologies to Human-Computer Interaction for Healthcare

Edited by
B. Sundaravadivazhagan, Balasubramaniam S,
Pethuru Raj, and K. Shantha Kumari

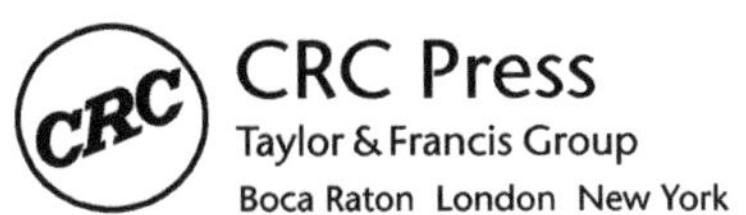

CRC Press
Taylor & Francis Group
Boca Raton London New York

CRC Press is an imprint of the
Taylor & Francis Group, an **informa** business

AN AUERBACH BOOK

Designed cover image: © Shutterstock

First edition published 2025
by CRC Press
2385 NW Executive Center Drive, Suite 320, Boca Raton FL 33431

and by CRC Press
4 Park Square, Milton Park, Abingdon, Oxon, OX14 4RN

CRC Press is an imprint of Taylor & Francis Group, LLC

© 2025 selection and editorial matter, B. Sundaravadivazhagan, Balasubramaniam S, Pethuru Raj, and K. Shantha Kumari; individual chapters, the contributors.

ISBN: 9781032792378 (hbk)
ISBN: 9781032793689 (pbk)
ISBN: 9781003491668 (ebk)

DOI: 10.1201/9781003491668

Typeset in Adobe Garamond
by KnowledgeWorks Global Ltd.

Contents

Preface

In the dynamic context of contemporary society, researchers are constantly engaged in the pursuit of achieving a state of balance between the virtual and physical domains. This endeavor involves the contemplation of several tangible aspects inside the digital realm. In this digital realm, individuals possess the capacity to participate in social exchanges and partake in many activities, including purchasing and consumption. The metaverse is an expansive virtual computer platform that encompasses a broad range of individual users, their own gadgets, and many platforms. The successful achievement of this goal is contingent upon the proficient execution of human–computer interaction (HCI) within the realm of metaverse advancement, particularly in the smooth translation of user activities into the virtual world. HCI is a systematic procedure that enables the transfer of information between individuals and computer systems in a manner that is tailored to accomplish predetermined objectives.

The essential premise of the metaverse centers around the elimination of boundaries between the virtual and physical domains, facilitating the seamless execution of real-world tasks through technology equipment within a virtual environment. Emerging from the field of HCI, the metaverse undergoes a transformative process, developing into a complex and interconnected digital network comprising multiple virtual realms. The metaverse possesses particular characteristics that render it well suited for a wide range of applications within the context of massively multiplayer online situations. These applications encompass multiplayer games, video chats, distance learning, remote work, and various other functionalities. The metaverse is a fusion of modern interactive technologies, necessitating the presence of technological infrastructure grounded in the principles of HCI. The provision of this support is crucial in facilitating the translation of human actions into computer input and effectively reintegrating them into the virtual domain. Extended reality (XR) is a crucial element of this support system, covering virtual reality (VR), augmented reality (AR), and mixed reality (MR) technologies. These technologies are specifically developed for interaction through wearable devices. By utilizing XR technology, the host computer receives real-time user actions and then displays them on the web platform through network connections. This feature facilitates the participation of multiple users in synchronous activities on the platform, hence promoting engagement and the establishment of a sense of community. In the present setting, the importance of VR and AR technology and gadgets is particularly emphasized.

The concept of the metaverse signifies the forthcoming stage of development for the Internet, wherein it will facilitate the creation of virtual worlds that are enduring, decentralized, and capable of providing immersive experiences in real time. The metaverse has vast potential for utilization in the domains of life sciences and healthcare, hence motivating us to investigate new trends, early adoption uses cases, and the forthcoming opportunities it presents. The metaverse possesses the capacity to fundamentally transform decentralized clinical trials through the elimination of physical and geographical constraints. This paradigm shift entails the relocation of clinical trials from conventional settings to the comfort and convenience of patients' residences, resulting in improvements in health behavior, medication adherence, remote monitoring, and other associated factors. When it comes to the treatment, management, and prevention of medical illnesses, immersive therapeutics is all about using medical interventions that utilize AR, VR, and MR. Applications such as cognitive therapy, support groups, psychiatric examinations, rehabilitation, and even physical therapy are emerging in the metaverse, with the use of haptic sensors. Within the metaverse, surgeons have the ability to fully engage themselves in an environment that facilitates the acquisition of knowledge, the development of intricate surgical strategies, and the refinement of their abilities with heightened accuracy and uniformity. By utilizing technology, it becomes possible to recreate the distinct pathology of individual patients in a three-dimensional manner, so enabling comprehensive practice and preoperative preparation for surgical procedures. In the current practice of radiology diagnosis, medical pictures are commonly observed in a sequential fashion, one slice at a time, on two-dimensional displays. Nevertheless, the progression of medical imaging visualization shows potential in augmenting the efficacy of disease analysis and surgical planning. The metaverse, characterized by its immersive and technologically advanced visualization capabilities, possesses the potential to offer enhanced interactivity and realism in the realm of medical experiences. The integration of extended reality tools within the metaverse offers a promising telehealth option. Healthcare practitioners have the capability to provide a variety of services, such as diagnosis, treatment, monitoring, and care, through the utilization of AR headsets and wearable devices in remote settings. Moreover, the immersive attributes of VR function as a proficient mechanism to divert patients' attention and mitigate tension during healthcare encounters. The continuous development of technology is expected to facilitate the growth and maturation of the metaverse, hence enabling substantial business benefits for the life sciences and healthcare industries. This evolutionary process is anticipated to effectively tackle some of the imminent issues within these sectors.

This book focuses on the current developments in the metaverse, investigates its applications in the life sciences and healthcare industry based on metaverse powered HCI, analyzes early adoption use cases that provide measurable commercial benefits, and anticipates future prospects in this rapidly evolving domain.

About the Editors

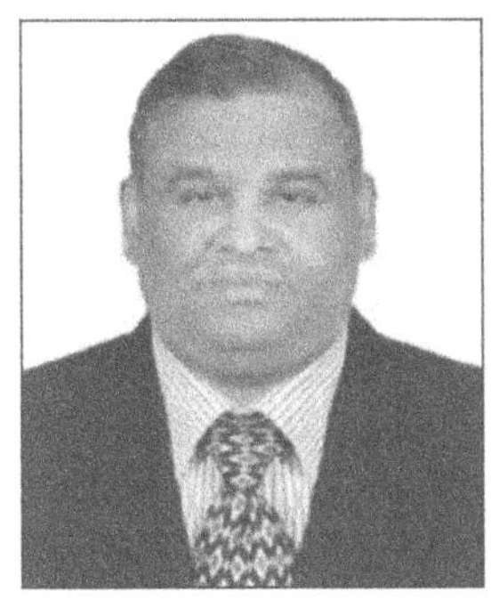

B. Sundaravadivazhagan, PhD, has obtained his PhD in computer science from Anna University, Chennai India. Currently, he is a faculty member in the Department of Information Technology at the University of Technology, and Applied Science—AL Mussanah in Oman. He has professional memberships in ISACA and the Indian Society for Technical Education (ISTE) and is a senior member of the Institute for Electrical and Electronics Engineers (IEEE). His academic and research background spans more than 23 years at many institutions. He is working on two financed research projects for the Ministry of Higher Education Research Innovation in Oman via The Research Council (TRC). His research interests include cybersecurity, artificial intelligence and machine learning, deep learning, and cloud computing. He has published more than 75 technical articles in journals and conferences throughout the world.

Orcid Id: https://orcid.org/my-orcid?orcid=0000-0002-5515-5769

Academic URL: https://www.utas.edu.om/mussanah/Academics/Information-Technology/IT_Faculty

LinkedIn: https://www.linkedin.com/in/dr-b-sundaravadivazhagan-a3562b136/

Google Scholar: https://scholar.google.com/citations?user=gWbzTjMAAAAJ&hl=en

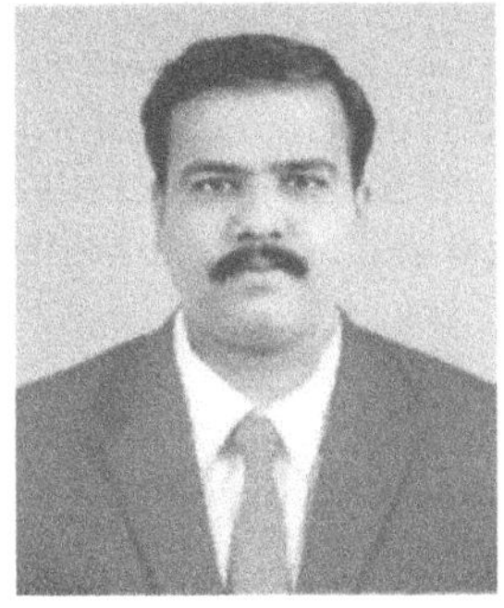

Balasubramaniam S, PhD, (IEEE Senior Member) is working as an assistant professor in School of Computer Science and Engineering, Kerala University of Digital Sciences, Innovation and Technology (Formerly IIITM-K), Digital University Kerala, Thiruvananthapuram, Kerala, India. Before joining Digital University Kerala, he served as a Senior Associate Professor at the School of Computer Science and Engineering, Vellore Institute of Technology (VIT), Chennai, Tamilnadu, India He has a total of over ten years of experience in teaching, research, and industry.

He has completed his postdoctoral research in the Department of Applied Data Science, Noroff University College, Kristiansand, Norway. He holds a PhD degree in computer science and engineering from Anna University, Chennai, India in 2015. He has published nearly 25+ research papers in the reputed *Science Citation Index* (SCI), *Web of Science* (WoS), and *Scopus* indexed journals. He has also granted with one Australian patent and two Indian patents and published two Indian patents. He has presented papers at conferences and contributed chapters to edited books and served as editor for few books published by international publishers. His research and publication interests include machine learning and deep learning–based disease diagnosis, federated learning, cloud computing security, generative AI, and electric vehicles.

Orcid Id: https://orcid.org/my-orcid?orcid=0000-0003-1371-3088

LinkedIn: https://www.linkedin.com/in/dr-balasubramaniam-s-6873533b/

Google Scholar: https://scholar.google.co.in/citations?user=1KGLST0AAAAJ&hl=en

Academic url: https://duk.ac.in/personnel/balasubramaniam-s/

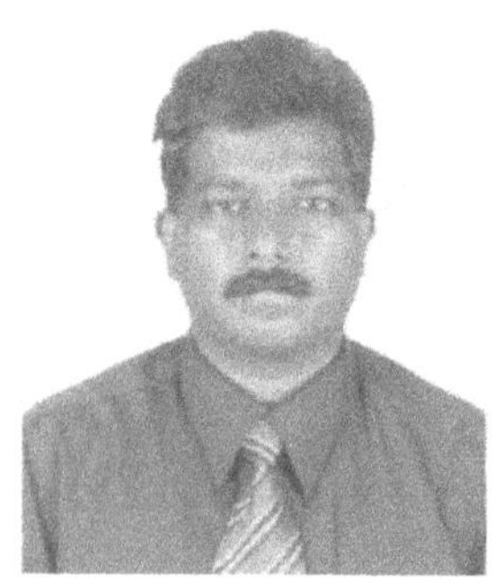

Pethuru Raj, PhD, is a chief architect at the Edge AI division of Reliance Jio Platforms Ltd. (JPL) Bangalore. Previously he worked at the IBM Global Cloud Centre of Excellence (CoE), Wipro consulting services (WCS), and Robert Bosch Corporate Research (CR). Raj has gained over 23 years of information technology (IT) industry experience and nine years of research experience. He finished the Council of Scientific and Industrial Research (CSIR)–sponsored PhD degree at Anna University, Chennai, and continued with the University Grants Commission (UGC)–sponsored postdoctoral research in the Department of Computer Science and Automation, Indian Institute of Science (IISc), Bangalore. After that, Raj was granted two international research fellowships (Japan Society for the Promotion of Science [JSPS] and Japan Science and Technology Agency [JST]) to work as a research scientist for 3.5 years at two leading Japanese universities.

Dr. Raj is focusing on some of the emerging technologies such as the Industrial Internet of Things (IIoT); Efficient, Explainable, and Edge AI; prompt engineering for large language models (LLMs); blockchain; digital twins; cloud-native and edge computing; green and generative AI; reliability and platform engineering for agile software engineering; 5G/6G; quantum computing; etc.

https://www.jio.com/platforms

Technology Books: https://peterindia.vercel.app/books

Google Scholar: https://scholar.google.co.in/citations?user=MgMlqAwAAAAJ&hl=en

LinkedIn Page: https://www.linkedin.com/in/sweetypeter/

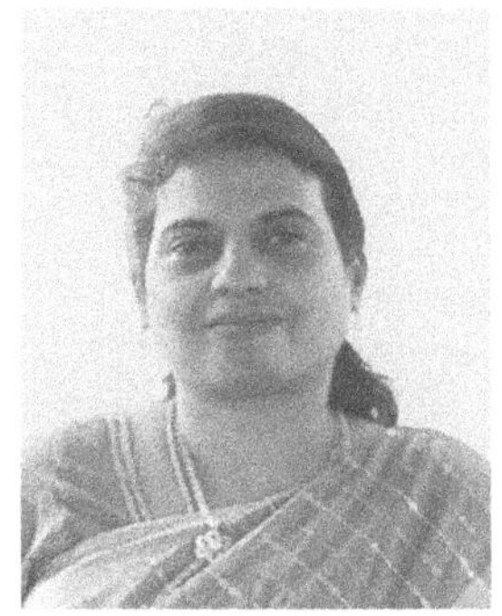

K. Shantha Kumari, PhD, is presently working in Department of Data Science and Business Systems, School of Computing, SRM Institute of Science and Technology, Kattankulathur, India. She received her PhD degree from Pondicherry University. She has 23 years of teaching and research experience supervising students in emerging technologies. She has published over 25 research papers in national and international journals and conferences. She has also filed a few patents. She has also delivered technical talks on artificial intelligence, data science, cryptography, blockchain, and other emerging areas and handled many special sessions at international conferences. Her research interests include information security, data science, blockchain technology, Web 3.0, and digital healthcare.

Academic url: https://www.srmist.edu.in/faculty/dr-k-shantha-kumari/

Google Scholar: https://scholar.google.com/citations?user=30zycjAAAAAJ&hl=en

List of Contributors

Ashwini A
Department of Electronics and
  Communication Engineering
Vel Tech Rangarajan Dr. Sagunthala
  R&D Institute of Science and
  Technology
Avadi, Chennai, Tamil Nadu, India

Sayed Sayeed Ahmad
Rochester Institute of Technology
Dubai Campus
Dubai, UAE

Hariharan B
Department of Computational
  Intelligence
SRM Institute of Science and
  Technology
Kattankulathur, Tamil Nadu, India

N. Bindu
Department of Computer Science
Sree Narayana College
Cherthala, Alappuzha, Kerala, India

Preethika Immaculate Britto
Department of Biomedical Engineering
  College of Engineering (Women)
King Faisal University
Kingdom of Saudi Arabia

Radha Raman Chandan
Department of Computer Science
School of Management Science
Varanasi, Uttar Pradesh, India

Rahul D
Department of Futures Studies
University of Kerala
Thiruvananthapuram,
  Kerala, India

Joshua R. Dalrymple
Purdue University Global
West Lafayette, Indiana, United States

Anupama C. G
Department of Computational
  Intelligence
SRM Institute of Science and
  Technology
Kattankulathur, Tamil Nadu,
  India

Vadivu G
Department of Data Science and
  Business Systems SRM Institute of
  Science and Technology
Kattankulathur, Chennai, India

Susan George
Department of Futures Studies
University of Kerala
Thiruvananthapuram, Kerala, India

Shamini G. I
Department of Electronics and
    Communication Engineering
Sathyabama Institute of Science and
    Technology
Chennai, Tamil Nadu, India

Priyanka Gupta
Guru Ghasidas Central University
Bilaspur, India

Celestine Iwendi
School of Creative Technologies,
    University of Bolton
Bolton, United Kingdom

Seifedine Kadry
Noroff University College
Oslo, Norway

Naresh Kumar Kar
GITAM (Deemed to be University)
Hyderabad, India

V. Kavitha
Department of Computational
    Intelligence, School of Computing,
    SRM Institute of Science and
    Technology
Kattankulathur, Tamil Nadu, India

K. Satheesh Kumar
School of Digital Sciences
Digital University Kerala
Mangalapuram, Thiruvananthapuram,
    Kerala, India

Rajesh Kumar
School of Law UPES
Dehradun, India

R. Ajith Kumar
Kerala University of Digital Sciences,
    Innovation and Technology
    Technocity Campus
Thiruvananthapuram, Kerala, India

Rishi Kumar
Division of Cyber Security and Digital
    Forensics, School of Computing
    Science and Engineering
VIT Bhopal University
Madhya Pradesh, India

T. K. Manoj Kumar
Kerala University of Digital Sciences,
    Innovation and Technology
    Technocity Campus
Thiruvananthapuram, Kerala,
    India

Suggala Lohitha
Department of Biomedical
    Engineering
Kalasalingam Academy of Research
    and Education
Krishnankoil, Tamil Nadu, India

Abinaya M
Department of Data Science and
    Business Systems SRM Institute of
    Science and Technology
Kattankulathur, Chennai, India

Meera Mathew
School of Law
CHRIST (Deemed to be University)
Delhi NCR, India

Abolfazl Mehbodniya
Department of Electronics and
    Communication Engineering
Kuwait College of Science and
    Technology (KCST)
Doha, Kuwait

Ratnakumari Neerukonda
Department of Computational
    Intelligence
SRM Institute of Science and
    Technology
Kattankulathur, Tamil Nadu, India

Yatish Pachauri
School of Law
UPES
Dehradun, India

Manoj Kumar Pandey
Pranveer Singh Institute of Technology
Kanpur, India
and
Chandigarh University
Chandigarh, Punjab, India

Sheetal Pawar
Department of Electronics and
    Telecommunication Engineering
Dr. D. Y. Patil Institute of Technology
Pimpri, Pune, India

S. Poonkodi
Department of Computing
    Technologies
School of Computing, SRM Institute
    of Science and Technology
Kattankulathur, Tamil Nadu, India

Banu Priya Prathaban
Department of Networking and
    Communications
School of Computing, SRM Institute
    of Science and Technology
Tamil Nadu, India

Amritha P. S
Department of Futures Studies
University of Kerala
Thiruvananthapuram, Kerala,
    India

T. Radhakrishnan
Kerala University of Digital Sciences
Innovation and Technology Technocity
    Campus
Thiruvananthapuram, Kerala,
    India

Pankaj Rahi
Department of Health Information
    Technology Management
Institute of Health Management
    Research
Bangalore, Karnataka. India

Jayaraj Ramasamy
Botho University
Gaborone, Botswana

Shaik Reena
Computer Science and Engineering
Kalasalingam Academy of Research
    and Education
Krishnankoil, Tamil Nadu, India

Balasubramaniam S
School of Computer Science and
    Engineering
Kerala University of Digital Sciences,
    Innovation and Technology, Digital
    University Kerala
Thiruvananthapuram, Kerala, India

Hariharasitaraman S
Division of Cyber Security and Digital
    Forensics
School of Computing Science and
    Engineering, VIT Bhopal University
Madhya Pradesh, India

Sakthivel Sankaran
Department of Biomedical Engineering
Kalasalingam Academy of Research
    and Education
Krishnankoil, Tamil Nadu, India

Sagar Shinde
Faculty of Engineering
Lincoln University College
Malaysia

R. Subash
Department of Computing
    Technologies
School of Computing, SRM Institute
    of Science and Technology
SRM Nagar, Kattankulathur, Chennai,
    India.

B. Sundaravadivazhagan
Department of Information
    Technology
University of Technology and Applied
    Science-AL Mussanah
Al-Mussanah, Oman

K. Suresh
Department of Computational
    Intelligence
School of Computing, SRM Institute
    of Science and Technology
Tamil Nadu, India

Jyoti Upadhyay
G.D. Rungta College of Science and
    Technology
Bhilai, Chhattisgarh, India

Kavitha V
University College of Engineering
Kancheepuram, Tamil Nadu, India

Mithra Venkatesan
Department of Electronics and
    Telecommunication
    Engineering
Dr. D. Y. Patil Institute of
    Technology
Pimpri, Pune, India

Lalit Kumar Wadhwa
Department of Electronics and
    Telecommunication Engineering
Dr. D. Y. Patil Institute of
    Technology
Pimpri, Pune, India

Julian L. Webber
Department of Electronics and
    Communication Engineering
Kuwait College of Science and
    Technology (KCST)
Doha, Kuwait

Chapter 1

Introduction to the Metaverse

Yatish Pachauri, Rajesh Kumar,
and Joshua R. Dalrymple

1.1 Introduction

It is challenging to anticipate the appearance of our future in the digital realm. What will be the subsequent digital upheaval and how will it impact our daily existence? These are fundamental inquiries that are continually being contemplated by not just scientists, but also by the industry, politics, and a portion of the populace. The implementation of a metaverse has the potential to revolutionize the digital landscape by eliminating the economic and political obstacles that now exist on the Internet [1]. Metaverse is a comprehensive term that refers to digital three-dimensional realms [2]; recently, companies have made substantial expenditures in their own metaverse projects [3]. Figure 1.1 shows investment in the metaverse, including other sectors, from the years 2022 to 2030 based on current trends, as per the data published by Statista.

This market would be reaching to its new valuation from $46.1 billion in 2022 to $74.4 billion United States by 2024. This is not going to be restricted here and projected to around $507.8 billion by 2030.

According to some investors, the metaverse has the potential to become the next iteration of the Internet, potentially leading to the establishment of Web 3.0 or at the very least being integrated into it [4, 5]. Furthermore, an additional objective of the metaverse is to create a navigable rendition of the Internet, leading to the emergence of novel business sectors [6]. Among the companies globally, Facebook

DOI: 10.1201/9781003491668-1

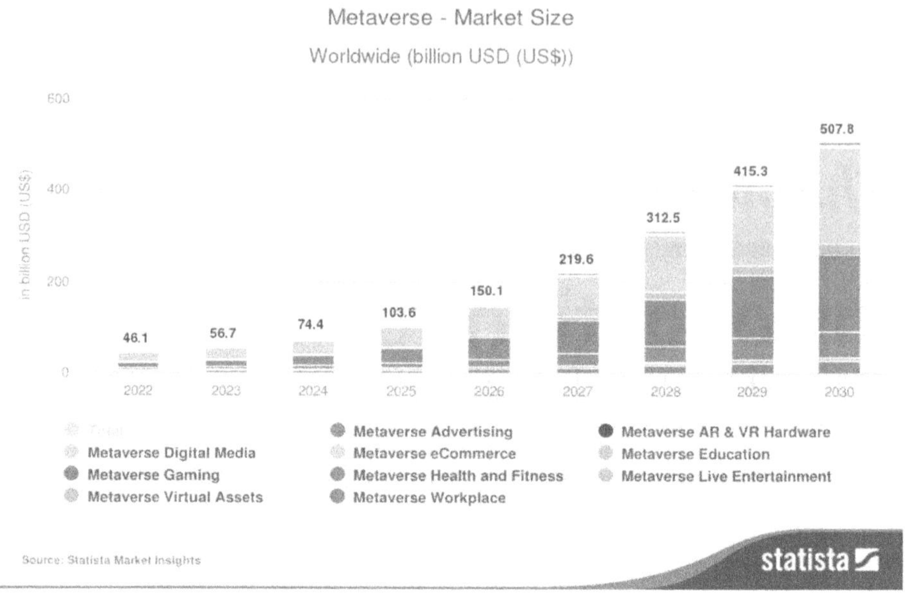

Figure 1.1 **Metaverse Market revenue, 2022–2030. (From Statista Market Insights.)**

revealed its plans in 2021 to lead the digital transformation with their metaverse initiative and later rebranded their corporation as Meta [7]. This event sparked a newfound push for the term metaverse, extending far beyond the confines of the scientific community. Within the realm of research and practical application, there exists a wide array of diverse interpretations on the definitions of the concept known as the metaverse. Hence a clear and universally accepted scientific definition has yet to be established. Definitions are subject to change over time, have continually evolved throughout history, and are subject to varied interpretations by distinct individuals or groups. The concept of the metaverse mentioned as an entity represents the evolution of the online world. It allows individuals to interact with each digital application in a setting using avatars. Over time, the idea of the metaverse is moving toward becoming more inclusive. This involves creating a vast metaverse with a focus on features.

This introduction specifically examines the substance of the publications and provides a comprehensive evaluation in terms of their range and methodology. The chapter centers around the subsequent research inquiries:

■ The metaverse articles primarily consist of the subject matter and information contained inside them.
■ What are some instances of applications in the metaverse?
■ The metaverse reality presents several obstacles.

1.1.1 Background

Neal Stephenson initially coined the term metaverse [8] in his science fiction novel Snow Crash, which presents the idea of the metaverse and set the stage for the term and its fundamental concept. Nevertheless, a comprehensive understanding of the technical process is involved in transforming a metaverse [9]. Second Life is an online platform where users can create their avatar and interact with each other in multiverse realm. But, it was unable to make a significant impact due to inherent technical constraints and its limited potential audience. The platform's lack of economic success was hindered by both information technology (IT) infrastructural issues and the then-underdeveloped technology of virtual reality (VR) glasses. The platform continues to exist but caters to a specific and limited audience in the era of widespread social media connectivity [9]. Throughout this entire period, there has been a complete transformation and significant growth in the comprehension and utilization of the Internet and media. The term metaverse has been a topic of dispute and has continually been subject to attempts at redefinition [10, 11]. The definitions succinctly encapsulate the attributes of the metaverse in a repetitive manner, highlighting both common and contrasting features. These shared and contrasting attributes can be utilized to assess the frequency of these traits in all definitions, resulting in an overall determination of their importance. Following Meta's statement in 2021 about the construction of its own metaverse, the term gained significant prominence once again. Meta aims to combine its presence in VR and augmented reality (AR) with its prominent position in the social media landscape. This refers primarily to system immersion [12]. The technology is distinguished by its ability to replicate human perception using multimodal displays and tracking technologies, which provide both feedback and feedforward. The system immerses users by employing VR tech along with mixed reality (MR) and AR technologies. In recent years, significant progress in technologies has sparked increased attention from both consumer and business sectors. Within the scientific world, there are various interpretations and explanations of the metaverse. However, there is currently a lack of a comprehensive assessment of the scientific definitions of the metaverse, highlighting a gap in study. To tackle the existing research shortfall, this chapter introduces a research question (RQ1) for exploration: What are the current scientific and academically inclined definitions of "metaverse"? Additionally, a notable gap is identified in the lack of a critical evaluation of these definitions, where they are not only compared but their characteristics are also weighted. Conducting such an analysis could greatly aid in crafting a more thorough definition of the metaverse, one that improves upon earlier versions by incorporating all essential aspects highlighted in previous definitions.

1.1.2 Focus on the Articles

This section provides a concise overview of the chosen articles, arranged in chronological order, with regard to their scope and methodology. Much literature introduced the concept of the metaverse, as another study explored challenges in designing and building the metaverse [13]. It examined existing research on online games with large, global user bases interacting through avatars [14]. These games raise questions about the metaverse's social, political, economic, and ethical implications, especially regarding how users represent themselves virtually. Focusing on Volkswagen, [15] categorize them into online games and the metaverse. They define essential characteristics of these virtual environments, including multimodal input methods, diverse client devices, scalable servers, network limitations, object encoding schemes, physics engines, security measures, privacy considerations, and fairness mechanisms. In a 2009 study, the concept of virtual collaboration and teamwork within immersive online environments was explored. To better grasp the potential advantages and drawbacks, a new framework is suggested that identifies five critical elements.

- The metaverse in general.
- Human users and their virtual representations (avatars) within the metaverse.
- Technological functionalities and capabilities within the metaverse.
- The actions and conduct of avatars within the metaverse.
- The outcomes and results produced.

This delves into virtual collaboration and teamwork within the metaverse, exploring how these aspects can influence its success [16]. They propose a conceptual model with five key constructs to understand the potential benefits and risks [17].

Furthermore, in a 2009 study, this also investigated the impacts of marketing products and services, particularly on the Volkswagen (VW) online platform utilized by both individuals and businesses. They carried out a comparison between traditional in-store retailing, e-commerce, and metaverse-based retail strategies. Several key questions were raised during their analysis, including the following: What requirements must be met for retail operations in a virtual environment? Which governing body will oversee the pricing of products? Is it possible to convert virtual currencies from metaverse transactions into real-world money? [18] explored the impact of journalism in a simulated environment and the ways in which the interaction between real life and Second Life (SL) affects and molds news material. Moreover, an evaluation was undertaken on the Alphaville Herald, Metaverse Messenger, and SL newspapers that originated within the VR environment. This evaluation yielded some conclusions that can be used to future journalistic applications. In other research, [19] developed a three-dimensional user interface for a VR home automation system. However, the study also demonstrated the capability of remotely monitoring and controlling home gadgets through the Internet using this interface, regardless of location or time.

[20] is another study that delved into the transformative and introspective effects of metaverse services, exploring avenues such as life journaling, mirror worlds, augmented reality (AR), and virtual worlds. Data regarding IP traffic and

iPhone sales volume were gathered for the websites twitter.com, maps.google.com, and secondlife.com, spanning from the first quarter of 2008 to the last quarter of 2009. This was conducted to evaluate the popularity of Twitter, Google, iPhone, and products associated with SL. The data were analyzed using the Bass model, which is a time series–based modeling approach. The study demonstrated that each service exhibits distinct values for both innovation and reflection coefficients. Furthermore, it was found that the reflection effects surpass the innovation effects for all metaverse services [20]. Furthermore, another study probed the correlation between the religious aspects of the physical world and the hereafter via the lenses of the sociology and psychology of religion [21]. The potential of utilizing metabots equipped with movement features in intricate virtual worlds was investigated [22]. In addition, a learning model was constructed using evolutionary computing approaches to enhance the performance of fuzzy controllers utilized by metabots for navigation within a simulated environment [22]. Another study explored "the notion of philosophers' islands as a metaphor in literature and philosophy" [23]. The author contends that "utopic" islands serve as a fictional arena for conducting experiments to create "real" state territories. He thoroughly analyzed the notions of Utopia, Endotopia, and Xenotopia in the study, approaching them from a similar standpoint. Another study reviewed the necessary considerations for transitioning from a collection of separate virtual worlds to a unified network of virtual worlds, known as the metaverse, which serves as an alternate environment for human socio-cultural engagement [24].

The primarily focus of the study [24] is based on below mentioned factors which are as follows:

1. Realism.
2. Omnipresence.
3. Interoperability.
4. The ability to scale as essential components of an authentic metaverse.

Crespo et al. [25] further explored the use of educational virtual environments and how knowledge is shared via free courses within the metaverse. They carried out a simulation to evaluate the properties of objects created in the metaverse with GNU tools. The authors particularly highlighted the importance of Open Sim for various engineering fields. Furthermore, the autoregressive integrated moving average (ARIMA) model was used to predict the server load resulting from students accessing online course registration, showing that this method produced favorable results.

Hassouneh and Brengman [26] researched the 27 virtual shops within SL and created a system to categorize these stores using atmospheric types. This research outlines a framework for investigating consumer behavior within virtual retail environments. Research was conducted focusing on SL to explore cultural interactions within virtual environments and to analyze the reasons behind the diminishing interest in SL. The research initially examined the technical aspects but found them to be of minor importance. The author deduced that the difficulty in defining SL strictly as a game or a form of social media leads to reduced interest among users, who then move on to platforms that offer genuine interactions with their peers. The paper outlines various elements that cause user disengagement in SL, including the portrayal of societal flaws and issues through idealistic elements, the lack of a unified story, difficulties in making connections with other participants, and an absence of erotic content. However, it was anticipated that these challenges would be quickly addressed, allowing for an improved approach to engaging users in SL.

In another study, the communication, interaction, and collaboration of students in virtual learning settings that incorporated three-dimensional (3D) simulations was examined [27]. The article examined the interplay between the participant and the 3D object, as well as the resulting interaction among participants, which serves as a catalyst for student learning.

The creation, development, and implementation of a virtual or metaverse environment tailored for educational purposes, employing the Scrum methodology, were presented in [28]. Additionally, the provision of both synchronous and asynchronous information serves as an alternative method for sharing and acquiring knowledge through technological means. This metaverse is crafted to emulate an authentic university setting for systems engineering students, integrating both hybrid and mobile learning strategies that accommodate flipped and collaborative classroom methodologies [29]. VR is presented as a medium that advances media traditions by enabling ongoing involvement and immersion, rather than being viewed as a mystical technology. He presented VR not as an unavoidable and deceptive metaverse, but as a simulated environment that constantly necessitates the deliberate manufacture of belief.

The impact of personal connection in virtual worlds on collective creativity was investigated in [30]. The essay explored the impact of the metaverse environment on creativity, specifically focusing on the formation of unique symbolic connections among participants. An example of this is the Avatar Orchestra. Research has found that virtual environments that lack face-to-face interaction and eliminate obstacles such as age, race, and geographical variation in the real world are conducive to fostering collective innovation.

A virtual museum encounter by linking a pointer positioned within a physical exhibition hall to an HMD (head-mounted display) is described in [31]. The metaverse, a fusion of AR and virtual worlds (VWs), enhanced the user experience by providing diverse information and narratives related to the artworks in the museum display.

Ayıter [32] explored the metamorphosis of a miniature 3D artwork made within the meta realm, drawing inspiration from Jorge Luis Borges' narrative, Aleph. Further, the author provided a philosophical reinterpretation of Aleph, defining it as a time machine for avatars.

According to other authors, "the concept of the Metaverse is not novel" [33]. Furthermore, technology has the potential to serve as a democratizing force in education, allowing individuals from all over the world to participate on an equal basis without being limited by geographical boundaries.

The literature has identified several difficulties, including metaverse privacy and various uses in fields such as medicine, education, and security. Both metaverse games and graphics have undergone evaluation. This evaluation has been bolstered by an analysis of the evaluated articles, considering several criteria such as the date when it was published, journal statistics, and the themes covered by articles. Regarding the obstacles encountered by academics, developers, and policymakers in the metaverse, a multitude of challenges are raised and noted and thoroughly debated. Finally, some significant and intriguing aspects of the metaverse have been addressed, encompassing crucial subjects like privacy in the metaverse, energy usage, the expenses of metaverse-related products, improvements in graphic design, and a few other themes. A total of 192 students in their first term enrolled in the mathematics fundamentals course engaged in the research conducted between August and December 2018. The study was conducted utilizing a computerized survey. The findings demonstrated a substantial enhancement in student performance when augmented reality was implemented in mathematics instruction.

Some authors also explored research on a mobile AR application specifically designed for utilizing escape games as an educational tool [34]. AR escape games can be readily implemented in overcrowded classes without the teacher and without the need for extensive planning. This examines the benefits and constraints of these instruments. Evidence has demonstrated that the suggested method is successful in enhancing motivation among the students involved in the trials.

In [35], the topic of discussion was the utilization of digital twin and mixed reality technologies in the metaverse for Boeing 737 maintenance training. The paper proposes the implementation of a practical training setting for aspiring engineers. This setting enables the management of aircraft by ensuring adherence to social distancing protocols using virtual resources and voice-activated instructions, particularly in the context of the ongoing pandemic. They implemented a metaverse platform to facilitate training and instruction for Boeing 737 aircraft maintenance. This platform includes legacy manuals, 3D models, 3D simulations, and aircraft maintenance information. The system utilizes the Neuro-Symbolic Speech Executor (NSSE) as a speech comprehension module, which distinguishes it from conventional speech recognition techniques. NSSE utilizes neurosymbolic artificial intelligence (AI), a technique that merges neural networks and traditional symbolic reasoning to comprehend user queries and provide contextually informed responses using aircraft-specific data. The model was trained using synthetic data. The performance was evaluated using automatic voice recognition measures on real user information. The model has demonstrated a generalization ability with an average accuracy of 94.7% and a word error rate (WER) of 7.5%.

The various challenges in inspiring distinct groups of players were investigated in [36]. This investigation involved 91 university students who participated in a class featuring gamification elements. This highlighted the importance of creating settings that allow players from varied backgrounds to develop their own gaming experiences, including the creation of rules and strategies, as an essential aspect of gamification design. The study determined that gamification positively impacts motivation, yet it did not identify significant challenges in inspiring among various players. Furthermore, a study was conducted to determine the elements that can influence how users perceive personalized virtual avatars [36]. These factors include likeness, familiarity, beauty, liking, and engagement. The avatars were developed as per face traits and expression of users. The familiar facial expressions expressed by the avatars of the participants exhibited a greater resemblance to the participants and evoked a stronger sense of familiarity compared to other avatars.

another study suggested an innovative AR method for enhancing traditional sport climbing training [37]. This method involves a teacher sequentially demonstrating the locations of the hands and feet to a rookie athlete. The climbing actions and positions are demonstrated to the student in real-time through character animations on a simulated climbing structure. Additionally, within this system, the student has the freedom to choose their desired learning path and can participate in multiple study sessions independently, without the need for instructor guidance. Research findings suggest that the utilization of AR in climbing instruction yields results comparable to those of traditional teaching methods.

1.2 Different Application of Metaverse

The digital world is undergoing a revolution with the rise of the metaverse. This immersive virtual space, fueled by advancements in VR, is capturing the imagination of people worldwide. It's a new frontier for social interaction, offering unique platforms for connection. People are flocking to virtual spaces to meet friends, attend events, and explore uncharted digital territories. The ability to craft personalized avatars, shedding the limitations of the physical world, is another major draw. This virtual identity empowers self-expression in exciting new ways. But the metaverse isn't just about socializing. It holds vast potential for entertainment, education, and even commerce, making it a magnet for a curious and engaged audience. This can be seen in Figure 1.2. Investment in sectors in collaboration with the metaverse is increasing every year. More investment is available in health and fitness gadgets, then in the education, gaming, virtual assets, gaming, and live entertainment sectors, followed by e-commerce, AR, and VR hardware.

1.2.1 Metaverse Games

Many individuals are currently engaged in Internet-based role-playing games [39]. These involve many participants who interact with each other [39].

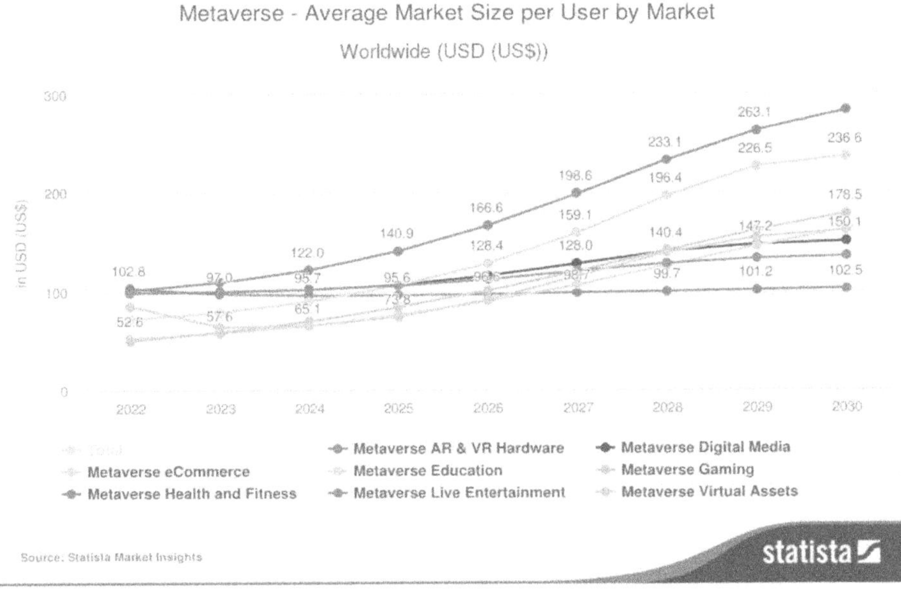

Figure 1.2 Market value per user (Target) as of October 2023 (From Statista Market Insights [38].)

They can do this by using their real-life personas or by creating new virtual identities that are not linked to their actual names [40]. The rate of subscriber growth is exhibiting a nonlinear pattern, indicating the potential for significant innovation comparable to the World Wide Web. The commercial opportunities and challenges posed by a digital environment such as SL have been discussed [41].

An examination has been conducted on the subsequent impacts of corporate social responsibility, with a specific focus on ethics and policies [41]. The study reflects how metaverse games might incorporate several modes of interaction based on the affordance theory. Specifically, the study focuses on the affordances of physiological experiences that players can have when playing these games. An investigation of the impact of players' affordances in minimum viable products (MVGs) on individuals' experience could be conducted by examining the perception and utilization of talents within a broader context. The primary focus is on the aptitudes of MVG players. The metaverse has been analyzed using a combination of experimental methods to identify important affordances and understand its dual nature. A player's perception of emotional talents is manifested through a heuristic process that selects affordances based on underlying cues in an immersive manner. Regarding affordance duplexity, it is suggested that the incorporation of social cues may potentially elucidate how users are able to establish and limit themselves in connection to the metaverse, which also functions as a framework that influences and restricts individual behaviors. When designing MVGs, designers must harness the potential offered by each platform and familiarize themselves with the capabilities of those platforms [42]. When creating MVGs, it is crucial to not only develop features that are instantly noticeable, but also to discover hidden potential. This can be achieved by developing games that effectively convert concealed features and functionalities into tangible skills. The research has constructed an enhanced model of affordances by establishing a framework that precisely outlines the process by which characteristics can be generated.

1.2.2 *Medical Applications*

Medical patients and clinicians in cardiovascular care have always depended on direct personal touch as a fundamental aspect of their connection [43]. The unique nature of this interaction has been scrutinized due to the recent pandemic, which has heightened the risks to the quality of healthcare services and created additional barriers between medical workers and patients. Due to the prevailing paradigm, there has been a significant increase in the usage of new technology in several aspects in everyday life, such as social interactions, entertainment, and healthcare services. In an unprecedented global health landscape, telemedicine, AR, and VR have thrived, pushing the boundaries of cardiology by integrating technology advancements. The aim is to deliver the highest possible quality of care to patients [43]. Despite anticipated challenges in security, technology, and legality, leveraging nonfungible tokens (NFTs) as a secure asset for patient records seems to be a viable option [43]. Recently, there has been a significant increase in the recognition and significance of the latest technological breakthroughs referred to as the metaverse [44]. This scientific breakthrough holds the potential to bring about a revolutionary technological transformation that can impact all aspects of our lives, beyond just healthcare [45]. The ongoing pandemics have led to a significant increase in the use of telemedicine by cardiovascular specialists.

Furthermore, it has spurred the emergence of technological innovations like the metaverse, a unique way to interaction in virtual worlds that integrates AR and VR [46]. This article introduces a theoretical framework for integrating metaverse technology in the field of cardiology. It offers boundless possibilities, including challenges in the field and bringing fresh insights into the study of illness, disease prevention, and disease diagnosis. It has several applications, with the most significant ones being enhancing medical visualizations, aiding in cardiovascular treatments, and transforming medical education delivery [47].

1.2.3 *Security Applications*

To foster the autonomous development of a metaverse, it's crucial to integrate safe digital twins' technology alongside parallel intelligence [48]. A metaverse represents a virtual realm existing alongside reality. Blockchain's inbuilt security, though still under development in other areas, offers a reliable way to store digital data for the Internet of Things (IoT). This approach secures the digital mapping process. Additionally, the proposed multidimensional hash geocoding method tackles challenges in handling complex geographic data.

1.2.4 Education-Related Metaverse Applications

To effectively interact with virtual objects in the 3D environment, spoken communications must be contextually aware of their surroundings [49]. A study proposes leveraging a metaverse for educational purposes in Boeing 737 aviation maintenance. This entails utilizing historical materials, 3D simulations [50], and specialized knowledge in aviation maintenance. An AI system in this metaverse trainer combines machine learning and symbolic reasoning to understand user questions in context, even with accents. It replaces expensive physical aircraft with customizable virtual ones for training, and acts as a virtual maintenance expert with hands-on guidance. Eye-tracking further enhances the immersive learning experience [35]. It identifies a correlation between rapid eye movements and emotional responses to certain issues, advocating for users' concerns promptly.

Three college students took part in an experiment where they discussed both a simple and a difficult problem. The teachers proposed assigning arithmetic homework to them for online work. Each session had a duration of ten minutes. The frequency of eye flickers for each participant was monitored during the session using specialist software. After the learning modules ended, the participants were provided with surveys to fill out. Subsequently, a comprehensive examination of the results was conducted. The findings suggest that the problematic issue can result in individuals experiencing unstable emotions, potentially leading to an elevated occurrence of eye flickering. By employing this method, instructors were able to thoroughly analyze the responses of their students, resulting in enhanced outcomes in the online project-based learning (PBL) course [51].

Researchers in the medical profession propose defining the metaverse as medical IoT (MIoT), which might be facilitated by the utilization of both AR and VR glasses [52]. Within the realm of the metaverse, a group of specialists from several disciplines, such as health and information technology, did a thorough study and examined published materials to ascertain the level of consensus among professionals regarding MIoT. Put simply, the metaverse enables various medical activities such as medical education, scientific communication, consultation, assessment and prognosis, medical trials, and even comprehensive medical therapy. These activities involve connecting with online specialists and endpoint physicians using cloud-based platforms. This can be achieved through the utilization of cloud computing. Examples of these services encompass disease management [53], healthcare [54], medical tests [47], diagnosis of illnesses, and therapy [47]. Services provided include first aid, outpatient care, consultation, and more.

Moreover, it is essential to underscore the importance of safety when utilizing the metaverse in the medical field. A dependable safety framework is crucial to ensure the seamless functioning of the metaverse. In the era of Society 5.0, the IoT facilitates collaboration among individuals from diverse countries, enabling them to offer solutions to our daily challenges.

[55] proposes a concept for an education system within the metaverse, highlighting its significance. The utilization of the metaverse enabled the implementation of a hybrid education model, integrating online learning with practical, interactive activities. The focus was on education regarding radiation, nuclear safety, and the fields of science, technology, engineering, and mathematics (STEM). Six competitors, all in the fifth and sixth grades, participated by actively engaging in the SL metaverse environment [56]. Following this, an instructor oversaw the practical application of radiation experiments in real-life scenarios, with another instructor present in person. Survey results clearly indicated that the proposal effectively met its initial objectives in STEM and nuclear safety education at the presecondary stages.

1.2.5 Exhibition Content Metaverse Applications

The metaverse can facilitate the creation of a diverse range of applications. Currently, there are significant transformations taking place in the methods that museums employ to exhibit their holdings. Smart glass approaches utilize several digital platforms to present exhibition content in a manner that facilitates a complete understanding of the shown goods [57]. This is accomplished while prioritizing the enhancement of the museum experience for visitors. However, most of these methods simply entail transmitting information in one direction. The disparity in illumination and lack of interaction with visiting tourists have made museums unsuitable as experiential destinations.

The paper outlines a plan for implementing content services aimed at enriching museum visitors' experiences. The proposed solution introduces an innovative service concept enabling users to immerse themselves in a virtual world. This is facilitated by establishing a connection between a physical beacon, typically positioned in a real-world location such as an exhibition room, and a head-mounted display [58]. Additionally, the service offers information about artifact characteristics and accompanying stories to enrich the user's experience, incorporating a narrative component. Designed with the specific goal of enhancing museum visits, whether online or in-person, this service aims to make the experiences more meaningful for visitors. The paper showcases exhibition content exclusively tailored for the metaverse exhibition [58], seamlessly integrating augmented reality with a virtual world in a highly effective manner [59].

1.3 Challenges

i. In the metaverse, new users aren't automatically connected. If you focus solely on building your virtual persona within a single platform, you risk being isolated and confined to outdated realms akin to Myspace or Friendster. This presents a significant concern [59].

ii. Prior to the realization of a fully-fledged metaverse, two critical hurdles must be overcome. Building high-quality 3D experiences and optimizing multimedia delivery are key for the future of immersive content. It's crucial for virtual reality and augmented reality platforms, along with device manufacturers and systems, to implement thorough privacy protections to safeguard the privacy of all participants in the metaverse. Despite the existing array of approaches and procedures, the proposed privacy methods are equitable and straightforward [60]. When users access the vast virtual worlds of the metaverse, they face the potential threat of privacy infringement in several forms, such as the possibility of other platform users eavesdropping on their discussions [61].

iii. The continued growth of the metaverse is primarily impeded by security and privacy issues. Concerns include cyber threats, data privacy issues, and potential bias in AI results. These extend to protecting physical infrastructure and personal information [61].

a. Due to its incorporation of cutting-edge technologies and their underlying methodologies, the metaverse is susceptible to inheriting the associated risks and inherent flaws of these technologies and methods. Emerging methodologies have already been associated with several scenarios, such as the illicit utilization of wearable devices or cloud-based storage, the pilfering of virtual currency, and the exploitation of AI to fabricate misinformation.

b. Furthermore, the interconnection of various technologies in virtual worlds might amplify and escalate the potential threats, leading to more severe repercussions. Simultaneously, novel hazards can emerge that are not present in either physical or cyberspace domains, such as virtual stalking and virtual espionage. More precisely, the private information contained within the metaverse may have been very detailed and exceptionally widespread to create a doppelganger of physical world. This introduces fresh avenues for perpetrating offenses through the utilization of personal big data.

Furthermore, given that individuals in the metaverse must be uniquely identified, it suggests that headsets and VR glasses might potentially be utilized to unlawfully track users' physical locations [62].

However, a significant number of the existing security mechanisms are inadequate and cannot be modified to suit the diverse applications. These features, such as the feeling of being fully engaged, the ability to exist in multiple spaces and times simultaneously, the ability to with stand challenges, and the ability to work well with other systems, may provide several challenges in effectively safeguarding these rights [63].

The metaverse provides not only the enjoyable experience of a seamlessly immersive virtual world but also pose challenges in securely integrating vast amounts of personal data of users while interacting with avatars [64].

   a. In the metaverse, the highly dynamic spatial and temporal characteristics certainly heighten the challenges of trust management and its inherent complexity. As these two realms increasingly converge, the metaverse could significantly complicate the differentiation between truth and fiction, particularly evident in cases involving deep fake occurrences. This presents specific challenges for legal and forensic research.
   b. The diverse hardware implementations, networking technology, and applications inside the large-scale metaverse provide substantial compatibility issues.

AR utilizes lightweight gadgets that are suitable for short interactions, but VR generally necessitates heavy and expensive technology for prolonged sessions. Certain techniques integrate the benefits of both AR and VR into a single device, enabling seamless switching between the two as needed. While this approach may be more expensive and less convenient compared to a single-model gadget, it offers the advantage of leveraging AR and VR in diverse ways. Holograms are not widely employed [65].

Privacy becomes a significant concern that must be handled due to the metaverse's collection of highly precise user activity data, surpassing mere user interactions, and browsing history. Implementing two-factor authentication for avatars is crucial, just like ensuring the security of sent data. Furthermore, the implementation of surveillance measures in response to the significant rise in user population, such as inadequate monitoring of chat rooms, censorship, and subsequent evaluation, highlights the necessity for organizations that fulfill similar roles as the government and law enforcement agencies in the physical world. Instances have occurred where individuals with unblemished records in the physical world have engaged in unlawful activities in the virtual realm due to the ability to remain anonymous online. A significant portion of metaverse participants consists of younger individuals who possess diverse viewpoints on various societal matters. To create a metaverse that can cater to different avatars and possesses a clear vision and ethical consciousness, it is necessary to move away from the notion of the metaverse as a physical place [65].

Engaging in research interviews with entrepreneurs or subscribers, researchers interact with individuals who may be either avatars or individuals using avatars as a disguise. This ongoing conversation between these two issues may influence subscriber behavior. There could potentially be a shift in behavior, and if so, it's crucial to understand how attitudes have changed. The overall impact on our culture and community is also significant to consider. Will new social trends emerge due to this behavior? Considering online games like role playing and SL as intricate social systems, not just games, also unveils deeper challenges. These complexities become significant later when seeking practical solutions [40].

1.4 Conclusion

The metaverse reimagines online interaction by merging social media connectivity with the immersive power of VR and AR. By unlocking the potential of this convergence, it could revolutionize various fields, including education. Meta-education, built on the metaverse's capabilities, offers diverse and immersive learning experiences. Imagine online 3D campuses that seamlessly blend formal and informal education. Metaverse-based learning can bridge the social interaction gap, making physical classrooms no longer the sole option. Virtual participation through telepresence, expressive avatars, and high-fidelity interactions can be equally effective. Additionally, social MR within the metaverse can fuel the adoption of active learning pedagogies, leading to deeper knowledge retention.

Furthermore, this technology holds the potential to democratize the education sector, enabling worldwide participation regardless of location. However, concerns remain, including metaverse privacy and its diverse applications across medicine, education, and security. This analysis evaluated both metaverse games and graphics, considering factors like publication date, journal data, and explored themes.

By comprehensively addressing the challenges faced by academics, developers, and policymakers, this work sheds light on key concerns and opportunities within the metaverse. Future trends and directions influencing its development and use have been explored. Additionally, critical aspects like privacy, energy consumption, costs of related products, graphic design advancements, and other relevant themes have been addressed.

References

1. Dionisio, J. D. N., Burns, W. G., & Gilbert, R. (2013a). 3D virtual worlds and the metaverse. *ACM Computing Surveys*, *45*(3), 1–38. https://doi.org/10.1145/2480741.2480751
2. Ball, M. (2022, June 10). *The metaverse: what it is, where to find it, and who will build it – MatthewBall.co*. MatthewBall.co. https://www.matthewball.co/all/themetaverse
3. Announcing a 1 billion funding round to support Epic's long-term vision for the metaverse. (2021, April 13). Epic Games. https://www.epicgames.com/site/en-US/news/announcing-a-1-billion-funding-round-to-support-epics-long-term-vision-for-the-metaverse
4. Cheng, R., Wu, N., Chen, S., & Han, B. (2022). Will metaverse be NextG Internet? Vision, hype, and reality. *IEEE Network*, *36*(5), 197–204. https://doi.org/10.1109/mnet.117.2200055
5. Newton, C. (2021, July 22). Mark Zuckerberg is betting Facebook's future on the metaverse. *The Verge*. https://www.theverge.com/22588022/mark-zuckerberg-facebook-ceo-metaverse-interview
6. Lee, L., Braud, T., Zhou, P., Wang, L., Xu, D., Lin, Z., Kumar, A., Bermejo, C., & Hui, P. (2021, October 6). *All One Needs to Know about Metaverse: A Complete Survey on Technological Singularity, Virtual Ecosystem, and Research Agenda*. arXiv.org. https://arxiv.org/abs/2110.05352

7. Isaac, M. (2021, October 28). Facebook renames itself Meta. *The New York Times.* https://www.nytimes.com/2021/10/28/technology/facebook-meta-name-change.html

8. Ritterbusch, G. D., & Teichmann, M. (2023). Defining the metaverse: A systematic literature review. *IEEE Access, 11,* 12368–12377. https://doi.org/10.1109/access.2023.3241809

9. Berge, Z. L. E. (n.d.). *Multi-user virtual environments for education and training? A critical review of.* https://eric.ed.gov/?id=EJ792161

10. Dionisio, J. D. N., Burns, W. G., & Gilbert, R. (2013b). 3D virtual worlds and the metaverse. *ACM Computing Surveys, 45*(3), 1–38. https://doi.org/10.1145/2480741.2480751

11. Jaynes, C., Seales, W. B., Calvert, K. L., Fei, Z., & Griffioen, J. (2003). The metaverse. *ACM Digital Library.* https://doi.org/10.1145/769953.769967

12. Nilsson, N. C., Nordahl, R., & Serafin, S. (2016). Immersion revisited: A review of existing definitions of immersion and their relation to different theories of presence. *Human Technology, 12*(2), 108–134. https://doi.org/10.17011/ht/urn.201611174652

13. Jaynes, C., Steele, R. M., & Webb, S. (2005). Rapidly deployable multiprojector immersive displays. *Presence, 14*(5), 501–510. https://doi.org/10.1162/105474605774918723

14. Papagiannidis, S., Bourlakis, M., & Li, F. (2008a). Making real money in virtual worlds: MMORPGs and emerging business opportunities, challenges and ethical implications in metaverses. *Technological Forecasting and Social Change, 75*(5), 610–622. https://doi.org/10.1016/j.techfore.2007.04.007

15. Kumar, S., Chhugani, J., Kim, C., Kim, D. H., Nguyen, A. D., Dubey, P., Bienia, C., & Kim, Y. (2008). Second Life and the new generation of virtual worlds. *Computer, 41*(9), 46–53. https://doi.org/10.1109/mc.2008.398

16. Davis, A., Murphy, J. D., Owens, D., Khazanchi, D., & Zigurs, I. (2009). Avatars, people, and virtual worlds: Foundations for research in metaverses. *Journal of the Association for Information Systems, 10*(2), 90–117. https://doi.org/10.17705/1jais.00183

17. Bourlakis, M., Papagiannidis, S., & Li, F. (2009). Retail spatial evolution: Paving the way from traditional to metaverse retailing. *Electronic Commerce Research (Print), 9*(1–2), 135–148. https://doi.org/10.1007/s10660-009-9030-8

18. Brennen, B., & Dela Cerna, E. (2010). Journalism in Second Life. *Journalism Studies, 11*(4), 546–554.

19. Han, J., Yun, J., Jang, J., & Park, K. (2010). User-friendly home automation based on 3D virtual world. *IEEE Transactions on Consumer Electronics, 56*(3), 1843–1847. https://doi.org/10.1109/tce.2010.5606335

20. Lee, S. G., Trimi, S., Byun, W. K. et al. (2011). Innovation and imitation effects in metaverse service adoption. *Service Business, 5,* 155–172. https://doi.org/10.1007/s11628-011-0108-8

21. Leone, M. (2011). The semiotics of religious space in Second Life®. *Social Semiotics, 21*(3), 337–357. https://doi.org/10.1080/10350330.2011.564385

22. Arroyo, Á., Serradilla, F., & Calvo, O. (2011). Adaptive fuzzy knowledge-based systems for control metabots' mobility on virtual environments. Expert Systems, *28*(4), 339–352. https://doi.org/10.1111/j.1468-0394.2011.00595.x

23. Cameron, A. (2012). Splendid isolation: 'Philosopher's islands' and the reimagination of space. *Geoforum, 43*(4), 741–749. https://doi.org/10.1016/j.geoforum.2011.12.008

24. Dionisio, J. D. N., Burns, W. G., & Gilbert, R. (2013c). 3D virtual worlds and the metaverse. *ACM Computing Surveys, 45*(3), 1–38. https://doi.org/10.1145/2480741.2480751

25. Crespo, R. G., Escobar, R. F., Aguilar, L. J., Velazco, S. Y., & Sanz, A. (2013). Use of ARIMA mathematical analysis to model the implementation of expert system courses by means of free software OpenSim and Sloodle platforms in virtual university campuses. *Expert Systems with Applications, 40*(18), 7381–7390. https://doi.org/10.1016/j.eswa.2013.06.054

26. Hassouneh, D., & Brengman, M. (2015). Retailing in social virtual worlds: Developing a typology of virtual store atmospherics. *Journal of Electronic Commerce Research, 16*(3), 218–241. http://www.jecr.org/node/471

27. Byron, V. B., José, C. R., & Gallardo Echenique, E. E. (2016). The communication in simulated learning environments. *Revista Iberoamericana de Educación, 72*(2), 85–101. https://alicia.concytec.gob.pe/vufind/Record/UCON_f3d851a6ae12d7b661a3a88f5168b552

28. Díaz, J. E. M., Saldaña, C. a. D., & Ávila, C. a. R. (2020). Virtual world as a resource for hybrid education. *International Journal of Emerging Technologies in Learning/International Journal: Emerging Technologies in Learning, 15*(15), 94–109. https://doi.org/10.3991/ijet.v15i15.13025

29. Murray, J. H. (2020). Virtual/reality: How to tell the difference. *Journal of Visual Culture, 19*(1), 11–27. https://doi.org/10.1177/1470412920906253

30. Martín, G. F. (2018). Social and psychological impact of musical collective creative processes in virtual environments; the Avatar Orchestra Metaverse in Second Life. *Musica/Tecnologia, 12*(1), 73–85. https://doi.org/10.13128/music_tec-23801

31. Choi, H., & Kim, S. (2017a). A content service deployment plan for metaverse museum exhibitions – Centering on the combination of beacons and HMDs. *International Journal of Information Management, 37*(1), 1519–1527. https://doi.org/10.1016/j.ijinfomgt.2016.04.017

32. Ayıter, E. (2017). Building a (virtual) Aleph: The visual transformation of a tiny cosmogony. *Technoetic Arts, 15*(1), 3–13. https://doi.org/10.1386/tear.15.1.3_1

33. Reyes, C. E. G. (2020). High school students' views on the use of metaverse in mathematics learning. *Metaverse, 1*(2), 9. https://doi.org/10.54517/met.v1i2.1777

34. Estudante, A., & Dietrich, N. (2020). Using augmented reality to stimulate students and diffuse escape game activities to larger audiences. Journal of Chemical Education, 97(5), 1368–1374. https://doi.org/10.1021/acs.jchemed.9b00933

35. Siyaev, A., & Jo, G. (2021a). Neuro-symbolic speech understanding in aircraft maintenance metaverse. *IEEE Access, 9*, 154484–154499. https://doi.org/10.1109/access.2021.3128616

36. Park, S., Min, K., & Kim, S. (2021). Differences in learning motivation among Bartle's player types and measures for the delivery of sustainable gameful experiences. *Sustainability, 13*(16), 9121. https://doi.org/10.3390/su13169121

37. Kim, D. (2021). Effect of augmented reality affordance on motor performance: In the sport climbing. *scholarworks.bwise.kr.* https://scholarworks.bwise.kr/ssu/handle/2018.sw.ssu/41913

38. Statista. (n.d.). *Metaverse – Worldwide | Statista market forecast.* https://www.statista.com/outlook/amo/metaverse/worldwide#:~:text=The%20Metaverse%20market%20is%20projected,US%24507.8bn%20by%202030.\

39. Wiederhold, B. K. (2022). Ready (or not) player one: Initial musings on the metaverse. *Cyberpsychology, Behavior and Social Networking (Print), 25*(1), 1–2. https://doi.org/10.1089/cyber.2021.29234.editorial

40. Papagiannidis, S., Bourlakis, M., & Li, F. (2008b). Making real money in virtual worlds: MMORPGs and emerging business opportunities, challenges and ethical implications in metaverses. *Technological Forecasting & Social Change/Technological Forecasting and Social Change, 75*(5), 610–622. https://doi.org/10.1016/j.techfore.2007.04.007

41. Shahjalal, M., Roy, P. K., Shams, T., Fly, A., Chowdhury, J. I., Ahmed, M., & Liu, K. (2022). A review on second-life of li-ion batteries: Prospects, challenges, and issues. *Energy, 241*, 122881. https://doi.org/10.1016/j.energy.2021.122881

42. Shin, D. (2022). The actualization of meta affordances: Conceptualizing affordance actualization in the metaverse games. *Computers in Human Behavior, 133*, 107292. https://doi.org/10.1016/j.chb.2022.107292

43. Skalidis, I., Muller, O., & Fournier, S. (2023). CardioVerse: The cardiovascular medicine in the era of metaverse. *Trends in Cardiovascular Medicine, 33*(8), 471–476. https://doi.org/10.1016/j.tcm.2022.05.004

44. Yang, Y., Siau, K., Xie, W., & Sun, Y. (2022). Smart health. *Journal of Organizational and End User Computing, 34*(1), 1–14. https://doi.org/10.4018/joeuc.308814

45. Tan, T. F., Li, Y., Lim, J., Gunasekeran, D. V., Teo, Z. L., Ng, W. Y., & Ting, D. S. (2022a). Metaverse and virtual health care in ophthalmology: Opportunities and challenges. *Asia-Pacific Journal of Ophthalmology, 11*(3), 237–246. https://doi.org/10.1097/apo.0000000000000537

46. Thomason, J. (2021, December 31). *MetaHealth – How will the metaverse change health care?* https://dergipark.org.tr/en/pub/jmv/issue/67581/1051379

47. Marzouqi, A. A., Aburayya, A., & Salloum, S. A. (2022). Prediction of user's intention to use metaverse system in medical education: A hybrid SEM-ML learning approach. *IEEE Access, 10*, 43421–43434. https://doi.org/10.1109/access.2022.3169285

48. Nguyen, T. N. (2022). Toward human digital twins for cybersecurity simulations on the metaverse: Ontological and network science approach. *JMIRx Med, 3*(2), e33502. https://doi.org/10.2196/33502

49. Kye, B., Han, N., Kim, E., Park, Y., & Jo, S. (2021). Educational applications of metaverse: Possibilities and limitations. *Journal of Educational Evaluation for Health Professions, 18*, 32. https://doi.org/10.3352/jeehp.2021.18.32

50. Rauch, U., Cahodas, M., & Wang, T. (n.d.). *The Arts 3D VLE Metaverse as a network of imagination.* NSUWorks. https://nsuworks.nova.edu/innovate/vol5/iss6/1?utm_source=nsuworks.nova.edu%2Finnovate%2Fvol5%2Fiss6%2F1&utm_medium=PDF&utm_campaign=PDFCoverPages

51. Phungsuk, R., Viriyavejakul, C., & Ratanaolarn, T. (2017). Development of a problem-based learning model via a virtual learning environment. *Kasetsart Journal of Social Sciences, 38*(3), 297–306. https://doi.org/10.1016/j.kjss.2017.01.001

52. Jagadeeswari, V., Subramaniyaswamy, V., Ravi, L., & Vijayakumar, V. (2018). A study on medical Internet of Things and Big Data in personalized healthcare system. *Health Information Science and Systems, 6*(1). https://doi.org/10.1007/s13755-018-0049-x

53. Han, Y., & Oh, S. H. (2021). Investigation and research on the negotiation space of mental and mental illness based on metaverse. *2021 International Conference on Information and Communication Technology Convergence (ICTC).* https://doi.org/10.1109/ictc52510.2021.9621118

54. Tan, T. F., Li, Y., Lim, J., Gunasekeran, D. V., Teo, Z. L., Ng, W. Y., & Ting, D. S. (2022b). Metaverse and virtual health care in ophthalmology: Opportunities and challenges. *Asia-Pacific Journal of Ophthalmology, 11*(3), 237–246. https://doi.org/10.1097/apo.0000000000000537

55. Suzuki, S., Kanematsu, H., Barry, D. M., Ogawa, N., Yajima, K., Nakahira, K. T., Shirai, T., Kawaguchi, M., Kobayashi, T., & Yoshitake, M. (2020). Virtual experiments in metaverse and their applications to collaborative projects: The framework and its significance. *Procedia Computer Science, 176*, 2125–2132. https://doi.org/10.1016/j.procs.2020.09.249
56. Rymaszewski, M., Au, W. J., Wallace, M., Winters, C., Ondrejka, C., & Batstone-Cunningham, B. (2006). Second Life: The Official Guide. 1st ed. 2006 Wiley.
57. Siyaev, A., & Jo, G. (2021b). Towards aircraft maintenance metaverse using speech interactions with virtual objects in mixed reality. *Sensors, 21*(6), 2066. https://doi.org/10.3390/s21062066
58. Narin, N. G. (2021, December 31). *A content analysis of the metaverse articles.* https://dergipark.org.tr/en/pub/jmv/issue/67581/1051382
59. Choi, H., & Kim, S. (2017b). A content service deployment plan for metaverse museum exhibitions — Centering on the combination of beacons and HMDs. *International Journal of Information Management, 37*(1), 1519–1527. https://doi.org/10.1016/j.ijinfomgt.2016.04.017
60. Bermejo Fernandez, C., & Hui, P. (n.d.). Life, the metaverse and everything: An overview of privacy, ethics, and governance in metaverse.Cornell University, Journal-article, Mar. 2022. https://doi.org/10.48550/arXiv.2204.01480
61. Park, S. M., & Kim, Y. (2022). A metaverse: Taxonomy, components, applications, and open challenges. *IEEE Access, 10*, 4209–4251. https://doi.org/10.1109/access.2021.3140175
62. Tseng, W., Bonnail, E., McGill, M., Khamis, M., Lecolinet, É., Huron, S., & Gugenheimer, J. (2022). The dark side of perceptual manipulations in virtual reality. *CHI Conference on Human Factors in Computing Systems.* https://doi.org/10.1145/3491102.3517728
63. Wang, Y., Su, Z., Zhang, N., Xing, R., Liu, D., Luan, T. H., & Shen, X. (2023). A survey on metaverse: Fundamentals, security, and privacy. *IEEE Communications Surveys and Tutorials/IEEE Communications Surveys and Tutorials, 25*(1), 319–352. https://doi.org/10.1109/comst.2022.3202047
64. Nguyen, C. T., Hoang, D. T., Nguyen, D. N., & Dutkiewicz, E. (2022). MetaChain: A novel blockchain-based framework for metaverse applications. *arXiv (Cornell University).* https://doi.org/10.48550/arxiv.2201.00759
65. Nevelsteen, K. J. L. (2017). Virtual world, defined from a technological perspective and applied to video games, mixed reality, and the metaverse. *Computer Animation and Virtual Worlds, 29*(1). https://doi.org/10.1002/cav.1752

Chapter 2

Exploring Technologies Needed for the Metaverse

Abinaya M, Vadivu G, Balasubramaniam S, and Seifedine Kadry

2.1 Introduction

Metaverse is the term for the innovative and latest technologies for changing the style of working together, socializing and interacting in virtual environments, and also communicating with each other. In the metaverse, the Internet is revolutionized by the real-time and the virtual environment: immersive technology, interconnected networks, and shared digital spaces. The innovative metaverse is understandable from the chapter based on the dynamics and ethical challenges [1]. This chapter deals with and covers all the exploring technologies in the metaverse. The foundational technologies are immersive technology and spatial computing [2]. These systems are highly ethical. The first section focuses on the technologies behind the metaverse. Immersive environments and new, innovative technologies like virtual reality (VR), spatial computing (SC), augmented reality (AR), and artificial intelligence (AI) create seamless interactions between smart and attractive avatars [3]. To support the social and ethical privacy of the metaverse, the privacy of data, the inclusivity of data, culture, and identity, rules have been created for the management of the community and content control for governance and regulation [4]. This book aims to highlight all the possibilities and challenges of the metaverse. It's perfect for technical geeks, budding entrepreneurs, academicians, or anyone interested in digital connection in the future. So, let's dive in together and explore the metaverse, where the combination of reality and virtual content starts to blur and the innovative solutions come from the intersection of technologies and humans.

DOI: 10.1201/9781003491668-2

2.2 Virtual Reality (VR)

Users of VR are navigated to virtual worlds giving a sense of real presence and immersion in an interactive digital environment. The VR headsets that we use for viewing the scenario are high-resolution display panels, motion tracking sensors, and highly integrated audio systems, which are important parameters in VR experiences [5]. These VR headsets are available in different kinds of configurations along with built-in processing power and tethered connectivity systems that link to PCs [6]. A simulation of a three-dimensional (3D) environment with computer-generated help to explore and interact in real time is an important factor of the technology of VR. Motion tracking of the user, spatial audio used according to the scenario, and graphics rendering of 3D data are important in the metaverse [7]. With the help of head-tracking sensors, users can naturally look around and navigate the virtual environment. By allowing users to interact with virtual objects through gloves or handheld controllers, the experience gains a tactile element [8].

VR has applications in many different industries and use cases. The technology offers immersive experiences in entertainment and gaming that take users to imaginary places and interactive journeys [9]. VR provides immersive learning environments for educational purposes, allowing students to perform experiments in simulated laboratories, dissect virtual organisms, and explore historical sites. VR is used in healthcare for medical education, pain management, and therapy [10]. It enables patients to have immersive experiences that support mental health and rehabilitation. [11] VR has the potential to change the world, but there are drawbacks as well, like motion sickness, discomfort, and the segregation of users from reality. Innovations in motion tracking algorithms, ergonomic design, and display technology are addressing these problems [11]. Furthermore, the expense and intricacy of virtual reality hardware have posed noteworthy obstacles to its extensive integration; however, the rise of more reasonably priced standalone gadgets and cloud-based VR systems is rendering VR increasingly available to both individuals and enterprises [12].

2.3 Augmented Reality (AR)

By superimposing digital content on top of the real world, AR enriches it and produces a hybrid experience where virtual and physical elements coexist [13]. To precisely position virtual content within the user's environment and identify objects and surfaces, AR technologies rely on computer vision, depth sensing, and spatial mapping [14]. AR experiences can be accessed via several devices, such as AR glasses, tablets, and smartphones. Users of AR glasses, like those from Google Glass and Microsoft's HoloLens, can see digital information superimposed on their field of vision while using them hands-free [15]. With the help of these glasses' transparent displays, which superimpose virtual content on the outside world, users can interact with virtual objects while still being aware of their immediate surroundings. AR applications for smartphones use the camera and sensors of the device to overlay digital content on the live camera feed. This allows for experiences like interactive gaming, shopping virtual try-ons, and navigational assistance [16].

AR has many broad and varied applications. It makes possible interactive marketing campaigns and immersive product experiences in retail that engage customers in novel and exciting ways. AR improves efficiency and accuracy in complex tasks by enabling hands-free access to digital instructions and visual aids in manufacturing and maintenance. AR in architecture and design enables clients and designers to see building projects at scale in the real world, improving communication and decision-making [17].

Occlusion is an important phenomenon in virtual objects for overlaying real-world surfaces. If occlusion occurs, it may feel unnatural, and lighting conditions also pose challenges to AR, potentially blending the virtual and the real world [18]. Advancements in high-configuration display technology are also addressing these issues. The field of view and resolution are also limiting factors in creating immersive experiences [19].

2.4 Spatial Computing

A group of technologies called "spatial computing" has been all about understanding and using 3D real and virtual spaces. It's about using spatial mapping tools to make detailed digital copies of physical places [20]. These tools help make super-accurate digital versions of the real world by taking pictures and using sensors to get info about the shapes and layouts of places. Once the digital copy is made, special algorithms can let people interact with it in a virtual space. To do this, the algorithms use the data from the sensors to figure out where the user is and what they're doing in the virtual environment. Then, they use that info to show the right virtual stuff at the right time and in the right spot [21].

This tech has a lot of different uses. In the field of architecture and engineering, spatial computing helps designers see how their building plans will look in the real world [22]. This makes it easier for them to work together and make better decisions. In marketing and retail, it lets people put virtual stuff like ads and products into real-world places, which helps customers interact with them more and gives them a more immersive shopping experience. In games and entertainment, spatial awareness algorithms let people interact with virtual stuff and environments in natural and intuitive ways [23, 24]. Spatial computing has the potential to be a game changer, but there are still obstacles in the way. These include the privacy issues for the use and collection of spatial data, the technical difficulties for high-quality configuration of sensors, and the potential processing power for handling the enormous amount of data and the spatial data in real time [25]. However, the field is developing quickly due to developments in edge computing, sensor technology, and hardware miniaturization. As a result, spatial computing is becoming more widely available and significant in a variety of industries [26].

2.5 Artificial Intelligence (AI)

The metaverse's experiences and capabilities are heavily influenced by AI, which allows virtual entities to interact with users in a smart and lifelike way. One of the main uses of AI in the metaverse is in the development of lifelike avatars and characters that can chat and interact with users in a natural way [27]. These AI-powered avatars use natural language processing (NLP) algorithms to understand and respond to user inputs, enabling super-immersive interactions in virtual environments [28]. Not only do AI-driven avatars provide realistic conversation, but they also power other metaverse applications like virtual assistants, content recommendation engines, and personalized experiences [29]. Virtual assistants, which are like digital concierges or guides, use AI algorithms to give users info, directions, and support in the metaverse. Content recommendation systems use machine learning algorithms to analyze user preferences and behavior and suggest content that they might like. Personalized experiences use AI to modify the virtual world and user interactions based on input from users, making the experience unique and responsive to how you interact with it [30].

AI is a big part of making stuff for the metaverse, like games and experiences. It helps with the whole process from brainstorming ideas to building and sharing them with people. It's like having a super-smart assistant who can get stuff done. Based on high-level specifications or design principles, generative AI algorithms can automatically create virtual environments, objects, and characters [29]. This speeds up the process of creating content and increases the scalability and diversity of virtual experiences. AI-driven animation tools can realistically and fluidly animate virtual objects and characters, giving virtual environments lifelike movements and interactions [31]. AI in the metaverse poses ethical and societal questions about data privacy, algorithmic bias, and the effects of AI-driven interactions on human behavior and relationships, despite its potentially transformative potential. To guarantee that AI improves human well-being and promotes positive interactions within virtual environments, it will be crucial to address these concerns through strong governance frameworks, transparent algorithms, and ethical guidelines as AI develops and permeates every part of the metaverse. It's especially useful for making interactions between users and virtual objects more interesting and immersive. The two main areas of AI in the metaverse we're focusing on here are NLP for communication and AI-powered avatars and characters [32].

2.6 AI-Powered Characters and Avatars for Lifelike Interactions

Avatars and characters are controlled by AI and are like digital people who can understand and react to what's going on around them in virtual worlds. They use smart algorithms to figure out what you're saying and do things that seem realistic and natural [33]. With AI, these avatars can act and feel like real humans, showing emotions and making expressions that make you feel like you're there in the metaverse. AI thus helps make your experience in these virtual worlds seem much more real and immersive [34].

Applications for these AI-powered avatars and characters can be found all over the metaverse, used for social meetings, gaming, education, and even entertainment. These AI-driven avatars help make virtual conversations and interactions feel more natural, with gestures and such, which helps when people in different places need to work together as a team [35]. AI-driven characters can be like companions or even nonplayer characters (NPCs) in games and movies, making the whole experience feel more dynamic and interactive [35]. AI-driven avatars are trained with a ton of data about people and how they act, like facial expressions and the way we talk. This lets the avatars learn how to act and respond in a way that feels realistic to us. Since these avatars are made from all these data, they can change and get better over time as they learn from the people using them and the feedback they get [36].

2.7 Natural Language Processing (NLP) for User–Virtual Entity Communication

The goal of AI's NLP is to help computers understand, interpret, and produce human language just like we do. This is especially important for the metaverse, where people use chatbots, virtual assistants, and AI-powered avatars to talk to each other [37]. To do this, NLP algorithms process the stuff we say to these virtual things, like voice commands or typed questions, and figure out what we mean and what we want.

To do this, NLP algorithms look at the structure of our language, like syntax and grammar, but they also focus on meaning, like what we're talking about (semantics) and how we're talking about it (pragmatics). This lets the AI in the metaverse respond to us in a way that makes sense and feels natural. It's like having a conversation with another person [38]. Without NLP, we cannot connect with the new interfaces, and we cannot learn new things to command the virtual settings. With the help of NLP, we can interact exactly as we do with someone who is beside us [39]. In the metaverse, NLP is used for the virtual assistant like the chatbot. We can interact with the new avatar characters to create realistic characters [40]. AI-powered avatars and the following characters are using NLP. The lifelike and realistic characters are created with the help of NLP. We might even be able to have completely new and amazing experiences in the metaverse [41].

2.8 Blockchain

In the realm of tech, blockchain has blown up and is now extremely influential. It's the foundation for the metaverse, which is changing how we think about ownership and governance in virtual spaces, as well as how we do transactions. One of the main ways blockchain is used in the metaverse is by giving people decentralized control over their virtual stuff. For example, you don't have to rely on some big company to manage your stuff [42]. Also, cryptocurrencies are a huge part of these transactions, because they let people trade and do economic stuff in both the real world and the virtual world. A major revolution in the generation, exchange, and control of digital assets within the metaverse is encapsulated by decentralized ownership and management [43]. Virtual resources such as digital collectibles, game materials, and real estate can be tokenized and represented on a blockchain network as separate digital tokens using blockchain technology. These tokens are protected by cryptographic techniques; thus, people can transact directly without involving intermediaries and enjoy irrefutable proof of ownership. Decentralized ownership eliminates fraud, censorship, and loss experienced from centralization with virtual assets since users are completely responsible for their own decisions [44]. The common form of payment in cyberspace is cryptocurrency, which facilitates financial transactions among virtual world participants. With the integration of cryptocurrencies into virtual economies, users can easily purchase or sell virtual goods and services by utilizing digital currencies that are exclusive to these environments. Cryptocurrencies are a preferred choice in virtual economies because they have lower transaction fees, faster settlement times, and provide user pseudonyms, which helps foster inclusivity for various stakeholders in such ecosystems [45]. Additionally, one of the new economic systems created using cryptocurrencies includes token-based governance systems and decentralized autonomous organizations (DAOs) that permit people to participate in the managing and decision-making processes of online communities and platforms [46].

The metaverse's architecture is based on blockchain technology that is redefining virtual world notions of ownership, governance, and transactional systems. Two significant applications of blockchain in the metaverse include decentralized ownership and management of virtual assets, as well as the integration of cryptocurrencies for real-world commerce and economies [47]. Decentralized ownership and management represent a paradigm shift in the creation, trading, and control of digital assets within the metaverse. By using blockchain technology, virtual assets such as digital collectibles, in-game items, or real estate can be tokenized to become distinct digital tokens on a blockchain network. Since these tokens are secured by cryptographic methods, users can transact with one another directly without intermediaries while having proof that can never be reversed [48]. Therefore, decentralized ownership enables users to have fraud-free transactions, unlike centralized platforms, where fraud cases are many.

The primary means of payment in virtual environments is cryptocurrency. In the metaverse, this enables users and other entities to pay comfortably and securely. By incorporating cryptocurrencies into virtual economies, consumers can easily purchase virtual products and services associated with native Virtual Economy Currencies (VECs). Considering the benefits of cryptocurrencies over traditional fiat monies like lower transaction fees instant settlements and pseudonymous transactions, they improve the efficacy and inclusivity of virtual economies [49]. Moreover, new economic models facilitated by cryptocurrencies, such as token-based governance and decentralized autonomous organizations, allow users to participate in the online community and platform management and decision-making. Decentralized ownership and cryptocurrencies make for a brand-new, unconstrained, digitally native economic system. The higher the number of users who can gain financial control of their lives and digital possessions, the more vibrant the digital environment. In the metaverse, the value of such a thriving virtual state of nature does not rely on community, commerce, or creativity. The period for disrupting the current system and introducing a new one in the current system is right around the corner [50]. As blockchain technology grows and matures, the chances of widespread adoption of decentralized digital economies and innovative financial models increase rapidly. This shift could usher in a third phase of decentralized digital encounters and economies.

2.8.1 Standards and Interoperability

Standards and working together are key for metaverse connection. They help things fit together and talk to each other. This happens through open rules for making and sharing stuff and through protocols for different things to work with each other. By making sure different worlds and systems can trade data and messages, folks can jump between places and take their stuff with them [51]. This helps make connected metaverse experiences that work well across platforms. Some examples of these rules are WebXR, OpenXR, and VRML. They let folks make cool experiences that work on lots of devices. Open rules for making and sharing stuff make sure that things made on one platform can be used on others. This helps to make things work well together. For 3D models, there's graphics library transmission format (glTF), and for real-time talks and sharing, there's HTTP and WebRTC. All this helps to make it easy for folks to move between different worlds, chat with others, and use lots of different stuff. As the metaverse grows, the need for these rules and working together will be even more crucial, bringing more people in to innovate and collaborate on more possible advances in the metaverse. File formats such as glTF for 3D models and protocols like HTTP and WebRTC for real-time communication and content distribution are examples of open standards for content creation and distribution [52]. A metaverse ecosystem that is networked and interoperable is based on open standards for content creation and distribution as well as cross-platform communication and compatibility protocols. These technologies enable users to interact with each other across different platforms, gain access to various content, including that suitable for different ages and such, and move between various virtual environments at will. The significance of open standards has the potential to grow further still in the metaverse's development phase leading to change inclusivity, accessibility, and creativity within the confines of cyberspace [53].

2.9 Cloud Computing

Moreover, the metaverse mainly relies on cloud computing, which provides the infrastructure that can be scaled to host massive virtual worlds and serve millions of users simultaneously. Equally important is edge computing, which is required to reduce delays in communication and enhance the interactivity experience in virtual environments [54]. The term "scalable infrastructure" means adaptable and as needed computing resources provided by cloud service vendors. These resources can be changed dynamically depending on user workload or demand changes. In the metaverse, scalable infrastructure enables developers to build incredibly large size virtual environments that support many users and intricate simulations without having to invest in expensive initial infrastructures or hardware [55]. Developers can use cloud computing resources for making VR including complex architectures, wide landscapes, and immersive experiences that make it comparable to the real world [56].

Edge computing brings computing closer to end users, thereby reducing latency and improving real-time interactions within virtual environments while at the same time enhancing the cloud's underlying infrastructure. The amount of time it takes for data to travel from a user's device through networks to reach the cloud server can also be reduced by developers [57].

A distributed computing ecosystem of cloud and edge computing powers the metaverse, enabling developers to create and deploy realistic virtual experiences at scale with user responsiveness and performance optimization intact. The metaverse's evolution will depend heavily on developments in cloud and edge computing technologies toward promoting innovation, inclusivity, and accessibility in virtual environments [58].

2.9.1 Edge Computing

In the metaverse, edge computing plays a role in reducing delays, enhancing the speed of real-time interactions. Data traveling between the user's device and the cloud server can introduce delays. Traditionally, cloud computing handles data processing on servers located in data centers. Edge computing addresses this issue by bringing resources to the user, typically at the network edge or even directly on the user's device [59]. By placing edge computing nodes at points within the network infrastructure, such as at the network edge or nearby data centers, developers can minimize data travel distance. This results in reduced latency and improved responsiveness for real-time interactions within environments. For example, in multiplayer gaming scenarios where split-second decisions are critical, edge computing can significantly decrease the time it takes for player actions to be processed and reflected in the game. This leads to enhanced immersion for players [60].

Edge computing is particularly beneficial for applications that rely on low-latency communication and real-time interaction like events, cooperative simulations, and

AR experiences. computing. Edge computing, on the other hand, presents the ideal technique for addressing low latency and high responsiveness because it processes data closer to where they are consumed, developing it in real time, even with low network bandwidth and intermittent network connections. This will not only produce a better user experience but will also pave the way for new applications and use cases that were previously unthinkable due to latency challenges. Edge computing is required to achieve the shortest latency and the quickest responsiveness while interacting in the metaverse at the moment. Since data do not need to travel far, there is very little latency, and interactions may occur smoothly.

Edge computing is a distributed computing concept where data get processed closer to the devices that create and use the data on the network. This could be useful for the metaverse, which is like a virtual world where people can hang out and interact with each other and digital stuff in real time. Here's how edge computing could be used in the metaverse:

1. **Reduce lag time:** Edge computing causes data to get processed faster when it's closer, so it could help make the metaverse feel smoother and more immersive, making our virtual experiences more realistic [61].
2. **Improve security:** Edge computing could also help keep our info safe by keeping it on our devices or at the outer edge of the network instead of sending it to some central server where it could be hacked or otherwise compromised [62].
3. **Increase bandwidth:** Basically, having devices do some of the computing work instead of servers could free up more room for everyone to do their thing in the metaverse. This is important cause it could support more people and complex virtual places, like virtual cities or huge virtual concerts [63].

2.10 Social Interaction Tool

In the metaverse, social tools are extremely important for building strong relationships and working together with other users in virtual worlds. They're the combination of everything together, making the whole experience way more fun and interactive. Social platforms and communication instruments are the two primary means, each with a specific function in promoting social interaction in virtual environments [64].

2.10.1 Social Platforms

These virtual spaces allow users to gather, connect, and work jointly in real time. Within these systems, individuals can simulate real-world settings where they can interact, explore, and navigate, such as virtual worlds, social hubs, or customizable areas. People can communicate with each other, participate in activities, and exchange experiences by using avatars to symbolize themselves, which promotes social presence and a sense of engagement. Social VR provides numerous possibilities for bringing people together through virtual experiences. Users can explore imaginative worlds, compete in lively competitions, exchange virtual goods in groundbreaking economies, and shape customizable digital representations of themselves [65]. Within these realms, a selection of communication methods fosters interaction. Voice allows natural, synchronous dialogue similar to face-to-face discussion, facilitating the seamless exchange of ideas. Beyond words, gesture and motion capture the nuances of body language, imbuing exchanges with added depth through implied sentiment and subtle cues. Facial simulation transfers even subconscious emotion, cultivating empathy and understanding among participants. Together, these techniques reconstruct the interpersonal richness of physical colloquy, if through an alternate medium, helping users form connections in novel ways [66].

The foundation of social interaction in the metaverse consists of social VR platforms and communication tools that enable users to interact, communicate, and work together within immersive virtual environments. These tools facilitate transcending geographical boundaries, promoting a sense of interconnectedness and belonging by establishing communities, sharing experiences collectively, and developing meaningful relationships within virtual spaces. The future of digital communication and socialization will be significantly impacted by advances in social interaction utilities, opening novel pathways for human connection and collaboration during the digital era as the metaverse progresses in fascinating complexity [67]. Social VR platforms are a useful tool for social interaction as they allow users to interact with others virtually. Face expressions, gestures, and voice chat are examples of communication tools.

2.10.2 ChatGPT Social Interaction Tools in the Metaverse

Social interaction tools are essential components of the metaverse that enable users to connect and build strong connections in 3D environments. There are two types of products: social VR platforms and communication tools, with each serving a distinct function in the social realm: Social VR platforms assist and encourage the user to meet, talk to others, and interact with other users in real time. Platforms were created in the metaverse to create virtual realities in which people could immobilize and communicate with one another. Platforms model atmospheres have been specifically designed to permit users to navigate, communicate, and interact. Social VR platforms let us hang out with friends in all sorts of ways, like playing games together, buying and selling stuff, dressing up our avatars, and even going to virtual parties [68]. When we're in these virtual worlds, we need ways to talk to each other, just like we would in real life. There are lots of tools to help us do that, and they make our interactions feel more natural and real. For example, voice chat lets us have real-time conversations with our buddies, just like we would if we were standing right next to each other. We can talk about anything we want, share our feelings, and even laugh together [69]. We can also use gestures and facial expressions to communicate better. Just like in real life, we can wave hello, give a thumbs up, or even roll our eyes at something funny. This makes our interactions more interesting and helps us understand each other better. And, just like in real life, seeing someone smile or frown can tell us a lot about how they're feeling without them having to say a word [70]. Overall, these communication tools help us have more fun and more meaningful relationships with our friends in virtual reality. It's like being at a big, awesome party where everyone can talk, laugh, and connect no matter where they are in the world. The foundation of hanging out with friends and meeting new people in the metaverse is basically just social VR platforms and communication tools. These things let us interact, talk, and work together in super-cool virtual worlds. And the best part is that we can use these tools to connect with people from all around the world, making us feel like we belong to a big, awesome community [71].

2.11 Security and Privacy

This section explores keeping users safe and making sure no one can access their info without permission.

2.11.1 Stopping Digital Harassment and Abuse

In the metaverse, safety and privacy are the important parameters for making the user feel safe and secure. The main two concerns for data protection are unauthorized users accessing another's data and the accessed data being used for harassment and abuse.

2.11.2 Protecting User Data and Preventing Unauthorized Access

Encryption and access controls are the two main parameters for making the data secure and safe in the metaverse. Encryption is the use of cipher text to disable other users from hacking a password. Access controls provide access only to certain people but not to everyone. For further protection, multifactor authentication is used, along with secret handshake algorithms and an additional password required to open a respective password. If there are any loopholes, the controls find and rectify them [72, 73]. This all helps keep our information safe and sound in the metaverse. It's important, because the Internet can be a pretty dangerous place sometimes. But with these security measures in place, we can at least have some peace of mind while we're exploring and doing our thing in the metaverse [71, 74, 75].

2.11.3 Stopping Virtual Harassment and Abuse

To make sure people feel safe and comfortable in the metaverse, there have to be systems in place to catch and stop harassment and abuse. They use AI to spot bad language and such, and report systems so users can tell someone if something's wrong. Also, community guidelines explain what's cool and what's not, and features like privacy controls and blocking enable users to choose who sees what [76, 77]. By putting all these things together, the metaverse can be a chill and safe place for people to hang out and do their thing. Everyone making and running the metaverse needs to take safety and privacy seriously, so users don't get to worry about getting hurt or having their stuff stolen. As the metaverse keeps growing, staying on top of safety and privacy is vital to make sure the metaverse is a place where people want to be. We can share experiences, have fun, and even make new friends through these virtual spaces. It is the new, innovative way to communicate once it is used day by day. It replaces all the new innovative social platforms with the metaverse for effective communication [78].

2.11.4 Inclusive Learning

Designing and developing a metaverse that's accessible and welcoming to users with disabilities is also critically important. A big part of that is using technology to make it inclusive for people with different needs. Another important part is creating user interfaces (UI) that work for a wide range of people. If we want people with disabilities to enjoy the metaverse, we need to use technology that helps them navigate and interact with virtual environments [79]. Visually impaired people can use screen readers and text-to-speech tools that read out text descriptions and other info to help them understand what's going on. Haptic feedback and audio cues can also help them interact with the environment. For people with motor disabilities, adaptable input methods like voice commands, gesture recognition, and alternate controllers can make it easier to navigate and interact with virtual objects. Even people with cognitive impairments can benefit from accessibility features like clear instructions and simplified interfaces [80].

The metaverse wouldn't be the same without inclusive UI design. It's important to think about users' abilities and preferences when creating virtual environments. This might include using large, easy-to-read fonts, high-contrast color schemes, and intuitive navigation patterns to help people with visual impairments. For people with motor limitations, having options like touch, speech, and keyboard shortcuts can be helpful [81]. To make sure the metaverse is accessible to everyone, designers can build customization options and make the interface easy to understand and use. It's also a good idea to test the designs with different user groups, including those with disabilities, to make sure everyone's needs are met. In the metaverse, users can interact with each other and digital entities in totally immersive online experiences. That means existing legal frameworks will need to change to cover things like virtual property rights, taxes, and jurisdiction. For example, virtual assets and transactions will need to be recognized as property, and tax laws will need to be updated to fit the unique characteristics of these transactions [82]. Platforms also need to set clear rules about jurisdiction to handle disputes that might involve users from all over the world. When it comes to content moderation, platforms need to have strong rules and tools in place to stop bad behavior like harassment and hate speech. This means clearly defining community standards and enforcing them strictly. Penalties for users who break these rules could include account suspension (temporary or permanent), warnings, or support for victims of abuse or harassment. Doing this will make the metaverse safer and more enjoyable for everyone.

2.12 Conclusion

To revolutionize technological growth, the metaverse plays a major role in the digital landscape, as new trending technologies are used for developing the metaverse, such as immersive technology, blockchain, spatial computing, and edge computing. Such technologies are revolutionizing the way we interact in real time with the 3D model. This chapter has addressed the issues and ethical concerns developers much consider to help develop the technology in the right way to create the metaverse effectively. Every decision we make now will influence how the digital world develops in the future, and we're all in this together, trying to figure out how to protect metaverse users' privacy and give everyone a chance to be heard. It would also be smart to establish clear guidelines to promote fairness and avoid chaos. We're all trying to understand together, to make the right choices so that everyone can have an interesting experience in the metaverse.

References

1. Mystakidis, S. (2022). Metaverse. *Encyclopedia*, *2*(1), 486–497.
2. Lee, L. H., Braud, T., Zhou, P., Wang, L., Xu, D., Lin, Z., … & Hui, P. (2021). All one needs to know about metaverse: A complete survey on technological singularity, virtual ecosystem, and research agenda. *arXiv preprint arXiv:2110.05352*.
3. Van der Land, S., Schouten, A., & Feldberg, F. (2011). Modeling the metaverse: A theoretical model of effective team collaboration in 3D virtual environments. *Journal of Virtual Worlds Research*, *4*(3), 1–18.
4. Bibri, S. E. (2022). The social shaping of the metaverse as an alternative to the imaginaries of data-driven smart cities: A study in science, technology, and society. *Smart Cities*, *5*(3), 832–874.
5. Wohlgenannt, I., Simons, A., & Stieglitz, S. (2020). Virtual reality. *Business & Information Systems Engineering*, *62*, 455–461.
6. Angelov, V., Petkov, E., Shipkovenski, G., & Kalushkov, T. (2020, June). Modern virtual reality headsets. In *2020 International Congress on Human-Computer Interaction, Optimization and Robotic Applications (HORA)* (pp. 1–5). IEEE.

7. Fang, W., Zheng, L., Deng, H., & Zhang, H. (2017). Real-time motion tracking for mobile augmented/virtual reality using adaptive visual-inertial fusion. *Sensors, 17*(5), 1037.

8. Benko, H., Holz, C., Sinclair, M., & Ofek, E. (2016, October). Normaltouch and texturetouch: High-fidelity 3D haptic shape rendering on handheld virtual reality controllers. In *Proceedings of the 29th Annual Symposium on User Interface Software and Technology* (pp. 717–728). ACM, NY.

9. Choi, S., Jung, K., & Noh, S. D. (2015). Virtual reality applications in manufacturing industries: Past research, present findings, and future directions. *Concurrent Engineering, 23*(1), 40–63.

10. Hernández-de-Menéndez, M., Vallejo Guevara, A., & Morales-Menendez, R. (2019). Virtual reality laboratories: A review of experiences. *International Journal on Interactive Design and Manufacturing (IJIDeM), 13*, 947–966.

11. Burdea, G. C. (2003). Virtual rehabilitation – benefits and challenges. *Methods of Information in Medicine, 42*(05), 519–523.

12. Iwendi, C. (2023). Innovative augmented and virtual reality applications for disease diagnosis based on integrated genetic algorithms. *International Journal of Cognitive Computing in Engineering, 4*, 266–276.

13. Craig, A. B. (2013). Understanding augmented reality: Concepts and applications. Elseiver.

14. Turk, M., & Fragoso, V. (2015). Computer vision for mobile augmented reality. *Mobile Cloud Visual Media Computing: From Interaction to Service*, 3–42. Springer Nature.

15. Tikander, M., Karjalainen, M., & Riikonen, V. (2008, September). An augmented reality audio headset. In *Proceedings of the 11th International Conference on Digital Audio Effects (DAFx-08), Espoo, Finland* (pp. 33–36). International Conference on Digital Audio Effects (DAFx), Espoo, Finland.

16. Nee, A. Y., Ong, S. K., Chryssolouris, G., & Mourtzis, D. (2012). Augmented reality applications in design and manufacturing. *CIRP Annals, 61*(2), 657–679.

17. Wloka, M. M., & Anderson, B. G. (1995, April). Resolving occlusion in augmented reality. In *Proceedings of the 1995 Symposium on Interactive 3D Graphics* (pp. 5–12). ACM, NY.

18. Mulder, J. D. (2005, March). Realistic occlusion effects in mirror-based co-located augmented reality systems. In *IEEE Proceedings. VR 2005. Virtual Reality, 2005.* (pp. 203–208). IEEE.

19. Greenwold, S. (2003). Spatial computing. *Massachusetts Institute of Technology, Master*.

20. Ghosh, S., & Lohani, B. (2013). Mining lidar data with spatial clustering algorithms. *International Journal of Remote Sensing, 34*(14), 5119–5135.

21. Li, H. (2016). *Evaluation of Multi-Level Cognitive Maps for Supporting between-Floor Spatial Behavior in Complex Indoor Environments*. The University of Maine.

22. Benford, S., & Fahlén, L. (1993, September). A spatial model of interaction in large virtual environments. In *Proceedings of the Third European Conference on Computer-Supported Cooperative Work 13–17 September 1993, Milan, Italy ECSCW'93* (pp. 109–124). Dordrecht: Springer Netherlands.

23. Chung, Y. C., Wang, J. M., Bailey, R. R., Chen, S. W., & Chang, S. L. (2004, December). A non-parametric blur measure based on edge analysis for image processing applications. In *IEEE Conference on Cybernetics and Intelligent Systems, 2004.* (Vol. 1, pp. 356–360). IEEE.

24. Deschênes, F., Ziou, D., & Fuchs, P. (1992). Simultaneous computation of defocus blur and apparent shifts in spatial domain. In *Actes de 15th International Conference on Vision Interface* (pp. 236–243).

25. Kang, S. B., Szeliski, R., & Chai, J. (2001, December). Handling occlusions in dense multi-view stereo. In *Proceedings of the 2001 IEEE Computer Society Conference on Computer Vision and Pattern Recognition. CVPR 2001* (Vol. 1, pp. I–I). IEEE.

26. Brown, M. Z., Burschka, D., & Hager, G. D. (2003). Advances in computational stereo. *IEEE Transactions on Pattern Analysis and Machine Intelligence, 25*(8), 993–1008.

27. Huynh-The, T., Pham, Q. V., Pham, X. Q., Nguyen, T. T., Han, Z., & Kim, D. S. (2023). Artificial intelligence for the metaverse: A survey. *Engineering Applications of Artificial Intelligence, 117,* 105581.

28. Solska, D. (2022). Traversing the metaverse: The new frontiers for computer-mediated communication and natural language processing. *Forum Filologiczne Ateneum, 1* (10), 1–20.

29. Kim, D. Y., Lee, H. K., & Chung, K. (2023). Avatar-mediated experience in the metaverse: The impact of avatar realism on user-avatar relationship. *Journal of Retailing and Consumer Services, 73,* 103382.

30. Lim, W. Y. B., Xiong, Z., Niyato, D., Cao, X., Miao, C., Sun, S., & Yang, Q. (2022). Realizing the metaverse with edge intelligence: A match made in heaven. *IEEE Wireless Communications, 30*(4), 110–117.

31. Alam, A., & Mohanty, A. (2022). Metaverse and Posthuman animated avatars for teaching-learning process: Interperception in virtual universe for educational transformation. In *International Conference on Innovations in Intelligent Computing and Communications* (pp. 47–61). Springer, Cham.

32. de Souza, V. B., de Andrade, R. C., & Da Silva, T. C. (2023). NLP applied to systematic review: Case study for the creation of a golden set for the metaverse. In *Future of Information and Communication Conference* (pp. 431–449). Springer, Cham.

33. Hou, J., Wang, X., Xu, F., Nguyen, V. D., & Wu, L. (2009). Humanoid personalized avatar through multiple natural language processing. *International Journal of Computer and Information Engineering, 3*(11), 2731–2736.

34. Hudon, A., Phraxayavong, K., Potvin, S., & Dumais, A. (2023). Comparing the performance of machine learning algorithms in the automatic classification of psychotherapeutic interactions in avatar therapy. *Machine Learning and Knowledge Extraction, 5*(3), 1119–1131.

35. Kao, D., & Harrell, D. F. (2015, August). Toward avatar models to enhance performance and engagement in educational games. In *2015 IEEE Conference on Computational Intelligence and Games (CIG)* (pp. 246–253). IEEE.

36. Butler, C., Subramanian, L., & Michalowicz, S. (2016, May). Crowdsourced facial expression mapping using a 3D avatar. In *Proceedings of the 2016 CHI Conference Extended Abstracts on Human Factors in Computing Systems* (pp. 2798–2804). ACM, NY.

37. Tewari, A., Chhabria, A., Khalsa, A. S., Chaudhary, S., & Kanal, H. (2021, April). A survey of mental health chatbots using NLP. In *Proceedings of the International Conference on Innovative Computing & Communication (ICICC)* (pp. 288–296). Springer Nature, Singapore.

38. Ng, H. T., & Zelle, J. (1997). Corpus-based approaches to semantic interpretation in NLP. *AI Magazine, 18*(4), 45–45.

39. Kann, K., Cho, K., & Bowman, S. R. (2019). Towards realistic practices in low-resource natural language processing: The development set. *arXiv preprint arXiv:1909.01522.*

40. Zhu, H. (2022). Metaaid: A flexible framework for developing metaverse applications via ai technology and human editing. *arXiv preprint arXiv:2204.01614.*

41. Pyaraka, S. C. R., Lanka, S. S., Konanki, P., Venu Gopalachari, M., Rakesh, S., & Jayaram, D. (2022, December). Review on 3D Model Generation through Natural Language and Image Processing. In *International Conference on Information and Management Engineering* (pp. 311–317). Springer Nature, Singapore.

42. Zheng, Z., Xie, S., Dai, H. N., Chen, X., & Wang, H. (2018). Blockchain challenges and opportunities: A survey. *International Journal of Web and Grid Services, 14*(4), 352–375.

43. Huynh-The, T., Gadekallu, T. R., Wang, W., Yenduri, G., Ranaweera, P., Pham, Q. V., … & Liyanage, M. (2023). Blockchain for the metaverse: A review. *Future Generation Computer Systems, 143*, 401–419.

44. Tredinnick, L. (2019). Cryptocurrencies and the blockchain. *Business Information Review, 36*(1), 39–44.

45. Zheng, Z., Xie, S., Dai, H., Chen, X., & Wang, H. (2017, June). An overview of blockchain technology: Architecture, consensus, and future trends. In *2017 IEEE International Congress on Big Data (BigData Congress)* (pp. 557–564). IEEE.

46. Wright, A., & De Filippi, P. (2015). Decentralized blockchain technology and the rise of lex cryptographia. *Available at SSRN 2580664.*

47. Zarrin, J., Wen Phang, H., Babu Saheer, L., & Zarrin, B. (2021). Blockchain for decentralization of Internet: Prospects, trends, and challenges. *Cluster Computing, 24*(4), 2841–2866.

48. Atzori, M. (2015). Blockchain technology and decentralized governance: Is the state still necessary? *Available at SSRN 2709713.*

49. Anderson, J. H., Korsun, G., & Murrell, P. (2000). Which enterprises (believe they) have soft budgets? Evidence on the effects of ownership and decentralization in Mongolia. *Journal of Comparative Economics, 28*(2), 219–246.

50. Liu, Y., & Tyagi, R. K. (2011). The benefits of competitive upward channel decentralization. *Management Science, 57*(4), 741–751.

51. Lee, E., Seo, Y. D., Oh, S. R., & Kim, Y. G. (2021). A survey on standards for interoperability and security in the Internet of Things. *IEEE Communications Surveys & Tutorials, 23*(2), 1020–1047.

52. Hasan, M. K., Habib, A. A., Shukur, Z., Ibrahim, F., Islam, S., & Razzaque, M. A. (2023). Review on cyber-physical and cyber-security system in smart grid: Standards, protocols, constraints, and recommendations. *Journal of Network and Computer Applications, 209*, 103540.

53. Yang, L. (2023). Recommendations for metaverse governance based on technical standards. *Humanities and Social Sciences Communications, 10*(1), 1–10.

54. Antonopoulos, N., & Gillam, L. (2010). *Cloud Computing* (Vol. 51, No. 7). London: Springer.

55. Núñez, A., Vázquez-Poletti, J. L., Caminero, A. C., Castañé, G. G., Carretero, J., & Llorente, I. M. (2012). iCanCloud: A flexible and scalable cloud infrastructure simulator. *Journal of Grid Computing, 10*, 185–209.

56. Khmelevsky, Y., & Voytenko, V. (2010, May). Cloud computing infrastructure prototype for university education and research. In *Proceedings of the 15th Western Canadian Conference on Computing Education* (pp. 1–5). Canadian Society for Computational Studies of Intelligence, Edmonton, Alberta, Canada.

57. Koo, J., & Qureshi, N. M. F. (2021). Fine-grained data processing framework for heterogeneous IoT devices in sub-aquatic edge computing environment. *Wireless Personal Communications, 116*, 1407–1422.

58. Lamport, L., & Lynch, N. (1990). Distributed computing: models and methods. In *Formal Models and Semantics* (pp. 1157–1199). H. D. Apt, K. R. Apt, and J. W. de Bakker (eds.). Elsevier.

59. Cao, K., Liu, Y., Meng, G., & Sun, Q. (2020). An overview on edge computing research. *IEEE Access, 8*, 85714–85728.

60. Pan, J., & McElhannon, J. (2017). Future edge cloud and edge computing for Internet of Things applications. *IEEE Internet of Things Journal, 5*(1), 439–449.

61. Beraldi, R., Canali, C., Lancellotti, R., & Mattia, G. P. (2022). On the impact of stale information on distributed online load balancing protocols for edge computing. *Computer Networks, 210*, 108935.

62. Xiao, Y., Jia, Y., Liu, C., Cheng, X., Yu, J., & Lv, W. (2019). Edge computing security: State of the art and challenges. *Proceedings of the IEEE, 107*(8), 1608–1631.

63. Wang, J., Feng, Z., Chen, Z., George, S., Bala, M., Pillai, P., … & Satyanarayanan, M. (2018, October). Bandwidth-efficient live video analytics for drones via edge computing. In *2018 IEEE/ACM Symposium on Edge Computing (SEC)* (pp. 159–173). IEEE.

64. Lee, J., Lee, T. S., Lee, S., Jang, J., Yoo, S., Choi, Y., & Park, Y. R. (2022). Development and application of a metaverse-based social skills training program for children with autism spectrum disorder to improve social interaction: Protocol for a randomized controlled trial. *JMIR Research Protocols, 11*(6), e35960.

65. Liang, H., Li, J., Wang, Y., Pan, J., Zhang, Y., & Dong, X. (2023). Metaverse virtual social center for elderly communication in time of social distancing. *Virtual Reality & Intelligent Hardware, 5*(1), 68–80.

66. Hennig-Thurau, T., Aliman, D. N., Herting, A. M., Cziehso, G. P., Linder, M., & Kübler, R. V. (2023). Social interactions in the metaverse: Framework, initial evidence, and research roadmap. *Journal of the Academy of Marketing Science, 51*(4), 889–913.

67. Lee, J. H., Lee, T. S., Yoo, S. Y., Lee, S. W., Jang, J. H., Jin Choi, Y., & Park, Y. R. (2023). Metaverse-based social skills training programme for children with autism spectrum disorder to improve social interaction ability: An open-label, single-centre, randomised controlled pilot trial. *EClinicalMedicine, 61*, 102072.

68. Balasubramaniam, S, Syed, M. H., More, N. S., & Polepally, V. (2023). Deep learning-based power prediction aware charge scheduling approach in cloud based electric vehicular network. *Engineering Applications of Artificial Intelligence, 121*, 105869.

69. Voinea, G. D., Gîrbacia, F., Postelnicu, C. C., Duguleana, M., Antonya, C., Soica, A., & Stănescu, R. C. (2022). Study of social presence while interacting in metaverse with an augmented avatar during autonomous driving. *Applied Sciences, 12*(22), 11804.

70. Tu, J. (2022). *Meetings in the metaverse: Exploring online meeting spaces through meaningful interactions in Gather.Town* (Master's thesis, University of Waterloo).

71. Maloney, D. (2021). A youthful metaverse: towards designing safe, equitable, and emotionally fulfilling social virtual reality spaces for younger users.

72. Di Pietro, R., & Cresci, S. (2021, December). Metaverse: Security and privacy issues. In *2021 Third IEEE International Conference on Trust, Privacy and Security in Intelligent Systems and Applications (TPS-ISA)* (pp. 281–288). IEEE.

73. Macpherson, I., & Puplampu, A. (2023). Better than the real you? VR, identity, privacy, and the metaverse. In *Virtual Identities and Digital Culture* (pp. 152–160). A. Puplampu (ed.). Routledge.
74. Choudhury, A., Balasubramaniam, S, Kumar, A. P., & Kumar, S. N. P. (2023). PSSO: Political squirrel search optimizer-driven deep learning for severity level detection and classification of lung cancer. *International Journal of Information Technology & Decision Making, 22*(4), 1–34.
75. Hadi Mogavi, R., Hoffman, J., Deng, C., Du, Y., Haq, E. U., & Hui, P. (2023, July). Envisioning an inclusive metaverse: Student perspectives on accessible and empowering metaverse-enabled learning. In *Proceedings of the Tenth ACM Conference on Learning@ Scale* (pp. 346–353). ACM, NY.
76. Song, J. (2023). Inclusive educational effectiveness through metaverse for the disabled students and policy suggestions. *Journal of Intelligence and Information Systems, 29*(1), 175–201.
77. Balasubramaniam, S, & Kumar, K. S. (2022). Fractional feedback political optimizer with prioritization-based charge scheduling in cloud-assisted electric vehicular network. *Ad Hoc & Sensor Wireless Networks, 52*(3–4), 173–198.
78. Far, S. B., & Rad, A. I. (2022). Applying digital twins in metaverse: User interface, security and privacy challenges. *Journal of Metaverse, 2*(1), 8–15.
79. Balasubramaniam, S, Kadry, S., & Kumar, K. S. (2024). Osprey gannet optimization enabled CNN based transfer learning for optic disc detection and cardiovascular risk prediction using retinal fundus images. *Biomedical Signal Processing and Control, 93*, 106177.
80. Chen, B. J., & Yang, D. N. (2022, October). User recommendation in social metaverse with VR. In *Proceedings of the 31st ACM International Conference on Information & Knowledge Management* (pp. 148–158). ACM, NY.
81. Kadry, S., Dhanaraj, R. K., & Manthiramoorthy, C. (2024). Res-Unet based blood vessel segmentation and cardio vascular disease prediction using chronological chef-based optimization algorithm based deep residual network from retinal fundus images. *Multimedia Tools and Applications, 83*(1), 1–30.
82. Ryu, J., Son, S., Lee, J., Park, Y., & Park, Y. (2022). Design of secure mutual authentication scheme for metaverse environments using blockchain. *IEEE Access, 10*, 98944–98958.

Chapter 3

Metaverse-Powered Human–Computer Interactions and Applications

Rahul D, Susan George, and Amritha P. S

3.1 Introduction

The metaverse differs from conventional online platforms in that it is immersive and everlasting. It is an innovative combination of blockchain technology, augmented reality, virtual worlds, and artificial intelligence that has created previously unheard-of opportunities for improving user experiences and encouraging new kinds of creativity and cooperation. This chapter discusses (1) interaction technology in the metaverse, (2) the impact of 5G communication, (3) the influence of 5G connectivity on the evolution of the metaverse, (4) blockchain technology in the metaverse, (5) the current state of human–computer interaction (HCI), (6) computer vision in metaverse HCI, (7) computer vision challenges and solutions, (8) metaverse applications in the gaming and entertainment industry, (9) cyberspace metaverse application status, and (10) opportunities and challenges for HCI in the metaverse's future development.

3.2 Interaction Technology in the Metaverse

Three-dimensional (3D) printing, extended reality (XR, including augmented reality [AR], virtual reality [VR], and mixed reality [MR]), holographic projection,

          DOI: 10.1201/9781003491668-3

and brain–computer interfaces (BCI) are examples of interaction technologies used in the metaverse. The technologies like 3D printing and holographic projection have already reached a stable stage. While XR equipment has been available for some time, it has not yet been widely accepted by the public. When a visual presentation is required, like during exhibition setup or wedding organizing, holographic projection is commonly employed. HCI is an important element of interface technology that uses the interactions and patterns of computer interfaces between humans and computers. HCI attempts to uncover areas that still need development while facilitating smooth communication between the user and the computer. The main elements of HCI are humans, computer, and their interaction. To design maximally appropriate systems and provide useful and functional interaction situations, developers need to understand their clients from various points of view.

3.3 Technological Advancements Enabling the Metaverse

The new technologies that power the 3D metaverse are depicted in Figure 3.1. They are artificial intelligence (AI), Blockchain, Internet of Things (IoT), AR, VR, 3D reconstruction, and edge computing.

AI: AI has been utilized in recent years for faster computing, face recognition, decision-making, and corporate strategy planning. AI experts have been researching the creation of immersive metaverses lately. AI can provide real-time data analysis and is capable of producing novel outcomes and insights through training from past iterations and historical data. AI can generate life-like metaverse avatars by analyzing 2D and 3D images [1].

Blockchain: Blockchain technology facilitates value transfer, digital collectability, and decentralized digital evidence of possession, transparency, and connectedness. With cryptocurrency, people may work and socialize while transferring wealth in three dimensions. One can purchase virtual lands in Decentral and with Bitcoin. Players can purchase 16 × 16 meter nonfungible tokens (NFTs) with the game's cryptocurrency. Blockchain technology offers protection for digital property rights. Cryptocurrency may in the future encourage people to engage with and contribute to the metaverse [1].

IoT: Communication in IoT systems is made possible by the usage of different types of sensor devices (i.e., for exchanging data from the different devices to the Internet). A unique identifier is provided to each of these sensors, and they can autonomously exchange data once they are connected. IoT gathers and transmits data to the metaverse, using different sensors connecting to speakers, thermostats, medical equipment, and other gadgets, which enhances digital precision. IoT data streams can influence how metaverse objects function in response to weather conditions or other variables [2].

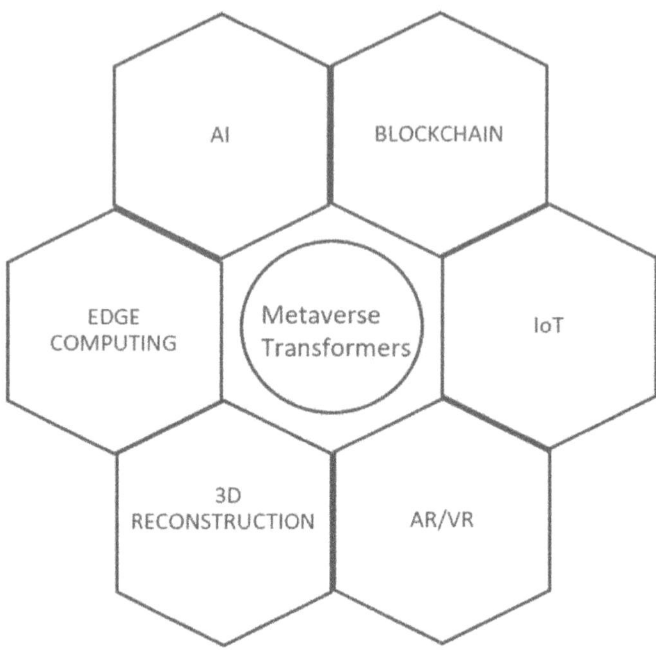

Figure 3.1   Top technologies for metaverse development.

AR and VR: AR modifies the real world by adding digital images and characters. It is compatible with almost any smartphone or digital camera, making it more accessible than virtual reality. VR already incorporates fake images. VR and AR together work like an early metaverse.

3D reconstruction: 3D reconstruction has been used more frequently (especially in the real estate industry) during the COVID pandemic, when lockdowns made it impossible for buyers to visit homes in person. Certain organizations offer virtual property tours through the use of 3D reconstruction. Similar to the metaverse, buyers may view new homes from anywhere and make purchases without going inside. A digital world that is as realistic as possible is created in the metaverse. Scenes with a life-like appearance are produced by 3D reconstruction. VR sites and objects are rendered with remarkable life-like 3D images using specialized 3D cameras.

Edge computing: Edge is essentially a formwork that is dispersed and comparable to cloud computing, with the exception that it is housed in a small data center nearby. On the edge, users can access cloud-like processing, storage, data, and application capabilities. For the user's experience to be comparable to the real thing, you must engage them and let them immerse themselves in the metaverse.

3.4 The Influence of 5G Connectivity on the Evolution of the Metaverse

Different technologies are used to create a sophisticated Internet application in the metaverse, and its structure is supported by technologies like networking and wireless communication [3]. The first-generation (1G) networks in digital communication could only provide voice services. Better text and voice messaging capabilities as well as modest data rate services were made possible by the introduction of the 2G network. However, it could not support mobile Internet access. However, the 3G network fixed this problem. Higher voice service capacity and faster data services were both made possible by the 3G standards. Later, high-capacity and high-speed data services for mobile multimedia were introduced by the relatively new 4G mobile communication networks. The introduction of the 5G communication system changed the entire Internet scenario by providing

- Enhanced mobile broadband services,
- Ultrareliable and low-latent communications, and
- Massive multiuser machine-type communication [4].

3.4.1 Enhanced Mobile Broadband (eMBB)

5G communication standards have enhanced broadband services to achieve uniform coverage with high data. This was made possible by an increase in data rates from 1 giga bytes per second (Gbps) in the 4G technology to 20 Gbps in IMT-2020 systems operating on 5G. So, 10 to 100 times higher data rate is possible by 5Gs and can provide a far faster and higher quality of experience (QoE) than 4G networks, owing to a tenfold increase in user-experienced data rate [4].

3.4.2 Ultrareliable Low-Latency Communications (uRLLC)

5G systems carry data at 300 Kps and provide services with a latency of less than 1 ms [5]. With a latency requirement of only 10 ms, this 4G technology represented a significant advancement. Numerous real-time technologies, including VR/AR and driverless cars, will succeed with this standard. The second aspect of this service is that even in the worst-case scenarios, 5G systems must be able to provide services with above 99.999% availability. These systems must have a system latency of less than 5 ms and be incredibly dependable. The goal of each of these is to contribute to an energy consumption reduction of above 90%.

3.4.3 Massive Multiuser Machine-Type Communications (mMTC)

The enhanced capacity for devices enabled by the wireless network is another feature of 5G services. It can efficiently transport modest payloads over a large number of devices thanks to its broader coverage area [4, 5]. XR gadgets and a multitude of sensors capture data from the surroundings. Examples include motion wristbands, gloves, light detection and ranging (LIDAR) sensors, volumetric capture cameras, haptic devices, and several other devices. The following are some basic needs shared by all of these devices for providing the required service at a reasonable cost and level of comfort:

- They require a safe and dependable network.
- The lowest possible latency must be used to connect these devices.
- To preserve equilibrium, computing tasks must be moved from these devices to the edge/cloud (computing).

This means that within a few milliseconds, data will be continuously flowing between AR/VR devices and the cloud at a high data rate and low latency. Therefore, it is crucial to have a wireless connection that is low-cost, secure, and dependable. The only technology that can accomplish these is 5G. Additionally, a few wireless connectivity options exist, including cellular technology, Bluetooth, and wireless fidelity (Wi-Fi). None of these include some essential components needed for universal access. Wi-Fi can deliver the required data rate, but when multiple devices are linked together, network congestion occurs, leading to very high latency. Comparably, Bluetooth's dependability, data rate, and range are lacking. Wi-Fi7 claims to alleviate Wi-Fi congestion, although its range is nowhere near as great as that of cellular technology. 5G also offers significantly more latency, range, and dependability of data [6].

Wireless communication networks will be subject to increased demands due to three distinct elements of the metaverse. Low latency, immersion, and anytime-anywhere are a few of these [5]. This means that in addition to improving device performance, wireless communication between the edge, cloud, and device must also be accomplished, posing unique demands on the current 5G network. This will necessitate a very latency-free and dependable network that supports large connectivity. The 5G eMBB, massive multiuser machine-type communications (mMTC), and ultrareliable and low-latency communication (uRLLC) solutions can handle them. A highly dedicated Internet communication network is a must for achieving the synchronization of both worlds. The 5G network's ability to deliver uRLLC makes this feature crucial.

The metaverse promises to dismantle the limitations imposed by place and time by enabling anyone to access it with ease from anywhere at any time. To do so, the metaverse must always be linked to the network. Due to this spatiotemporal aspect, a highly dependable, massively connected, and latency-free network is needed. The 5G solutions uRLLC, mMTC, and eMBB can handle this demand. To properly deploy and gain widespread usage of the metaverse, the following nonconnectivity concerns must also be addressed:

- Developers must be able to use 5G thanks to application program interfaces (APIs), and business logic must seamlessly integrate with APIs.

- Telecom companies need to follow global guidelines for the rollout of 5G and the creation of metaverse ecosystem standards; they should learn from the Internet's smooth standardization procedure [5, 7].

3.5 Blockchain Technology in the Metaverse

Blockchain is a secure method that works well for e-commerce sites since it uses proof of work as its consensus mechanism. Blockchain is the indispensable tool that the metaverse uses to impose accountability on the digital ecosystem. Its main goal is to secure the digital content that is owned by every metaverse user. Blockchain technology can operate without a central authority on data from decentralized ledgers [8]. Digital assets like homogenized tokens based on ERC-20 and nonhomogenized tokens based on ERC-721 or ERC-1155 are among the key services provided by the blockchain. The metaverse relies heavily on blockchain technology to maintain its smooth economic operations.

By enabling the exchange of virtual products for real money, blockchain technology allows users to integrate into the cryptocurrency market from within the metaverse. In the metaverse, virtual assets may be bought and sold using Bitcoin and other cryptocurrencies thanks to blockchain technology. Any kind of asset, including money, can be moved and utilized in any virtual world inside the metaverse. Furthermore, blockchain opens up the metaverse as a decentralized, open-source public platform where users can develop apps and conduct online transactions.

Blockchain technology can provide secured and efficient healthcare services in the metaverse by offering a distributed ledger (that is, it can safely store private information, including medical records). Furthermore, automatic payments between providers and insurers could be made possible by blockchain-based smart contracts, thereby eliminating the middlemen. Individuals will get more privacy over their health data via decentralized identity procedures on blockchains like Ethereum, while simultaneously ensuring that only those with permission can access medical records [9]. However, a breach of privacy on sensitive data is a huge risk in the metaverse when shared on centralized data exchange platforms [10]. High latency and scarcity of reliable data are the main limitations of the traditional sharing environment (due to the high degree of mutability) [11]. Compatibility is further limited by the stark disparities in consensus processes and transaction architecture between these virtual worlds [12]. Even one human mistake, like misplacing a private key, might compromise the security of blockchain technology. Because third-party apps frequently employ insufficient security measures, hackers can readily target them in the metaverse and compromise personal data in the process [13–15]. A centralized approach to storing data is not desirable in such situations. Intervirtual world data sharing depends heavily on IoT devices' cross-platform capabilities [16].

Blockchain creates secure records of shared interactions in simulated universes by enabling data flow across IoT devices in the metaverse via cross-chain networks [17].

Transactions within the metaverse are verified and recorded to remove any potential conflicts and boost trust among participants. IoT-enabled blockchain allows real-time data storage in the metaverse. All parties involved may rely on the facts and take prompt, efficient action because blockchain transactions are irreversible [18]. Blockchain technology can only be used in the metaverse for digital twin applications if issues with scalability, privacy, and standardization are fixed. By combining federated learning, XAI, and blockchain technologies, user data privacy will be ensured and decisions made using sensor data will become explicable. It also improves the digital twin quality of the metaverse [19, 20].

3.6 Current State of HCI

HCI contributes to the design of intuitive interfaces, immersive interactions, and engaging virtual environments that enhance collaboration, communication, entertainment, and exploration within digital spaces.

It mainly focuses on the interactions and patterns of computer interfaces between humans and computer applications (shown in Figure 3.2). A reliable and user-friendly interactive interface can be developed by building a seamless interaction between the user and the computer through the use of HCI. HCI research, which examines how users interact with virtual environments inside the metaverse, places a strong emphasis on understanding human behaviors, preferences, and cognitive processes as they navigate through immersive digital settings. In the new

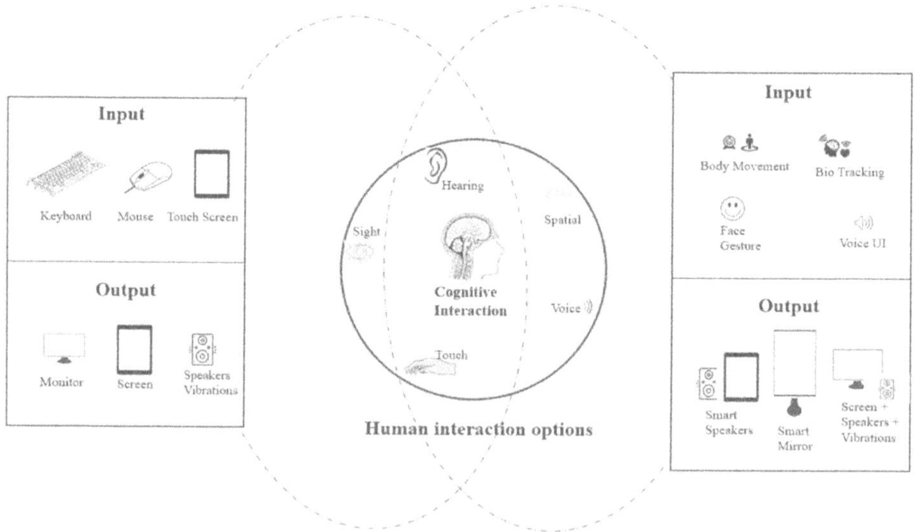

Figure 3.2   Human interaction options.

metaverse experience, current human engagement techniques like computer mouse clicks and keyboard typing could not be obvious. Understanding human behavior is crucial to designing interfaces that are user-friendly, efficient, and enjoyable. The design of interfaces that enable smooth interaction inside the metaverse is a critical responsibility of HCI specialists. This involves the development of user-friendly navigation systems, interactive menus, and responsive controls.

To increase the precision and speed of gesture recognition (GR), for instance, research into many algorithms is necessary for vision-based GR. Human characteristics such as lip reading, eye iris, handwriting, stride, voice, palm, and facial traits are also being researched and employed. HCI in the metaverse encompasses various aspects, such as AR/VR, voice interaction technology, and somatosensory interaction technology. Naturally, further technologies like blockchain, 5G communication, digital twins, and cloud computing are needed to make a true metaverse a reality. The following requirements are essential to accomplish this:

- Possess a solid understanding of how consumers interact with computing systems.
- Create strategies, tactics, and resources that let user access systems according to their needs.
- Make necessary changes, test, improve, validate, and make sure users can effectively communicate or engage with the systems.
- Always put end users first and establish a solid basis for HCI.

To fulfill the aforementioned points, developers must concentrate on two important areas: usability and user experience. HCI relies heavily on usability since it makes sure that users of all backgrounds can pick up and use computer systems rapidly. The following features define an HCI system that is useful and practical:

Safe: A safe system protects users against unfavorable and potentially dangerous situations. Users can feel more at ease navigating the system or interface when the system offers error recovery programs.

Utility: The term *utility* describes the different features and resources that the system offers to accomplish the desired goal. An integrated development environment (IDE) that occasionally makes suggestions to programmers or users is a prime example of a sound utility system. User experience is concerned with the feelings that people get when interacting with a computing system. Here, user emotions are examined on an individual basis to help developers and support teams target specific users to elicit good sensations during system usage. Based on the patterns they identify, HCI systems further enhance the system by classifying user interaction patterns into the following categories:
- Desirable traits: fulfilling, entertaining, inspiring, or surprising.
- Undesirable traits: annoying, unpleasant, or frustrating.

3.7 Computer Vision in Metaverse HCI

The metaverse will become a commercially viable reality through the use of AI, especially computer vision [21]. The key to portraying virtual worlds seamlessly is spatial computing, which makes use of sophisticated computer vision algorithms and intelligent 2D/3D sensors to map the real world precisely and construct realistic 3D metaverse environments [22]. Computer vision principles such as gesture identification, human-pose tracking, and mood and expression analysis will enable gadgets to interpret human behavior in their surroundings and utilize that information to create intuitive and incredibly lifelike sensory experiences in the metaverse. For instance, everyone who has ever used an Instagram or Snapchat filter is aware that face recognition technology has the ability to instantly process your image and transform it into a 3D animated figure, which is used to generate avatars [23, 24].

The production of highly immersive experiences will be made possible by advancements in machine vision, which will also make technology simpler and more accessible for devices such as smartphones. As the metaverse develops and becomes more complex, an increasing number of computer vision apps will become available online [25]. As it is, the metaverse is a fully realized virtual environment where users can connect, mingle, trade money, make digital art, and conduct hyperrealistic shopping and selling. With the exception of avatars, which let you be whatever you choose to be in the metaverse, nothing about it differs significantly from our physical plane of reality. But in this world, unlike the "real" one, technology is necessary [26]. Allied Marketing Research estimates that the supporting areas of computer vision will grow to a value of 41 billion by 2030 [27, 28]. This is because users need headsets, haptic gloves, apps, and connected equipment to see, hear, and feel the metaverse. Computer vision acts as the unseen infrastructure that makes these interfaces comprehensible [29].

The application of computer vision in the metaverse aids content preservation by utilizing algorithms that can recognize and remove inappropriate content. As such, this makes it easier to create virtual spaces that are courteous and safer [30]. It is imperative to acknowledge that this specific industry is seeing swift development, and these applications are expected to expand in tandem with technological breakthroughs and the increasing recognition of metaverse. It is essential to acknowledge that this specific industry is seeing swift development, and these applications are expected to expand in tandem with technological breakthroughs and the increasing recognition of the metaverse. Table 3.1 includes a summary of the key metaverse strategies of substantial importance.

3.8 Computer Vision Challenges and Solutions

The important challenges and problems associated with computer vision in the metaverse include the following.

Table 3.1 Different Metaverse Techniques

No	Technique	Description
1	VR	Users can interact with a computer-generated 3D virtual space with immersive technology. This technology often uses headsets and motion tracking.
2	AR	Uses tools like AR glasses or smartphones to overlay digital data into the physical world, improving the user's view of their surroundings.
3	Blockchain	Distributed ledger technology enables digital asset ownership and verifiable transactions in the metaverse by offering safe and transparent transactions.
4	AI	Enhances the realism and interaction of the metaverse by imitating human behavior, enabling intelligent agents and nonplayer characters (NPCs), and aiding dynamic content development.
5	Haptic feedback	Technology that gives users tactile sensations so they can interact and feel virtual items improves the user's experience of presence in virtual surroundings.
6	Decentralized identity	By granting individuals autonomy over their digital identities and belongings and safeguarding user security and privacy, this technology reduces the likelihood of centralized control in the metaverse.
7	Social VR platforms	Develops a sense of community within the metaverse by promoting social interactions through shared virtual places and avatars.
8	Gamification	Incorporates aspects of games like achievements and rewards into metaverse nongaming environments to boost motivation and engagement.

Realism and accuracy: One of the primary concerns when using computer vision algorithms in a metaverse environment is generating a high level of realism and accuracy. The metaverse is a virtual world, and the images and videos captured by the computer vision algorithm must represent information similar to virtual environments [31].

Transparency and interoperability: High-quality annotated datasets from machine learning models are necessary for improved computer vision to guarantee that metaverse hardware and software can cross boundaries between real and virtual worlds. Realistic rendering and tracking of objects, people, and settings in real time is a must for providing an immersive and lifelike experience to the users [1].

Computational power and scalability: Performance problems come from the need for large amounts of processing power required by many computer vision systems, especially those involving real-time analysis. Optimizing computer vision algorithms to reduce their processing requirements is one possible strategy. Moreover, it has been demonstrated that the metaverse's computer vision systems operate more efficiently when advanced hardware accelerators like graphics processing units (GPUs) are used [2].

Privacy and security: The metaverse is an intricate network of interconnected systems that necessitates the smooth operation of various platforms and gadgets. Interoperability and communication with other technologies, including AR, VR, and IoT, are critical for computer vision. The metaverse's dynamic structure poses challenges for computer vision systems. Computer vision algorithms that lack adaptability may face difficulties due to the dynamic nature of content and interactions inside the metaverse [32].

Environmental impact: The computational power required for computer vision algorithms can have a significant environmental impact, especially if the algorithms are run on energy-intensive hardware [33].

3.9 Metaverse Application in the Gaming and Entertainment Industry

Virtual worlds function through the network virtualization of human behavior, human endowments, the economy, and other elements necessary for life. Building the virtual world's infrastructure and regulations and finishing the virtual world line, characters, real players, and virtual people are some of the unseen components of this process. The creation of content, virtual money, interactive platforms, and dominating economic commodities are all made possible by the digital infrastructure. Using physical gestures, voice cues, visual cues, and other senses directly is known as somatosensory interaction [34, 35]. AR is required for the metaverse to fulfill its goal of enabling this kind of smooth communication due to the limitations of current technology. XR allows users to seamlessly travel between two worlds by using a computer to build a virtual world [36]. An extensive degree of anthropomorphic, immersive experience is necessary for the metaverse. The desktop and mobile gadgets that are currently on the market cannot accurately replicate the sense perception of experiencing the actual scenario. Enhancing realism and user experience is VR's main goal, and game design reflects this as well.

In 2019, Krompiec and Park aimed to provide consistent and realistic player interactions for first-person shooter games. In order to make physical equipment match with VR filming gear, they designed and changed the existing mapping ways between the virtual and physical/real worlds. It is essential to have devices that support HCI and collaboration, and interactive features are the only way to make this possible. Wearable interactive gadgets are becoming possible with recent developments in electronics, mechanical design, and materials science. To create wearable electronics, ultrathin stretchy electronics made from indium-zinc oxide semiconductor nanofilms made on sol−gel polymers can be used [37]. Additional advantages include a robust interface, undetectable wear, and adaptability. Wearable technology might be utilized to provide intelligent feedback by both robots and humans.

Surface electromyography (sEMG)−based GR and deep learning (DL) techniques are becoming more and more crucial to interpersonal communication in virtual environments. The benefits of augmenting conventional therapeutic techniques with multiuser virtual reality (MUVR) remote psychotherapy are being studied among patients with body image issues. The study revealed the efficacy of exposure treatment, play therapy, and acceptance and commitment therapy [38]. Common methods of interacting with VR environments include game controllers, motion tracking systems (MTSs), and data gloves. However, some users, such as those who have limb paralysis, may find them annoying or uncomfortable.

A music-on-demand system for a VR environment was also developed by the researchers using electro-oculography (EOG)−based HCI. (Select the appropriate song from the list, skip to the next one in the playlist, play a particular selected theme, or jump to the desired song in the library). Experiments ultimately demonstrated the method's efficacy. In a VR environment, patients with movement impairments will benefit immensely from this kind of interaction [39].

Despite the advancements in XR technology, consumers' experiences are nevertheless impacted by particularly complex wearable devices. Consequently, wearable-free tangible engagement techniques are rapidly becoming more commonplace, while they still need technology assistance for precise touch, motion detection, and feedback. A quick eye-tracking system was described by [19] to address situations requiring high processing speed but low precision. The low-resolution (640 × 480) webcam used in this experiment greatly reduced the hardware cost. The corresponding algorithms were developed to handle different quality levels of photographs. To lessen the computational load, an efficient pupil detection technique based on color intensity fluctuations is employed, providing a rapid and low-cost means of tracking eyes.

A metaverse system for AR distant collaboration in VR was presented by [7] regarding haptic feedback (HF). Through concrete encounters between in-person employees and virtual expert assistants, the technology offers tactile input. An internal user research comparing two interfaces for remote collaboration between skilled assistants and local staff was conducted using this system. Tangible physical mapping and free mapping in midair were the two interfaces that were being considered. The authors' assessments of operating error and performance time did not show any statistically significant variance. However, according to users, remote experts in VR can have a significantly better user experience with actual, physical sketching interfaces that support passive HF. Robotic design has also made use of tangible interaction. An experimental investigation of tactile and tangible interaction in a dual-reality setting was provided by [10].

AR has been applied to a variety of industries, including education, entertainment, and HCI. Nevertheless, tangible interactions with virtual and physical entities are not possible with current AR devices, particularly when it comes to direct manipulation and interior accessibility of virtual and physical/real elements inside a cube. As a result, [15] introduced AR Shell, a brand-new, inventive variation of the AR cube. AR Shells, in contrast to typical AR devices, provide natural, hands-on interactions with AR items. One important feature is the AR Shell's ability to use physics tools. This method of building AR Shells allows for a variety of viewpoints and real-world interactions through openings.

A nostalgic-themed interactive somatic sensory rehabilitation game was created by [40] for older patients suffering from mild cognitive impairment (MCI), drawing influence from the Tetris game. To find out whether adding a tangible game to rehabilitation improved the motivation and willingness of people with motor cognitive impairments to use restoration, an interactive, intuitive gesture-controlled game was deployed. According to the findings, new sensory rehabilitation activities can spark older persons' interest and boost their will to keep going through therapy. Only the motor and tangible systems can be consciously used to move the human body. The physical reaction and brain activity related to sensory perception are controlled by the motor execution system. [41] created an HCI environment with a game prototype which is handled by the game engine. The experiment's findings demonstrated that allowing mice to freely explore the system is a more straightforward method of interaction than other ways, and that tactile contact helps to strengthen and stretch muscles. Creating emojis for virtual characters makes it simple for users to comprehend the feelings and comfortable distances of other users.

3.10 Cyberspace Metaverse Application Status

The price and the size of integrated VR BCI devices can be reduced thanks to recent advancements in hardware and software for BCI applications in VR and XR. For instance, Galea and Cognixion ONE, headsets developed by OpenBCI and Cognixion, respectively, use six to eight dry electroencephalogram (EEG) electrodes in conjunction with an eye-tracking module and transmission module (such as Bluetooth and Wi-Fi). Galea is an AR-based headset, whereas Cognixion ONE is a VR-based headset.

Galea is dedicated to converting EEG signals into digital commands for usage in VR applications and gaming. In contrast, Cognixion ONE allows users to engage with augmented worlds and operate digital devices using a combination of facial expressions, eye movements, and EEG signals. All things considered,

Galea and Cognition ONE are both cutting-edge and fascinating devices that are expanding the field of BCI technology. The user's needs and preferences will determine which device they choose, though, as they are both have unique applications and strengths. For instance, Cognition ONE is better suited for healthcare metaverse applications, whereas Galea is more promising for gaming applications in the BCI-enabled metaverse, where each user can control their players with their thoughts [42].

3.11 Opportunities and Challenges for HCI in the Metaverse's Future Development

There are many controversial questions about the metaverse, of which the most critical is the issue of privacy. Huge amounts of user data will be generated in the metaverse, and the security of that data is a major concern. The development company may be able to augment VR devices and biometric data of users to collect personal data for other purposes. For example, before Facebook changed its name, it was revealed that Facebook used the personal information of users for targeted advertising. It was pointed out that the volume of data collected on the metaverse was dwarfed by the amount of data previously collected on the Internet. The amount of information leaked is extremely high, and it is still increasing every year. Since the metaverse is a social media platform, it will experience addiction, much like other social media platforms. A person suffering from this addiction may experience psychological and physical side effects. Sedentary behavior has been linked to several health problems, including obesity and cardiovascular disease. With excessive use, it has also been linked to behavioral issues, including anxiety and depression [43]. Some of the main challenges include the following:

Security and privacy of information: The exchange of personal data to various devices poses a major risk to users' security and privacy.

Identity hacking: Since bots can mimic human behavior and personality with ease, using avatars can make it more difficult to verify someone's identity. Therefore, to verify the user's identity, a variety of authentication processes, including voice recognition and biometric scans, are required.

Interoperability: Further difficulties arise when integrating wearable technology in a virtual setting with a variety of hardware and software components, as is the case with the metaverse. It is crucial to set up proper communication standards and data adoption procedures to ensure the security and consistency of sensitive data and prevent any negative consequences.

Legal complexity: Novel legal and regulatory frameworks will be required for the metaverse to ensure proper security, given its immense potential for virtual wrongdoing and regulatory complications.

Time synchronization: The primary obstacle encountered during the analysis of the metaverse system was the synchronization of time. The precision performance of the session would be greatly enhanced by proper time synchronization. In addition to being a difficulty for the metaverse, time synchronization is a typical issue in distributed computing systems that use wireless sensor networks [44–47].

3.12 Conclusion

The idea of the metaverse marks a new era in the advancement of HCI. In HCI, intelligent machines need to understand the communication between humans and the environment in a meaningful way. We need advanced intelligent machines, tools, and network protocols to make communication between humans and the environment work in a secure way. On the other side, the applications of HCI in domains like social networking, commerce, travel, education, the workplace, banking, and healthcare will also develop further as the underlying architecture continues to grow. At that time, it will bring huge investment opportunities to related fields. To extend the next level of development, the underlying technology, processing power of machines, storage capacity, and application effects involved all require extensive scientific research and the backing of numerous national policies, societal factors, laws, and regulations.

References

1. Buolamwini, J., & Gebru, T. (2018). Gender Shades: Intersectional Accuracy Disparities in Commercial Gender Classification. In Conference on fairness, accountability and transparency (pp. 77–91). Proceedings of Machine Learning Research.
2. Xu, M., Ng, W. C., & Lim, W. Y. B., et al. (2023). A full dive into realizing the edge-enabled metaverse: Visions, enabling technologies, and challenges. IEEE Communications Surveys & Tutorials, 25(1): 656–700.
3. Nezami, Y., Dohler, M., Shirazipour, M., & Blomquist, E. (2021). What is the metaverse and why does it need 5G to succeed? The metaverse 5G relationship explained, in The Ericsson Blog, 21 April.
4. Chowdhury, M. Z., Shahjalal, M., Hasan, M. K., & Jang, Y. M. (2019). The role of optical wireless communication technologies in 5G/6G and IoT solutions: Prospects, directions, and challenges. Applied Sciences, 9(20), 4367.
5. Morocho-Cayamcela, M. E., Lee, H., & Lim, W. (2019). Machine learning for 5G/B5G mobile and wireless communications: Potential, limitations, and future directions. IEEE Access, 7, 137184–137206.
6. Minoli, D., & Occhiogrosso, B. (2019). Practical aspects for the integration of 5g networks and IoT applications in smart cities environments. Wireless Communications and Mobile Computing, 2019(57108345), 1–30.
7. Wang, P., Bai, X., Billinghurst, M., Zhang, S., Han, D., Sun, M., Wang, Z., Lv, H., & Han, S. (2020). Haptic feedback helps me? A VR-SAR remote collaborative system

with tangible interaction. International Journal of Human–Computer Interaction, 36(13), 1242–1257.

8. Ynag, Q., Zhao, Y., Huang, H., & Zheng, Z. (2022). Fusing blockchain and AI with metaverse: A survey. arXiv preprint arXiv:2201.03201.

9. Chengoden, R., Victor, N., Huynh-The, T., Yenduri, G., Jhaveri, R. H., Alazab, M., Bhattacharya, S., Hegde, P., Maddikunta, P. K. R., & Gadekallu, T. R. (2022). Metaverse for healthcare: A survey on potential applications, challenges and future directions. arXiv preprint arXiv:2209.04160

10. Merrad, W., Habib, L., Heloir, A., Kolski, C., & Krueger, A. (2019). Tangible table-tops and dual reality for crisis management: Case study with mobile robots and dynamic tangible objects. Procedia Computer Science, 151(10), 369–376.

11. Yu, K., Tan, L., Aloqaily, M., Yang, H., & Jararweh, Y. (2021). Blockchain-enhanced data sharing with traceable and direct revocation in IIoT. IEEE Trans. Ind. Inform, 17(11), 7669–7678.

12. Wibowo, S., & Sandikapura, T. (2019). Improving data security, interoperability, and veracity using blockchain for one data governance, case study of local tax big data, in: International Conference on ICT for Smart Society, ICISS, Vol. 7, pp. 1–6.

13. Hassan, M. U., Rehmani, M. H., & Chen, J. (2019). Privacy preservation in block-chain-based IoT systems: Integration issues, prospects, challenges, and future research directions. Future Gener. Comput. Syst, 97, 512–529.

14. Kanter, T. G. (2021). The metaverse and extended reality with distributed IoT. IEEE IoT Newsletter, 2021(November).

15. Kim, M., Park, K. B., Choi, S. H., & Lee, J. Y. (2020). Inside-reachable and see-through augmented reality shell for 3D visualization and tangible interaction. Multimedia Tools and Applications, 79(9–10), 5941–5963.

16. Hajjaji, Y., Boulila, W., Farah, I. R., Romdhani, I., & Hussain, A. (2021). Big data and IoT-based applications in smart environments: A systematic review. Comp. Sci. Rev, 39, 100318.

17. Majeed, U., Khan, L. U., Yaqoob, I., Kazmi, S. A., Salah, K., & Hong, C. S. (2021). Blockchain for IoT-based smart cities: Recent advances, requirements, and future challenges. J. Netw. Comput. Appl, 181, 103007.

18. Dorri, A., Luo, F., Karumba, S., Kanhere, S., Jurdak, R., & Dong, Z. Y. (2021). Temporary immutability: A removable blockchain solution for prosumer-side energy trading. J. Netw. Comput. Appl, 180, 103018.

19. Cheng, Q., Zhang, S., Bo, S., Chen, D., & Zhang, H. (2020). Augmented reality dynamic image recognition technology based on a deep learning algorithm. IEEE Access, 8(2020, July), 137370–137384.

20. Wang, S., Qureshi, M. A., Miralles-Pechuaán, L., Huynh-The, T., Gadekallu, T. R., & Liyanage, M. (2021). Explainable AI for B5G/6G: technical aspects, use cases, and research challenges. arXiv preprint arXiv: 2112.04698.

21. Szeliski, R. (2022). Computer Vision: Algorithms and Applications. Springer Nat.

22. Sharma, H. K., & Choudhury, T. Hand gesture recognition. Available online: https://services.igiglobal.com/resolvedoi/resolve.aspx?doi=10.4018/978-1-7998-9434-6.ch003 (accessed on 2 Feb 2024).

23. Lee, H. M., Ham, S. M., & Moon, H., et al. (2023). A metaverse emotion mapping system with an AIoT facial expression recognition device. In: Proceedings of the 2023 IEEE International Conference on Metaverse Computing, Networking and Applications (MetaCom). 26–28 June; Kyoto, Japan. pp. 704–707.

24. He, S., Zhao, H., & Yu, L. (2023). The avatar facial expression reenactment method in the metaverse is based on overall-local optical-flow estimation and illumination difference. In: Proceedings of the 2023 26th International Conference on Computer Supported Cooperative Work in Design (CSCWD); 24–26 May; Rio de Janeiro, Brazil. pp. 1312–1317.

25. Jang, J. Y. (2023). Analyzing visual behavior of consumers in a virtual reality fashion store using eye tracking. Fashion and Textiles, 10(1), 24.

26. Hendrikx, M., Meijer, S., & Van Der Velden, J., et al. (2013). Procedural content generation for games. ACM Transactions on Multimedia Computing, Communications, and Applications, 9(1), 1–22.

27. Kipper, G., & Rampolla, J. (2013). Augmented reality. In: Augmented Reality: An Emerging Technologies Guide to AR, 1st ed. Elsevier. pp. 1–20.

28. Furukawa, Y., & Hernández, C. (2015). Multi-view stereo: A tutorial. Foundations and Trends® in Computer Graphics and Vision, 9(1–2), 1–148.

29. Elhagry, A. (2023). Text-to-metaverse: Towards a digital twin-enabled multimodal conditional generative metaverse. In: Proceedings of the 31st ACM International Conference on Multimedia; 29 October–3 November; Ottawa, Canada. pp. 9336–9339.

30. Wang, Y., Su, Z., Zhang, N., & Liu, D., et al. A survey on metaverse: Fundamentals, security, and privacy. Available online: https://arxiv.org/abs/2203.02662 (accessed on 2 June 2023).

31. Cheng, R., Wu, N., & Varvello, M., et al. (2022). Are we ready for the metaverse? In: Proceedings of the 22nd ACM Internet Measurement Conference. 25–27 October; New York, United States. pp. 504–518.

32. Chang, Y. T. Kernel-wise difference minimization for convolutional neural network compression in the metaverse. Available online: https://www.frontiersin.org/articles/10.3389/fdata.2023.1200382/full (accessed on 20 Feb 2024).

33. Yaqob, M., & Hafez, M. M. (2023). Metaverse – An overview of daily usage and risks. In: Proceedings of the 2022 OPJU International Technology Conference on Emerging Technologies for Sustainable Development (OTCON); 8–10 February; Raigarh, Chhattisgarh, India. pp. 1–6.

34. Zhou, K., Yang, J., Loy, C. C., & Liu, Z. (2022). Learning to prompt for vision-language models. International Journal of Computer Vision, 130(9), 2337–2348.

35. Yang, Z., Zeng, Z., Wang, K., Wong, S. S., Liang, W., Zanin, M., & He, J. (2020). Modified SEIR and AI prediction of the epidemics trend of COVID-19 in China under public health interventions. Journal of Thoracic Disease, 12(3), 165.

36. Gong, L., Seoderlund, H., Bogojevic, L., Chen, X., Berce, A., FastBerglund, Å, & Johansson, B. (2020). Interaction design for multiuser virtual reality systems: An automotive case study. Procedia CIRP, 93(53), 1259–1264.

37. Sim, K., Rao, Z., Zou, Z., Ershad, F., Lei, J., Thukral, A., Chen, J., Huang, Q.-A., Xiao, J., & Yu, C. (2019). Metal oxide semiconductor nanomembrane–based soft unnoticeable multifunctional electronics for wearable human–machine interfaces. Science Advances, 5(8), eaav9653.

38 Matsangidou, M., Otkhmezuri, B., Ang, C. S., Avraamides, M., Riva, G., Gaggioli, A., & Karekla, M. (2022). "Now i can see me" designing a multi-user virtual reality remote psychotherapy for body weight and shape concerns. Human–Computer Interaction, 37(4), 314–340.

39. Balasubramaniam, S, Kadry, S., & Kumar, K. S. (2024). Osprey gannet optimization enabled CNN based transfer learning for optic disc detection and cardiovascular risk prediction using retinal fundus images. Biomedical Signal Processing and Control, 93, 106177.
40. Chang, C. H., Yeh, C. H., Chang, C. C., & Lin, Y. C. (2022). Interactive somatosensory games in rehabilitation training for older adults with mild cognitive impairment: Usability study. JMIR Serious Games, 10(3), e38465.
41. Wu, J., Liu, Z., Xu, H., Liu, T., Wang, J., & Chai, Y. (2019). Serious game human−computer interaction design for rehabilitation training. Journal of System Simulation, 31(5), 909.
42. Zhao, H., Karlsson, P., & Chiu, D. et al. (2023). Wearable augmentative and alternative communication (wAAC): A novel solution for people with complex communication needs. Virtual Reality 27, 2441–2459.
43. Hassija, V., Chamola, V., Bajpai, B. C., & Zeadally, S. (2021). Security issues in implantable medical devices: Fact or fiction? Sustain. Cities Soc, 66, 102552.
44. Liu, L., Feng, J., Pei, Q., Chen, C., Ming, Y., Shang, B., & Dong, M. (2020). Blockchain-enabled secure data sharing scheme in mobile-edge computing: An asynchronous advantage actor−critic learning approach. IEEE Internet Things J, 8(4), 2342–2353.
45. Römer, K., Blum, P., & Meier, L. (2005). Time synchronization and calibration in wireless sensor networks. In Ivan Stojmenović (ed.), Handbook of Sensor Networks: Algorithms and Architectures. John Wiley & Sons, pp 199–237.
46. Kadry, S., Dhanaraj, R. K., & Manthiramoorthy, C. (2024). Res-Unet based blood vessel segmentation and cardio vascular disease prediction using chronological chef-based optimization algorithm based deep residual network from retinal fundus images. Multimedia Tools and Applications, 83, 87929–87958 (2024).
47. Wasaka, T., Kida, T., & Kakigi, R. (2021). Dexterous manual movement facilitates information processing in the primary somatosensory cortex: A magnetoencephalographic study. The European Journal of Neuroscience, 54(2), 4638–4648.

Chapter 4

The Role of 5G Communication in the Metaverse

Mithra Venkatesan, Sheetal Pawar,
Lalit Kumar Wadhwa, and Sagar Shinde

4.1 5G Technology

5G technology can offer enhanced data speed, reduced time delay, higher capacity, and enhanced service quality. To achieve this, the key technologies available are multiple input multiple output (MIMO) technology and communication between devices (D2D) communication to fulfill performance requirements. Moreover, there are emerging technologies, including interference management, cognitive radio for spectrum sharing, ultradense networks, association with multiradio access technology, full-duplex radios, and various short-range communication technologies like Wi-Fi, small cells, visible light communication, millimeter-wave solutions for 5G cellular networks, cloud technologies for radio access networks, and software-defined networks [1]. With the help of 5G, wireless carriers are able to expand their contributions beyond simple connectivity and services for businesses in a variety of industries. Fast connections with peak rates ranging from 2 to 20 Gbps, slower connections with a high device density (1 million devices per square meter) for sensing and actuating devices (such as the Internet of Things), a completely new category of connections that achieve minimal time delay (under 1 ms), and strong connection reliability (link outage of 99.999%) are all included in the 5G standards. When combined, these services result in a revolutionary class of applications. For the first time, 5G has expanded the use of wireless technology into entirely new

     DOI: 10.1201/9781003491668-4

economic sectors. Three different types of use cases are used to group 5G: ultrare-liable low-latency communications (uRLLC), massive machine-type communication (mMTC), and enhanced mobile broadband (eMBB). For large volume of data transfer and data rate, eMBB is used, while for machine-centric use cases, mMTC and URLLC are used [2].

5G provides higher speed up to 10 Gbps faster than 4G. This enables ultra-fast mobile communication and enhances media usages. Also, it provides high-speed Internet access, which enhances personalization, flexibility, and versatility in media usage. 5G supports wireless backhaul connections and high bandwidth, enabling efficient and effective wireless connections. 5G technology aims to pro-vide flexible, inclusive, user-focused services with abundant data capacity that aligns with user expectations [3]. While 5G technology offers several benefits, the complexities of its technology pose significant challenges. These include difficulties in penetrating building materials, the requirement for an extensive deployment of small antennas and cell towers, and challenges related to the radio spectrum. As a result, 5G signals face obstacles from structures, terrain, vegetation, and even the human body, especially in densely populated urban areas. Additionally, the air can absorb these waves over short distances, less than a kilometer, even without physical barriers [4].

In spite of its limited challenges, 5G technology has found applications in var-ied domains such as high-speed mobile networks, entertainment and multimedia, healthcare and mission critical applications, satellite Internet, the Internet of Things (IoT), etc. Also, it provides benefits to the IoT in applications such as smart cities, smart home, industrial IoT, smart farming, and autonomous driving [5]. 5G has been a great enabler for the metaverse whereby many of its requirements are being fulfilled by characteristic features of 5G. The next section details the fulfillment of requirements of the metaverse by 5G.

4.2 The Metaverse

The term *metaverse* refers to virtual reality (VR) driven by advanced technology, with various aspects of wireless communication systems being prominent concepts. It creates a virtual environment where users can work, play, and talk using portable devices like goggles and headsets [6]. The requirements of the metaverse are ful-filled by 5G technology. Significantly, the growth of the metaverse is closely tied to the capabilities offered by 5G wireless connectivity [7]. The metaverse needs to have minimal delays, high dependability, extensive connectivity, ample bandwidth, and energy efficiency [8]. As an advanced technology with various experimental platforms, the metaverse is contributing to the advancement of wearable and por-table devices. These devices feature 5G connectivity, providing a deeply immersive experience, whether used remotely or in real time with haptic devices and the tactile Internet (TI) [9].

By using the metaverse, augmented reality (AR) and VR technologies could potentially extend the real-world experience by allowing users to interact seamlessly in both physical and simulated environments, utilizing avatars and holograms [10]. The key features of the metaverse are realism, universality, interoperability, and integration of technologies. With the help of these, the metaverse can blur the boundaries in the physical and digital worlds by providing a platform where users can interact, engage in economic activities, and experience a sense of presence in a virtual environment that mirrors aspects of the real world. Industrial investment, regulation, industry integration, and technological breakthroughs play crucial roles in the further development of the metaverse. The technologies used are modeling and rendering technologies to create virtual items, interaction technologies to get real-time feedback, authentication technologies, smart wearable devices, avatars, nonplayer characters (NPCs), learning scenes, learning resources, learning logging, learning analysis (computing, databases, or AI), and learning authentication [11].

There is existing theoretical framework proposed contributing to understanding of the metaverse in the form of legal governance rules, guidelines for merging virtual and real elements, and regulations for technological partnerships. By incorporating these rules into the theoretical framework, a comprehensive perspective on the key aspects that govern the functioning and development of the metaverse is obtained. It offers a structured approach to understanding the complexities of this virtual environment and guides future research and decision-making processes within the metaverse industry [12]. The multidisciplinary perspectives such as comprehensive analysis, innovative solutions, user-centric design, ethical considerations, and interdisciplinary research have significant impact in enhancing the understanding of the metaverse by bringing diverse expertise and insights from various fields [13]. Industrial investment, regulation, industry integration, and technological advances play crucial roles in the further development of the metaverse. Industrial investment is in the form of capital layout and diversification, and regulation establishes rules and addresses challenges. Industry integration includes collaboration and technology synergy and technology breakthroughs such as supporting infrastructure for AR/VR, blockchain, edge computing, and innovation. By leveraging industrial investment, regulatory frameworks, industry collaboration, and technological innovations, the metaverse can continue to develop, offering users enhanced experiences, new opportunities for interaction, and a more integrated virtual environment that creates a seamless transition between the real and digital domains [14]. The technology faces challenges in the form of equipment available, privacy and data security, ethics and morality, addition, and social interaction. The following section briefs on the research trends in the metaverse [15–17].

4.3 Research Trends in the Metaverse

In order to understand the research tends in the metaverse, the Scopus database was chosen, as it has the best collection of referred articles. The broad range of search phases based on current trends in the metaverse was used [18–20]. A systematic process was used to reach 4,549 articles, as shown in Table 4.1. Data collected from the Scopus database contain inaccurate or garbage data due to incorrect entries, missing fields, or repeated entries in different documents. Search keywords taken were "Metaverse," subject area ("Computer Science," "Engineering," "Decision Science," "Mathematics"), document type (article and review paper), and language (English). As a result, the dataset was cleaned to avoid any error in the extracted data before proceeding with the analysis. The first search was carried out using keywords, and 459 articles were obtained. Then data were filtered as recent year from 2020 to 2024, and 4,382 articles were taken [21–22]. Then the subject areas were taken, and 1,627 articles were obtained. Then search by document type as article and review papers and got 701, and the applied filter of language (English) got 663 articles.

Figure 4.1 indicates that research in the metaverse started from 2020 to 2024, wherein the total number of publications mapped with the year. The most productive years are 2023 (453 articles), 2022 (120 articles), 2020 (two articles), 2024 (80 articles), and ongoing research [23–25].

Figure 4.2 gives documents published per year from 2021 to 2024. The Scopus database is the source for the same period. In *The IEEE Journal on Selected Areas in Communication*, a total of seven articles were published, in *IEEE Network* 39 articles, *IEEE Access* 47 articles, *Electronics Switzerland* 32 articles, and *Applied Sciences Switzerland* 29 articles, and *Sensors* published 27 articles [26–28].

Table 4.1   Inclusion Criteria for Selection of Articles

Selection conditions	Discard	Take
Online search platform: Scopus		
Exploration date: 02/25/2024		
Keyword: ("Metaverse") Since 1995–2024	–	4,549
Year: 2020–2024	167	4,382
Subject area: Engineering	2,755	1,627
Document type: "Article," "Review"	926	701
Language: English	38	663

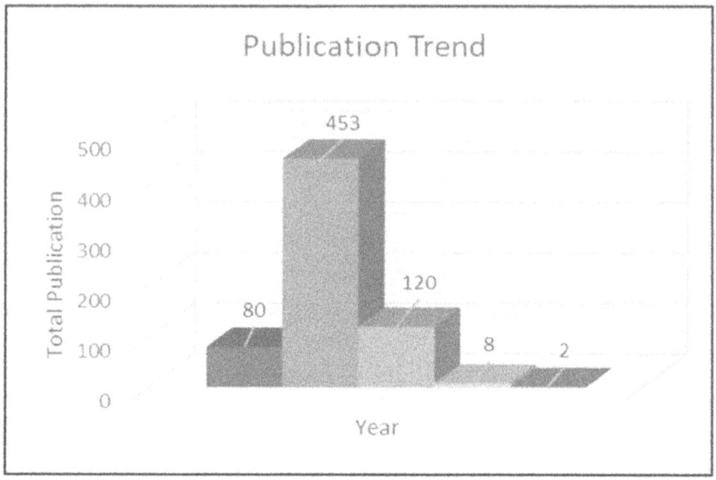

Figure 4.1 Publication per year (publication trend).

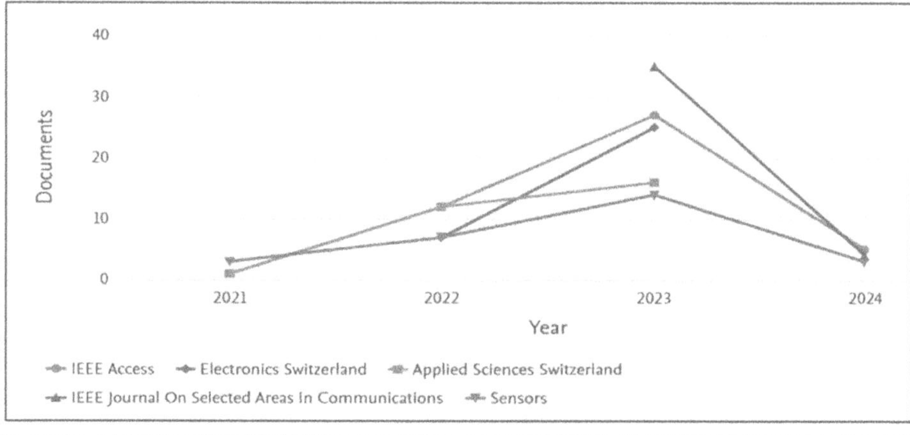

Figure 4.2 Document per year by source.

Table 4.2 gives top journals covering the metaverse, along with total citations and total publications. *IEEE Access* and *Applied Sciences* (Switzerland) are the top cited journals in this field. Citations are 1,089 and 422 respectively. The two most effective journals in the field of the metaverse are *IEEE Access* (45 research papers) and *Electronics* (Switzerland; 32 research papers). In the years 2020–2021, *Sensors* published 27 papers. In 2022–2023, *IEEE Access and Electronics* (Switzerland) has published a good quantity of papers. In 2022–2023, *IEEE Access* has contributed more compared to other journals. The following section explains how 5G technology is utilized in the metaverse [29, 30].

Table 4.2 Top Journals of the Metaverse

Journals	Total citations	Total publications	Multidisciplinary	2020–2021	2022–2023	2024
IEEE Access	1,089	45	✓	1	39	5
Applied Sciences (Switzerland)	422	29	✓	1	28	–
Sensors	308	27	✓	4	20	3
IEEE Communications Surveys and Tutorials	283	4	✓	–	4	–
Electronics (Switzerland)	274	32	✓	–	32	–
IEEE Transactions on Systems, Man and Cybernetics: Systems	255	20	✓	–	20	–
Smart Cities	229	5		–	5	–
International Journal of Emerging Technologies in Learning	161	4		2	2	–
IEEE Transactions on Learning Technologies	127	19	✓	–	14	5
IEEE Wireless Communications	111	24		–	23	1
Mathematics	84	11		–	11	–

(Continued)

Table 4.2 (Continued) Top Journals of the Metaverse

Journals	Total citations	Total publications	Multidisciplinary	2020–2021	2022–2023	2024
IEEE/CAA Journal of Automatica Sinica	77	5	✓	–	4	1
IEEE Wireless Communications Letters	70	1		–	1	–
IET Intelligent Transport Systems	69	1		–	1	–
Signal Processing	66	1		–	1	–
Buildings	63	5		–	5	–
IEEE Consumer Electronics Magazine	61	17	✓	–	12	5
Telematics and Informatics	59	3		–	2	1
IEEE Multimedia	57	6	✓	–	6	–
Nano Energy	56	5		–	6	–

4.4 5G in the Metaverse

The role of 5G in the metaverse is illustrated in Figure 4.3. The different characteristics of 5G along with requirements and features of the metaverse help in transformation of the application realm from real world to virtual world. There are varied real-world applications such as education, military, and healthcare where the metaverse can be used. These real-world scenarios are realized virtually through VR and AR by digital users or by remote working through the able support provided by 5G characteristics. In fact, the 5G characteristics empower themetaverse and enable the realization of the metaverse in the virtual world [31–33].

There has been research on exploring this role of 5G in the metaverse. Toward understanding the research trends, the Scopus database was chosen, as it has the most good collection of referred articles. The broad range of search phases based on current trends in 5G in the metaverse was used. A systematic process was used

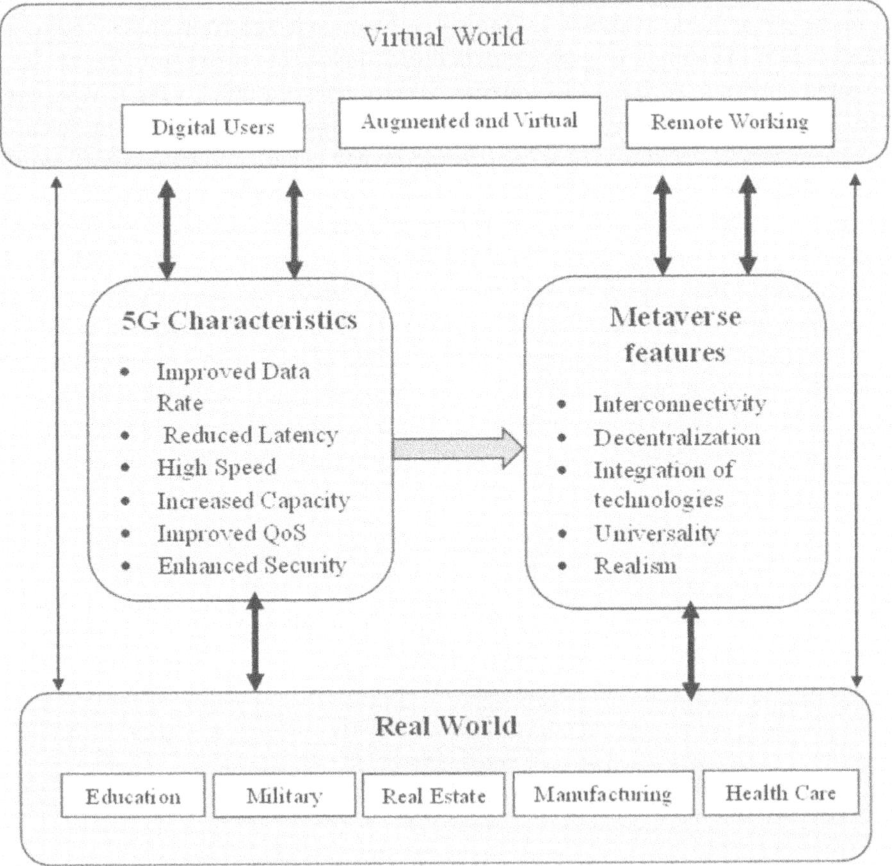

Figure 4.3   5G in the metaverse.

Table 4.3 Criteria Used for Searching and Selecting Articles

Criteria for filtering	Approve	Decline
Database: Scopus		
Timestamp: February 28, 2024		
Keyword: ("Metaverse") Since 2021–2024	----	151
Subject area: "Computer Science," "Engineering," "Decision Science," "Mathematics"	10	141
Document type: "Article," "Review"	92	49
Language: English	4	45

to reach 151 articles, as shown in Table 4.3. Data collected from the Scopus database contain inaccurate or garbage data due to incorrect entries, missing fields, or repeated entries in different documents. Search keyword taken were ("Metaverse" and "5G"), subject area ("Computer Science," "Engineering," "Decision Science," "Mathematics"), document type (article and review paper), and language (English). As a result, the dataset was cleaned to avoid any error in the extracted data before proceeding with the analysis. The first search was carried out using keywords, and 151 articles were obtained. Then the subject areas were taken and 141 articles was obtained. Then search by document type as article and review papers and got 49 articles, and the applied filter of language (English) got 45 articles [34, 35].

Figure 4.4 indicates that research in the role of 5G in the metaverse started from 2021 to 2024, with the total number of publications mapped with the year. From publication trends, research in the metaverse started from 1995, but the role of 5G in the metaverse was introduced recently around 2021. The most productive

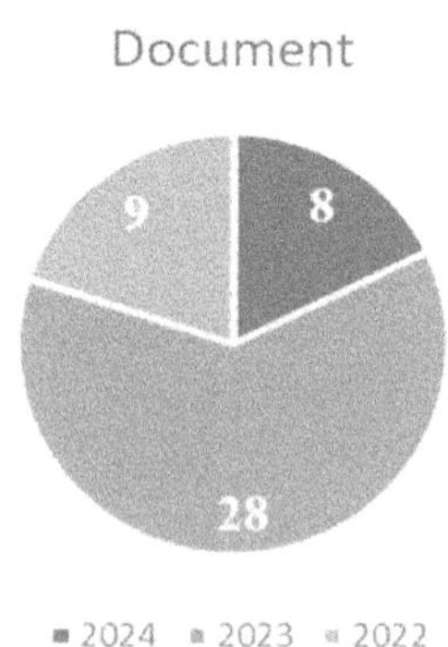

Figure 4.4 Documents per year.

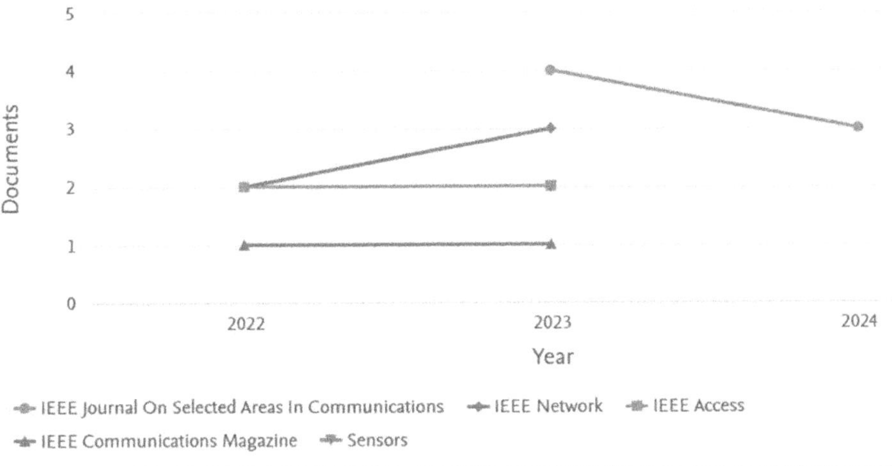

Figure 4.5   Documents per year by source.

years are 2023 (28 articles), 2022 (nine articles), 2024 (eight articles), and ongoing research [36–38].

Figure 4.5 gives the documents published per year from 2022 to 2024. The Scopus database again was used. In *The IEEE Journal on Selected Areas in Communication,* a total of seven articles were published, *IEEE Network* had five articles, *IEEE Access* four articles, *IEEE Communication Magazine* two articles, and in *Sensors* two articles were published.

Figure 4.6 depicts documents published by different authors. The figure shows that Chaudhary, Chen, Han, Hashemi-Dezaki, Jamshidi, Liyanage, Nouri, Rezaei, and Yahya contributed in the field of the role of 5G in the metaverse.

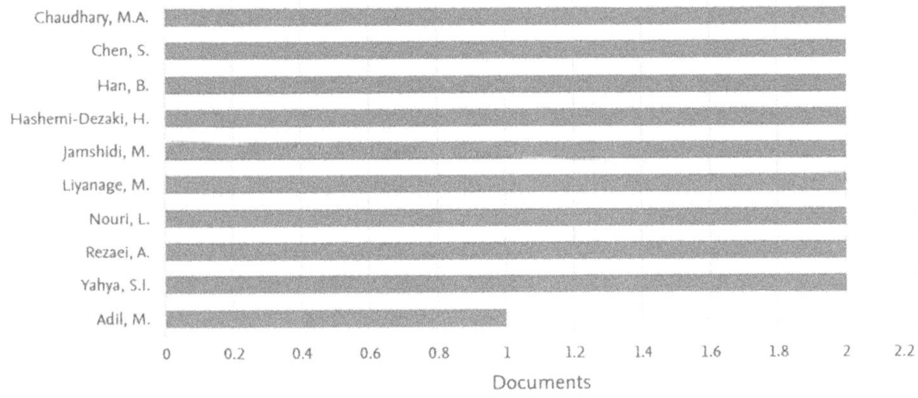

Figure 4.6   Documents per year by author.

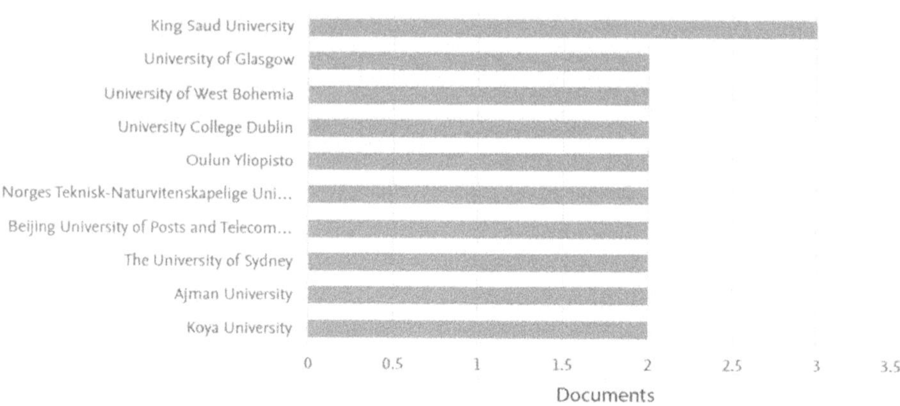

Figure 4.7 Documents by affiliation.

Figure 4.7 illustrates statistics of documents published by universities on 5G in the metaverse. King Saud University contributed more toward research as compared to other universities. This is because of its extensive collaboration with various research organizations around the globe in this area of specialization [39].

Figure 4.8 illustrates details of documents published by countries. From this, it is observed that China has contributed more to the field of 5G in the metaverse, as funding provided in China, as the figure shows, is huge. Funding and contribution of Luxembourg is much less compared to other countries [40].

Figure 4.9 details the number of documents published by subject area. It shows that research in the field of 5G in the metaverse is ideally applied in computer science, engineering, decision science, and mathematics [41].

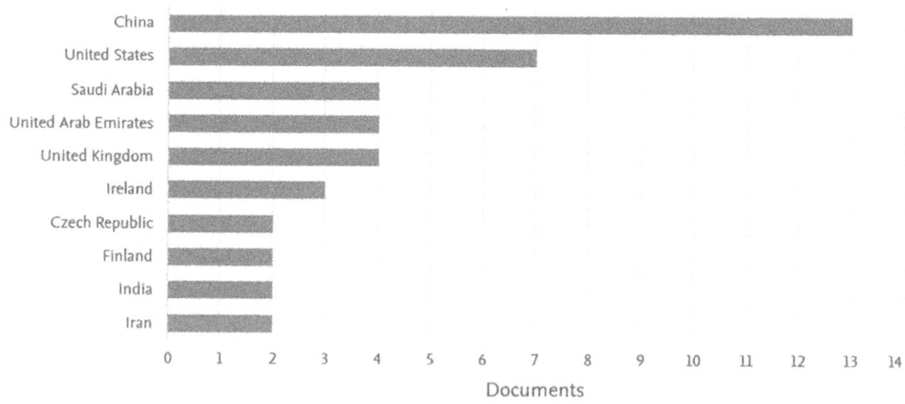

Figure 4.8 Documents by country.

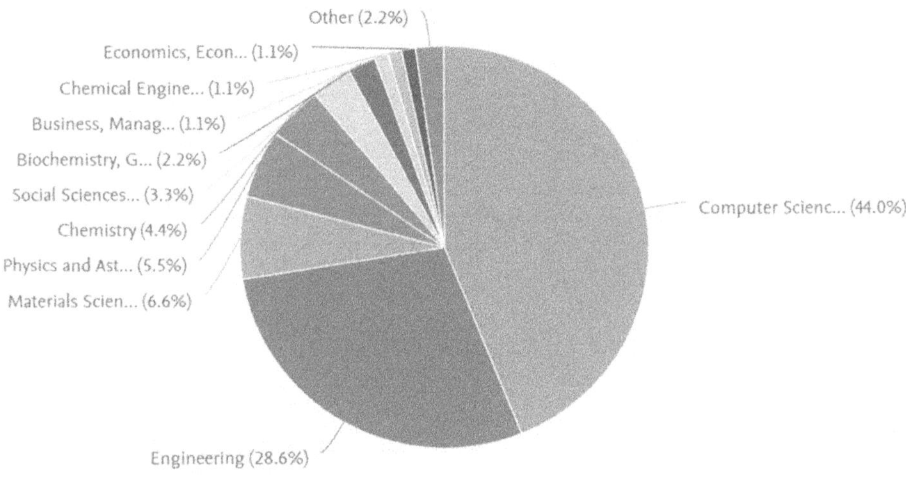

Figure 4.9 Documents by subject area.

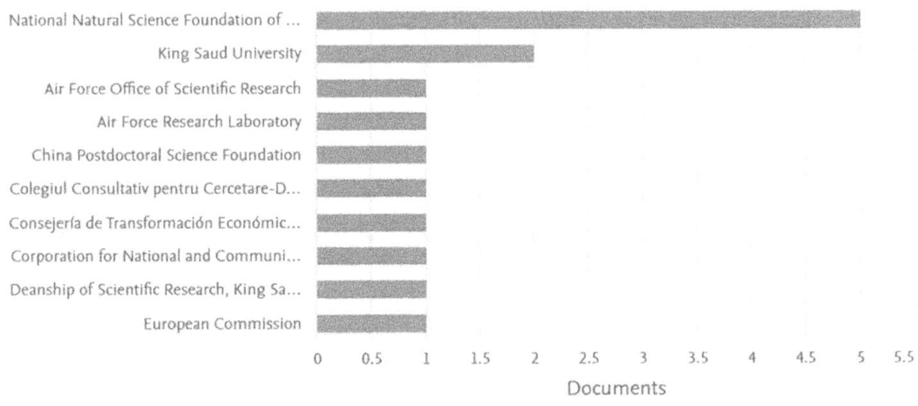

Figure 4.10 Documents by funding agency.

Figure 4.10 details funding available in the field of 5G in the metaverse. It shows that funding is largely available in countries like China and Saudi Arabia and are inadequate in Luxembourg [42].

The top countries in the field of 5G in the metaverse along with their institutions and countries are presented in Table 4.4.

Table 4.4 highlights the top countries in the field of 5G in the metaverse. The United States and China are the top countries, having 94 and 90 citations and a total of eight and 17 publications respectively in this field.

The knowledge foundation of a field is given by semantic linkages of references that are cited together, as identified through co-citation analysis. Co-citation

Table 4.4   Top Countries with High Citations

Total citation	Country	Total publication
94	United States	8
90	China	17
39	Saudi Arabia	5

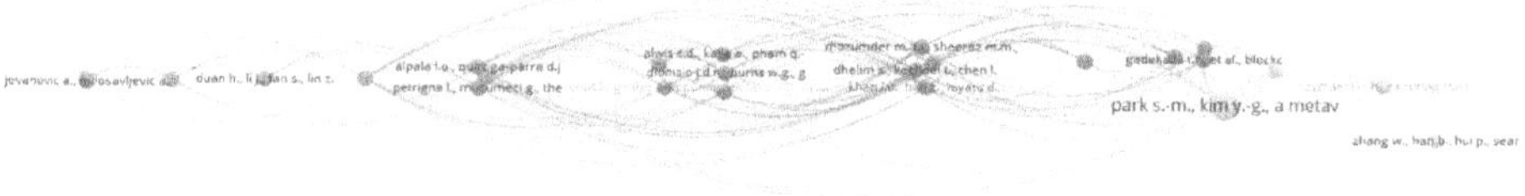

Figure 4.11   Co-citation analysis of reference cited by the article on 5G in the metaverse.

analysis of 5G in the metaverse is shown in Figure 4.11, which gives analysis of publications that are cited together [43]. Every point in the figure stands for a referenced source. The various shades of the points indicate groups of references that share similar themes and topics: 25 items, four clusters, 15 links, and 180 link strengths [44].

The size of the nodes indicates how much a source is cited locally, with bigger circles showing a higher level of local citations. The connections between the circles represent when sources are cited together. The thickness of these connections shows the strength of those co-citations, with thicker lines indicating a stronger connection between sources [45].

Figure 4.12 shows co-citation analysis of author, including a total of six items (number of papers), two clusters, and 15 links, and the total link strength is 543.

4.5 Future Scope of 5G in the Metaverse

The research trend and existing work exploring the role of 5G in the metaverse is at a very nascent stage, and there is a huge scope for work. There are varied avenues yet to be explored and hence offering avenues for research in the future. Toward understanding the future scope of 5G in the metaverse, thematic analysis of existing work is presented in Figure 4.13. Thematic analysis involves grouping of existing work and clustering them into themes based on keywords. These themes lay the roadmap for future work [46].

Thus, future research directions of 5G in the metaverse are identified by bibliographic exploration. From this exploration, five distinct thematic clusters have emerged, and all are tied to the concept of the role of 5G in the metaverse. These

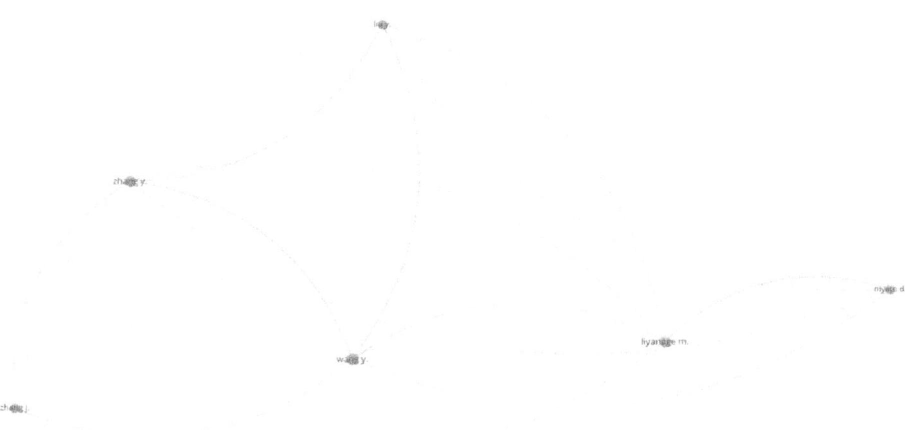

Figure 4.12 Co-citation analysis of author analysis.

clusters offer a roadmap for future exploration, areas such as usage of advanced intelligent technologies for realization of the metaverse, mobile edge technology for developing prototypes and to provide solutions, edge computing to overcome limitations of traditional cloud computing, and next-generation mobile networks with involvement of 5G, resulting in future research trends along with applications and prototyping. By exploring these thematic clusters, this bibliographic exploration not only enhances our understanding of the role of 5G in the metaverse but also sets the stage for an exciting and transformative journey within the domain metaverse [47].

Co-occurrence analysis has been used to further analyze thematic tendencies in the role of 5G technology in the metaverse by expanding the insights shown

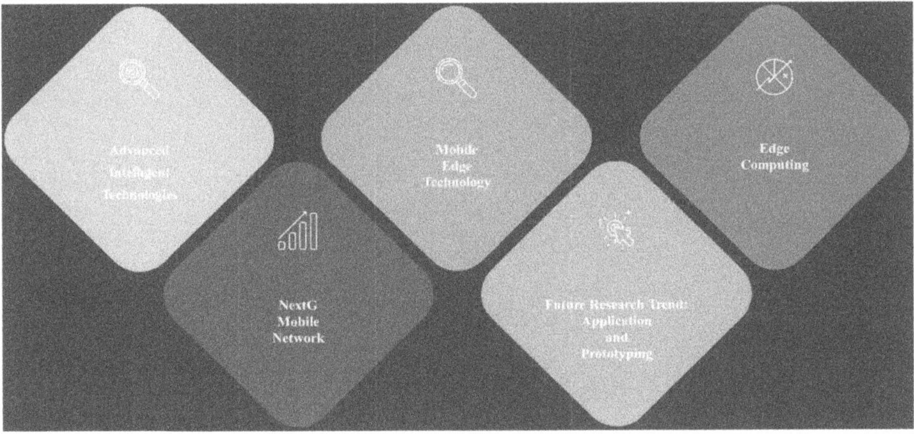

Figure 4.13 Thematic analysis.

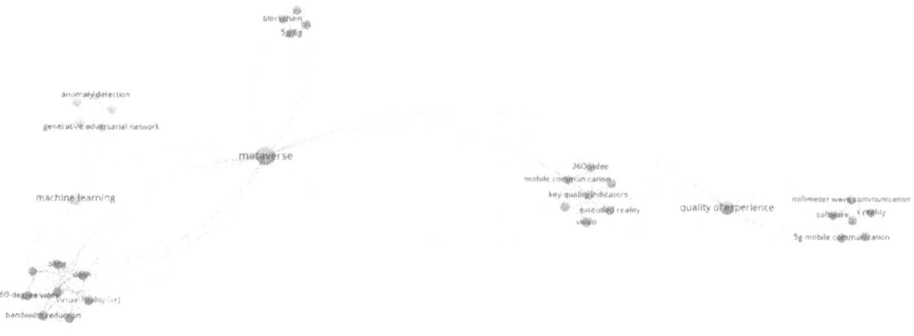

Figure 4.14   Thematic trends in 2022.

through analysis of co-citation and bibliographic coupling, building on the foundational elements and overarching themes. For co-occurrence analysis, author keywords are used. The evolution is described in Figure 4.13. All such figures show the top topics in research domain of the role of 5G technology in the metaverse during different periods [48].

Figure 4.14 represents research on 5G/6G in the metaverse, machine learning, extended reality, 5G mobile communication, and bandwidth reduction. Therefore, the most influential topics in the research of the role of 5G in the metaverse are 5G/6G in the metaverse, machine learning, extended reality, 5G mobile communication, and bandwidth reduction in the year 2022 [49].

Figure 4.15 presents research on 5G and beyond networks (purple node), 5G advanced (yellow node), AR (green node), task analysis (blue node), edge computing

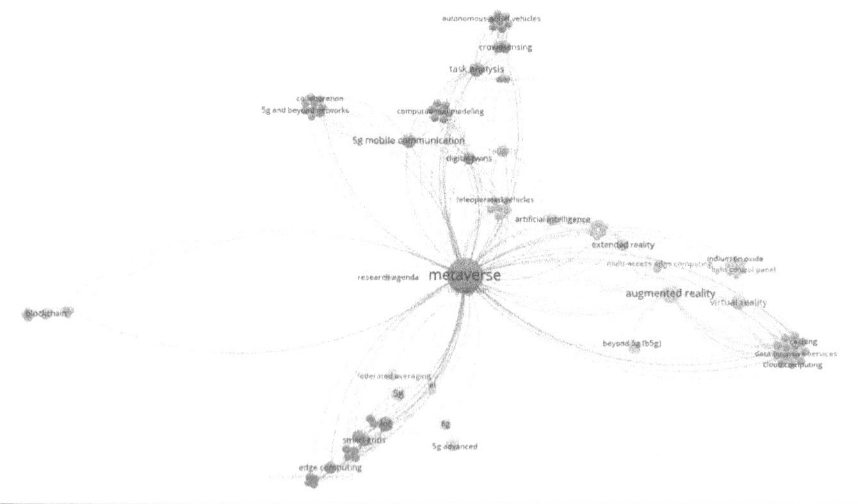

Figure 4.15   Thematic trends in 2023.

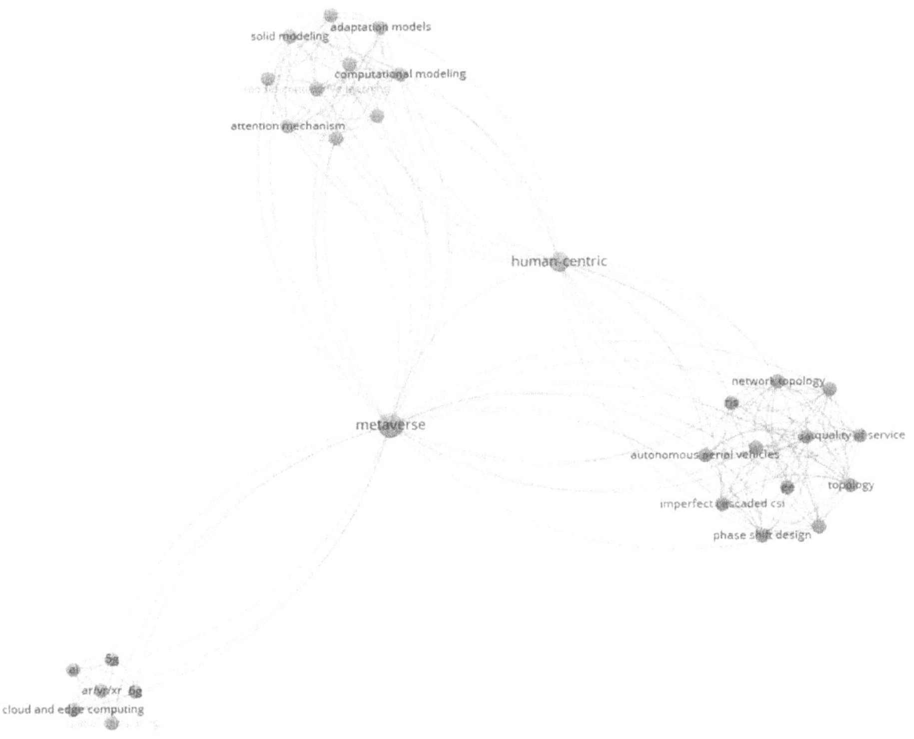

Figure 4.16   Thematic trends in 2024.

(red node), blockchain (pink node), artificial intelligence, computational modeling (brown node), and teleoperated vehicles (orange node). Therefore, the most influential topics in the research of the role of 5G in the metaverse are 5G and beyond networks, 5G advanced, AR, task analysis and edge computing, blockchain, artificial intelligence, computational modeling, and teleoperated vehicles in year 2023 [50].

Figure 4.16 gives research on computational modeling (green node), cloud and edge computing (blue node), and network topology (red node). Therefore, the most influential topics in the research of the role of 5G in the metaverse are computational modeling, cloud and edge computing, and network topology in the year 2024 [51–55].

4.6 Conclusion

5G technology has been key enabler in wireless communication domain because of its improvisation of various key parameters resulting in improved performance of networks and being relevant to emerging applications [9, 56]. The metaverse empowered through AR and VR is envisioned to make usage of many real-world applications possible in virtual world too. This chapter explores the amalgamation of these two technologies. The chapter details the research trends in the metaverse and 5G in the metaverse. The key features of 5G communication that are enablers for the metaverse are identified. Further, the future scope on the role of 5G in the metaverse is also investigated through thematic clustering and analysis. Thus, it is concluded that 5G will play a major role in realizing advanced applications of the metaverse.

References

1. Gupta, A., & Jha, R. (2015). A survey of 5G network: Architecture and emerging technologies. IEEE Access, 3, 1206–1232. https://doi.org/10.1109/ACCESS.2015.2461602
2. Bhawan., K. L. J. (2019). 5G-key capabilities & applications. FN Division. Telecommunication Engineering Centre, 1–26.
3. Jadhav, A., Mali, K., Jadhav, S., & Thorat, S (2022). 5G: Overview, challenges and benefits. International Journal for Science Technology and Engineering, 10(12), 1070–1073. https://doi.org/10.22214/ijraset.2022.48118
4. Abdel, S. (2021). 5G technology and the future of architecture. Procedia Computer Science, 182, 121–131. https://doi.org/10.1016/j.procs.2021.02.017
5. Dangi, R., Lalwani, P., Choudhary, G., & Pau, G. (2021). Study and investigation on 5G technology: A systematic review. Sensors (Basel), 22, 1–172. https://doi.org/10.3390/s22010026
6. Telecom Regulatory Authority of India. (2023). Digital transformation through 5G ecosystem (24/2023).
7. Njoku, J., Ifeanyi, C., & Kim, D. (2022). The role of 5G wireless communication system in the metaverse. 27th Asia Pacific Conference on Communications (APCC), Jeju Island, Republic of Korea, pp. 290–294. https://doi.org/10.1109/APCC55198.2022.9943778
8. 3GPP (Dec. 2021). Service requirements for the 5G system, V.18.5.0.
9. Tychola, K., Voulgaridis, K., & Lagkas, T. (2023). Tactile IoT and 5G & beyond schemes as key enabling technologies for the future metaverse. Telecommunication Systems, 84, 363–385. https://doi.org/10.1007/s11235-023-01052-y
10. Trunfio, M., & Rossi, S (2022). Advances in metaverse investigation: Streams of research and future agenda. Virtual Worlds, 1(2), 103–129. https://doi.org/10.3390/virtualworlds1020007
11. Zhang, X., Yuchen, C., Lailin, H., & Wang, Y. (2022). The metaverse in education: Definition, framework, features, potential applications, challenges, and future research topics. Frontiers in Psychology, 13, 1016300. https://doi.org/10.3389/fpsyg.2022.1016300
12. Song, C., Shin, S., & Shin, K (2023). Exploring the key characteristics and theoretical framework for research on the metaverse. Applied Science, 13(13), 1–21. https://doi.org/10.3390/app13137628
13. Dwivedi, Y. K., Hughes, L., Baabdullah, A. M., Ribeiro-Navarrete, S., Giannakis, M., Al-Debei, M. M., Dennehy, D., Metri, B., Buhalis, D., Cheung, C. M. K., Conboy, K., Doyle, R., Dubey, R., Dutot, V., Felix, R., Goyal, D. P., Gustafsson, A., Hinsch, C.,

Jebabli, I., Janssen, M., Kim, Y.-G., Kim, J., Koos, S., Kreps, D., Kshetri, N., Kumar, V., Ooi, K.-B., Papagiannidis, S., Pappas, I. O., Polyviou, A., Park, S.-M., Pandey, N., Queiroz, M. M., Raman, R., Rauschnabel, P. A., Shirish, A., Sigala, M., Spanaki, K., Wei-Han Tan, G., Tiwari, M. K., Viglia, G., & Wamba, S. F. (2022). Metaverse beyond the hype: Multidisciplinary perspectives on emerging challenges, opportunities, and agenda for research, practice and policy. International Journal of Information Management, 66, 102542. https://doi.org/10.1016/j.ijinfomgt.2022.102542

14. Huang, J., Pingjin, S., & Weijie, Z. (2022). Analysis of the future prospects for the metaverse. Proceedings of the 2022 7th International Conference on Financial Innovation and Economic Development (ICFIED 2022), pp. 1899–1904. https://doi.org/10.2991/aebmr.k.220307.312

15. Cheng, R., et al. (2022). Will metaverse be NextG internet? Vision, hype, and reality. IEEE Network, 36(5), 197–204. https://doi.org/10.1109/MNET.117.2200055

16. Lidan, H., Kexuan, L., Zehao, H., & Liangcai, C. (2023) Three-dimensional holographic communication system for the metaverse. Optics Communications, 526. https://doi.org/10.1016/j.optcom.2022.128894

17. Aloqaily, M., Bouachir, O., Karray, F., Ridhawi, I., & Saddik, A. (2023). Integrating digital twin and advanced intelligent technologies to realize the metaverse. IEEE Consumer Electronics Magazine, 12(6), 47–55. https://doi.org/10.1109/MCE.2022.3212570

18. Jagadeesha, R., Bhat, S., & AlQahtani, M (2023). FinTech enablers, use cases, and role of future internet of things. Journal of King Saud University – Computer and Information Sciences, 35(1), 87–101. https://doi.org/10.1016/j.jksuci.2022.08.033

19. Ding, S., Kou, L., & Wu, T. (2022). A GAN-based intrusion detection model for 5G enabled future metaverse. Mobile Networks and Applications, 27, 2596–2610. https://doi.org/10.1007/s11036-022-02075-6

20. Maksymyuk, T., Gazda, J., Bugár, G., Gazda, V., Liyanage, M., & Dohler, M. (2022). Blockchain-empowered service management for the decentralized metaverse of things. IEEE Access, 10, 99025–99037. https://doi.org/10.1109/ACCESS.2022.3205739

21. Wu, D., Yang, Z., Zhang, P., Wang, R., Yang, B., & Ma, X. (2023). Virtual-reality interpromotion technology for metaverse: A survey. IEEE Internet of Things Journal, 10(18), 15788–15809. https://doi.org/10.1109/JIOT.2023.3265848

22. Xiang, W., Yu, K., Han, F., Fang, L., He, D., & Han, Q. (2024). Advanced manufacturing in Industry 5.0: A survey of key enabling technologies and future trends. IEEE Transactions on Industrial Informatics, 20(2), 1055–1068. https://doi.org/10.1016/j.jii.2021.100257

23. Zikas, P., et al. (2023). MAGES 4.0: Accelerating the world's transition to VR training and democratizing the authoring of the medical metaverse. IEEE Computer Graphics and Applications, 43(2), 43–56. https://doi.org/10.1109/MCG.2023.3242686

24. Jamshidi, M., Yahya, S., Nouri, L., Hashemi-Dezaki, H., Rezaei, A., & Chaudhary, M. (2023) A super-efficient GSM triplexer for 5G-enabled IoT in sustainable smart grid edge computing and the metaverse. Sensors, 23, 3775. https://doi.org/10.3390/s23073775

25. Catak, F., Kuzlu, M., Catak, E., Cali, U., & Guler, O. (2022) Defensive distillation-based adversarial attack mitigation method for channel estimation using deep learning models in next-generation wireless networks. IEEE Access, 10, 98191–98203. https://doi.org/10.1109/ACCESS.2022.3206385

26. Wong, E., Wahab, N., Saeed, F., & Nouf, A (2022). 360-degree video bandwidth reduction: Technique and approaches comprehensive review. Applied Sciences, 12(15), 7581. https://doi.org/10.3390/app12157581

27. Jamshidi, M., Salah, Y., Leila, N., Hamed, H., Rezaei, A., & Chaudhary, M. (2023) A high-efficiency diplexer for sustainable 5G-enabled IoT in metaverse transportation system and smart grids. Symmetry, 15(4), 821–840. https://doi.org/10.3390/sym15040821

28. Wang, W., Yang, Y., Xiong, Z., & Niyato, D. (2023) Footstone of metaverse: A timely and secure crowdsensing. IEEE Network, 38(2), 1–8. https://doi.org/10.1109/MNET.134.2200598

29. Bhattacharya, P., Verma, A., Prasad, V., Tanwar, S., Bharat, B., Florea, B., Taralunga, D., Fayez, A., & Tolba, A. (2023). Game-o-Meta: Trusted federated learning scheme for P2P gaming metaverse beyond 5G networks. Sensors, 23(9), 4201–4226. https://doi.org/10.3390/s23094201

30. Morimoto, Y., Shiu, S., Huang, I., Fest, E., Ye, G., & Zhu, J. (2023). Optically transparent antenna for smart glasses. IEEE Open Journal of Antennas and Propagation, 4, 159–167. https://doi.org/10.1109/OJAP.2023.3238721

31. Chiang, J., Lin, C., Chiang, Y., & Su, Yushun (2022). Optimization of the spectrum splitting and auction for 5th generation mobile networks to enhance quality of services for IoT from the perspective of inclusive sharing economy. Electronics, 11(1), 3. https://doi.org/10.3390/electronics11010003

32. Penaherrera-Pulla, O., Carlos, B., Sergio, F., Eduardo, B., & Raquel, B. (2022). KQI assessment of VR services: A case study on 360-video over 4G and 5G. IEEE Transactions on Network and Service Management, 19(4), 5366–5382. https://doi.org/10.1109/TNSM.2022.3192762

33. Karunarathna, S., Wijethilaka, S., Ranaweera, P., Hemachandra, K., Samarasinghe, T., & Liyanage, M. (2023). The role of network slicing and edge computing in the metaverse realization. IEEE Access, 11, 25502–25530. https://doi.org/10.1109/ACCESS.2023.3255510

34. Chandramouli, D., Andres-Maldonado, P., & Kolding, T. (2023). Evolution of timing services from 5G-A toward 6G. IEEE Access, 11, 35150–35157. https://doi.org/10.1109/ACCESS.2023.3265213

35. Xiaoou, L., Xiaoyi, C., Bi, Qi, Liang, W., Li, J., & Zhang, Z. (2023). Blockchain-based distributed operation and incentive solution for P-RAN. Computer Communications, 198, 77–84. https://doi.org/10.1016/j.comcom.2022.11.008

36. Han, B., Pathak, P., Chen, S., & Yu, L. (2022) CoMIC: A collaborative mobile immersive computing infrastructure for conducting multi-user XR research. IEEE Network, 37(6), 124–131. https://doi.org/10.1109/MNET.126.2200385

37. Huang, Y., Zhu, Y., Qiao, X., Su, X., Dustdar, S., & Zhang, P. (2022). Towards holographic video communications: A promising AI-driven solution. https://doi.org/10.48550/arXiv.2210.06794

38. Chen, M., Liu, A., Xiong, N., Song, H., & Leung, V. (2024). SGPL: An intelligent game-based secure collaborative communication scheme for metaverse over 5G and beyond networks. IEEE Journal on Selected Areas in Communications, 42(3), 767–782. https://doi.org/10.1109/jsac.2023.3345403

39. Gao, H., Chong, A., & Bao, H. (2023). Metaverse: Literature review, synthesis and future research agenda. Journal of Computer Information Systems, 64(4), 533–553. https://doi.org/10.1080/08874417.2023.2233455

40. Zhihan, L. (2023). State-of-the-art human-computer-interaction in metaverse. International Journal of Human–Computer Interaction. 40(21), 6690–6708. https://doi.org/10.1080/10447318.2023.2248833

41. Zhou, X., Yang, Q., Zheng, X., Liang, W., Wang, K., Ma, J., Pan, Yi, & Jin, Q. (2024). Personalized federation learning with model-contrastive learning for multi-modal user modeling in human-centric metaverse. IEEE Journal on Selected Areas in Communications, 42(4), 817–831. https://doi.org/10.1109/JSAC.2023.3345431

42. Hande, P., et al. (2023). Extended reality over 5G – Standards evolution. IEEE Journal on Selected Areas in Communications, 41(6), 1757–1771. https://doi.org/10.1109/JSAC.2023.3276056

43. Zhang, X., Zhang, H., Sun, K., Long, K., & Li, Y. (2024). Human-centric irregular RIS-assisted multi-UAV networks with resource allocation and reflecting design for metaverse. IEEE Journal on Selected Areas in Communications, 42(3), 603–615. https://doi.org/10.1109/JSAC.2023.3345426

44. Xing, H., et al. (2023). Task-oriented integrated sensing, computation and communication for wireless edge AI. IEEE Network, 37(4), 135–144. https://doi.org/10.48550/arXiv.2306.06603

45. Meng, Z., et al. (2024). Task-oriented cross-system design for timely and accurate modeling in the metaverse. IEEE Journal on Selected Areas in Communications, 42(3), 752–766. https://doi.org/10.1109/JSAC.2023.3345398

46. Balasubramaniam, S, & Kumar, K. S. (2022). Fractional feedback political optimizer with prioritization-based charge scheduling in cloud-assisted electric vehicular network. Ad Hoc & Sensor Wireless Networks, 52(3–4), 173–198.

47. Zhang, X., Zhao, H., Zhou, J., Yang, F., Liu, S., & Xie, G. (2023). Remote collaborations in metaverse under 5G mobile networks. IEEE Communications Magazine. 61, 16–22. https://doi.org/10.1109/MCOM.003.2200624

48. Balasubramaniam, S, Kadry, S., & Kumar, K. S. (2024). Osprey Gannet optimization enabled CNN based transfer learning for optic disc detection and cardiovascular risk prediction using retinal fundus images. Biomedical Signal Processing and Control, 93, 106177. https://doi.org/10.1016/j.bspc.2024.106177

49. Huang, Z., & Friderikos, V (2023). Optimal mobility-aware wireless edge cloud support for the metaverse. Future Internet, 15(2), 1–20. https://doi.org/10.3390/fi15020047

50. Zhu, P., Yoshida, Y., Akahane, K., & Kitayama, K (2024). High-speed reach-extended IM-DD system with low-complexity DSP for 6G fronthaul. Journal of Optical Communications and Networking, 16(1), A24–A32. https://doi.org/10.1364/JOCN.499108

51. Pan, Y., Luo, K., Liu, Y., Xu, C., Liu, Y., & Lin, Z. (2024). Mobile edge assisted multi view light field video system: Prototype design and empirical evaluation. Future Generation Computer Systems, 153, 154–168. https://doi.org/10.1016/j.future.2023.11.023

52. Kadry, S., Dhanaraj, R. K., & Manthiramoorthy, C. (2024). Res-Unet based blood vessel segmentation and cardio vascular disease prediction using chronological chef-based optimization algorithm based deep residual network from retinal fundus images. Multimedia Tools and Applications, 1–30. https://doi.org/10.1007/s11042-024-18810-y

53. Morin, D., Lopez-Morales, M., Perez, P., Armada, A., & Villegas, A (2023). FikoRE: 5G and beyond RAN emulator for application level experimentation and prototyping. IEEE Network, 37(4), 48–55. https://doi.org/10.48550/arXiv.2204.04290

54. Siddiqi, S., Jan, M., Basalamah, A., & Tariq, M. (2023). Secure teleoperated vehicles in augmented reality of things: A multichain and digital twin approach. IEEE Transactions on Consumer Electronics, 70(1), 956–965. https://doi.org/10.1109/TCE.2023.3329007

55. Balasubramaniam, S, Syed, M. H., More, N. S., & Polepally, V. (2023). Deep learning-based power prediction aware charge scheduling approach in cloud based electric vehicular network. Engineering Applications of Artificial Intelligence, 121, 105869. https://doi.org/10.1016/j.engappai.2023.105869

56. Huang, Y., Sun, Q., Li, N., Chen, Z., Huang, J., Ding, H., & Lin, I. (2023). Validation of current o-RAN technologies and insights on the future evolution. IEEE Journal on Selected Areas in Communications, 42(2), 487–505. https://doi.org/10.1109/JSAC.2023.3336180

An Overview of the Significance of Cloud Computing in the Realm of the Metaverse

Hariharan B, Anupama C. G, Ratnakumari Neerukonda, and B. Sundaravadivazhagan

5.1 Introduction

Cloud computing is an evolving generation that lets in users to get right of entry to a shared cluster of computing sources, inclusive of servers, garage, databases, networking, and software remotely without the need of physical infrastructure or protection. The offerings are in far-flung information centers and can be used online; this is made possible by virtualization of computing gadgets. Cloud companies use infrastructure as a service (IaaS) to offer virtualized laptop assets to customers over the Internet. Users can lease and function digital machines (VMs), storage, and networking infrastructure as an alternative of purchasing and preserving real system. With virtualization, one-of-a-kind working structures (OS) and applications can operate on the same hardware, taking into account the efficient utilization of computing sources. Users and organizations can employ the various alternatives provided by the cloud in terms of the one-of-a-kind ranges of memory, computing sources, and protection alternatives. Cloud computing has a wide range of applications across various industries thanks to its flexibility, scalability, cost-effectiveness, and accessibility. Industries and sectors such as e-commerce, banking, finance,

DOI: 10.1201/9781003491668-5

healthcare, gaming, and entertainment have integrated cloud technologies with their business and continue to benefit from scaling their applications with the cloud. The technological advancements in cloud computing have opened up a new frontier for a shared digital space – the metaverse, where users can interact with each other and the virtual digital environment in real time and collaborate.

The metaverse has revolutionized the way we interact with virtual landscape and transformed the digital landscape. The metaverse consists of interconnected virtual worlds and immersion and is being driven by cloud computing. The use of cloud computing technologies has been rapidly increasing, with metaverse application developers and service providers expanding the use cases of the metaverse with the addition of new and engaging features. Using cloud architecture, the metaverse provides the benefits of shared computing resources, scalability, efficient data storage, content delivery, and management, thus providing a continuous and enjoyable experience for users. Recent cloud advancements are increasing performance, reliability, and security and are accelerating the adoption of the metaverse. Recent developments demonstrate how both the breadth and depth of cloud computing technologies used in the metaverse advance research in this area.

Augmented reality (AR), virtual reality (VR), and cloud computing applications in the metaverse reshape digital ecosystems. AR and VR technologies are widely used in a variety of industries, from gaming, healthcare, and entertainment to connecting cloud computing to create and enable an immersive, interactive environment and facilitate simple content delivery and data management. Cloud computing also expands the availability of metaverse applications as well as improving uptime to enable multiple metaverse applications to be served simultaneously by billions of users worldwide. This development opens up new possibilities for collaborative workspaces, events that have authenticity and entertainment experiences. Using cloud-based infrastructure enables developers to create and operate extensive, rich, and dynamic metaverse communities, transforming the way we interact with digital objects and each other.

This chapter presents a radical and comprehensive evaluation of the important role that cloud computing plays in shaping the improvement, operation, and destiny potentialities of the metaverse. The concept of the metaverse is explored as a collective digital shared area that breaks the bounds among physical and digital worlds, facilitating seamless interplay and collaboration among users. We discover the benefits that the integration of cloud computing technology brings to the metaverse, which includes improved collaboration, immersive gaining knowledge of stories, customized healthcare, digital occasion control, and the advent of the latest sales streams. We delve into the architecture of a metaverse cloud software and its additives. Additionally, we deal with the challenges confronted in leveraging cloud computing for metaverse applications, consisting of worries and roadblocks, including technical complexity, privacy issues, cybersecurity risks, intellectual belongings problems, and regulatory frameworks. Furthermore, we talk about emerging traits and future directions within the discipline, highlighting the importance of interoperability, synthetic intelligence integration, digital reality programs, decentralized structure, and moral concerns in shaping the evolution of the metaverse.

The chapter proceeds as follows: Section 5.2 covers present methodologies, whereas sections 5.3 and 5.4 detail the idea of the metaverse and outline the main advantages of the metaverse in cloud computing. Section 5.5 elucidates the cloud architecture of a metaverse application, and the challenges of the metaverse in cloud computing are explored in section 5.6, and the conclusion follows.

5.2 Related Works

Cai, Yang et al. [1] address the efficient delivery of real-time stream-processing applications in distributed cloud architectures like fog and mobile edge computing. These applications involve multicast traffic, where data packets are shared and consumed by multiple users/devices simultaneously. Existing technologies struggle to handle this multicast nature efficiently, leading to traffic redundancy and network congestion. The authors introduce a unified framework for distributed cloud network control with generalized (mixed-cast) traffic flows, optimizing packet processing, forwarding, and replication operations. A novel queuing system is designed to schedule data packets based on their current destinations, and a fully decentralized algorithm, GDCNC, is proposed for throughput- and cost-optimal multicast flow control. The paper's contributions include characterizing the multicast network stability region, devising decentralized control policies, and demonstrating performance gains through numerical experiments.

Cai, Yang et al. [2] discuss the transformational effect of metaverse packages on community infrastructure. The authors argue for the mixing of computing, caching, and communication (3C) technologies into NextG networks to satisfy the demands of real-time, immersive digital experiences. The authors illustrate the significance of surprisingly disbursed and densely incorporated computer and facts-intensive networks as regular structures for next-technology digital reports. The paper outlines the requirements of metaverse applications, describes the predicted infrastructure, and proposes a comprehensive cloud community with a mathematical framework for end-to-end optimization and control. This framework helps green operations with the aid of dynamically allocating sources, optimizing provider shipping, and ensuring low latency. The authors gift a holistic method to designing community infrastructure capable of supporting the diverse, stressful, and evolving needs of the metaverse. The authors introduce a mathematical framework for "Cloud Network Flow," which has been designed for the cease-to-end optimization of cloud systems. The authors discover the metaverse infrastructure and the diverse sectors in which the metaverse can be implemented to create and decorate immersive stories. The paper discusses the metaverse infrastructure and the various necessities, consisting of processing, storage, and communication. The authors offer numerical findings and information to support their conclusion that the framework has an advantage in producing green operations on metaverse networks [3].

Shokrnezhad, Masoud, et al. [4] introduce the idea of adaptable computing-network convergence (ACNC) as an option for the troubles of aid scarcity and dynamic person necessities in destiny 6G networks, particularly in eventualities along with the metaverse. ACNC uses machine learning (ML) in conjunction with computing-network convergence (CNC) to autonomously manipulate and allocate computing assets (computing gadgets) and community sources. Continual learning (CL) is used to deal with dynamic changes and context detection to categorize device states into predefined contexts. The ACNC framework consists of network and computing orchestrators, points of attachment (PoAs), and an end-to-end (E2E) orchestrator, which work together to optimize resource allocation and simplify complexity. ACNC targets to decrease the system states and installation context-conscious sellers and thus efficiently deal with the complex and dynamic interactions among the customers, offerings, and infrastructure. Hence, the quality of service (QoS) of the metaverse utility is ensured.

Chen, Ruxiao, and Shuaishuai Guo. [5] recommend a unique method to deal with demanding situations in offloading computation duties for multiuser mobile augmented reality (MAR) offerings in edge-cloud computing networks. The MAR carrier-orientated mission offloading scheme considers the assignment interdependency and uses a look-ahead offloading set of rules based totally on a changed Monte Carlo tree search (MMCT). The proposed scheme seeks to enhance QoS via efficiently scheduling offloading choices with attention to long-term outcomes and migration overheads. The system structure includes four layers: person, conversation, control, and computation layers, with more than one part and cloud servers presenting offloading paths. The MAR software model is improved upon, with directed acyclic graphs (DAGs) used to seize venture interdependencies appropriately. The trouble formula consists of an objective function that contains response time, energy usage, host traits, and service-level agreement (SLA) breaches, all of which are optimized to improve QoS. The MMCT framework presents real-time choice-making with the aid of quickly simulating multistep executions, resulting in reliable and scalable MAR offerings in risky environments.

Chang, Luyi, et al. [6] explore the integration of 6G-enabled edge artificial intelligence (AI) with the metaverse to overcome limitations in resources, computing power, and sensory devices. It introduces three edge-metaverse architectures leveraging 6G-enabled edge AI to address constraints. Challenges such as latency, stability, and security in edge AI are discussed, with 6G technology providing solutions for lower latency, stable connections, and enhanced security. The metaverse's immersive, multitechnology, interoperable, social, and lasting nature is outlined. Architectures including physical, virtual, and technical layers are depicted, utilizing technologies like digital twins, blockchain, network communication, decentralization, and computer vision. The paper underscores the importance of efficient integration between edge AI and the metaverse, paving the way for future research directions in realizing the metaverse's vision with 6G-enabled edge AI.

Farhoudi, Mohammad, Masoud Shokrnezhad, and Tarik Taleb [7] advocate a singular technique, known as water-filling of service placement (WISE), for QoS-conscious provider orchestration in part-cloud environments, focusing on Beyond 5G (B5G) networks. The foremost concept revolves around jointly optimizing service placement and aid allocation to meet dynamic consumer needs while minimizing average price and latency. The WISE method predicts user behavior using a double deep Q-learning (DDQL) agent, recurrent neural networks (RNNs), and the water-filling algorithm to manage resources and offerings times effectively. This method addresses the challenges of dynamic person behavior, ultralow latency requirements, and carrier continuity in B5G networks. Experimental outcomes show that WISE outperforms traditional techniques, supplying close to most fulfilling answers with scalable and efficient resource placement.

Yang, Liang, et al. [8] provide a complete analysis of interoperability within the rising idea of the metaverse. The authors talk about the problems and importance of interoperability in attaining the entire ability of the metaverse, which incorporates virtual, augmented, and mixed-fact settings. The authors use Urs Gasser's model to describe interoperability in virtual ecosystems, which covers technological, factual, human, and institutional additives. They highlight main topics, research findings, and limitations in metaverse interoperability with the aim of undertaking a comprehensive literature review and content analysis. The authors offer a systematic method to address the complexity of interoperability and establish criteria for future study.

Qian, Liangxin et al. [9] cope with the optimization of consumer connectivity and useful resource allocation in a blockchain-enabled metaverse, with a focus on nonfungible token (NFT) packages and 6G wireless communications. It introduces the agree-with-fee ratio (total capital ratio, or TCR), which compares user agreement with rankings to delay and strength fees. The proposed DASHF algorithm is based totally on the Dinkelbach set of rules, alternating optimization, semidefinite relaxation (SDR), the Hungarian approach, and functional programming. The DASHF algorithm improves personal venture offloading, resource allocation, and TCR through the usage of techniques consisting of quadratically constrained quadratic programming (QCQP), SDR, and the Hungarian method. The device version takes into account the conversation, computing, electricity utilization, and belief score. The key contributions are the usage of TCR, innovative optimization formulation, and the DASHF algorithm to handle complex issues in blockchain–metaverse integration over Wi-Fi networks. Extensive simulations show the usefulness of the proposed method, presenting vital insights for improving blockchain–metaverse programs, especially those using NFTs.

Ismail, Leila, and Rajkumar Buyya [10] delve into the evolving landscape of the metaverse, focusing on achieving real-time and scalable experiences while addressing security, privacy, and interoperability concerns. It begins by tracing the historical definitions of the metaverse and identifies key requirements such as immersive interaction, spatial temporality, interoperability, scalability, and quality of service/experience and what technical requirements and technologies are needed to achieve these goals. The paper then explores enabling technologies like AI, the Internet of Things (IoT), blockchain, VR/AR, edge/cloud computing, and spatial computing, each crucial for realizing the metaverse vision. A layered architecture is proposed, emphasizing infrastructure, distributed computing, platform, and application layers, to ensure scalability and flexibility. The paper also provides insights into development platforms, application domains, and critical challenges like real-time processing, energy consumption, security, and governance, offering potential solutions and future research directions. Overall, it presents a comprehensive roadmap toward building a green, dependable, and immersive metaverse experience.

Wang, Yitong, and Jun Zhao [11] speak of the evolution of cell computing paradigms impacted by utilizing IoT and 5G/6G technologies, specializing in mobile edge computing (MEC) as a strategy to the restrictions of conventional cloud computing for mobile gadgets. The MEC paradigm relocates computer-extensive processes to the network edge, improving storage, useful resource optimization, and computational efficiency. The confluence of MEC with new technology like the metaverse, 6G, AI, and blockchain is studied, with a focus on their capability synergies. The article explores MEC's use instances in MAR and its position in enabling the MEC-based total metaverse. It discusses the mixing of MAR with other surrounding technologies and packages. It additionally discusses problems and new traits in MEC, consisting of computing offloading and electricity consumption. The integration of MEC with 6G, AI, blockchain, and the metaverse is emphasized, paving the way for destiny studies instructions.

5.3 The Concept of the Metaverse

In this section, we discuss the concept of the metaverse and its use cases.

5.3.1 Metaverse

The metaverse is a virtual global universe, a virtual and digital vicinity where customers can engage with one another and with the digital surroundings, produce their fabric, and interact in a whole lot of sports. The metaverse blurs the difference between the bodily and digital worlds and introduces new opportunities for users to engage, cooperate, and talk. Users interact with the virtual global world with VR devices, which act as the interface between the user and the virtual space. The metaverse may be accessed through diverse gadgets, consisting of VR headsets, AR glasses, and smartphones. Several service vendors give customers get right of entry to the metaverse, and the user base of the metaverse has extended over the recent years. Users of the metaverse can participate in a wide variety of activities, which include socializing, developing content, gaming, attending digital events such as live shows, training, and accomplishing commercial enterprise. Users also can do specific kinds of multimedia and create and collaborate with the help of cloud technology. For instance, cloud object storage is used to store the exclusive content material that users produce in a stable and easily reachable manner. The real-time streaming made possible by employing the cloud infrastructure lets customers interact and collaborate [12].

The metaverse transforms the digital space by blurring the traces between bodily fact and virtual reality. It is mainly due to a shift in the way we consume media and hook up with each other. It develops a feel of a network and belonging by bringing humans from all backgrounds collectively to proportion studies, alternate ideas, and paintings on previously inconceivable projects. It offers a shared space for all of us to interact, talk, and for ideas and creations. Since the metaverse is built on decentralized technologies along with the blockchain, it permits peer-to-peer transactions and the creation of digital assets whose ownership is in the complete manipulation of the customers. This leads to new forms of creativity inclusive of digital exhibitions, performances, auctions, and digital marketplaces. Users can also purchase, promote, and trade virtual property in the metaverse, for this reason creating a virtual marketplace with new financial possibilities. As the metaverse evolves and expands, it can reinvent human connection and creativity in the digital age via transcending geographical borders and permitting global interactions, communications, and collaborations.

There is a need for a tremendously scalable, sturdy device that could serve tens of millions of concurrent users gaining access to the platform. Cloud computing and decentralization perform a pivotal function in the gadget infrastructure of the metaverse, providing the computational assets, storage and networking competencies needed to support its large digital landscapes and immersive experiences. Developers who wish to construct packages and offerings inside the metaverse can create scalable and reliable systems for websites hosting digital worlds using cloud computing technologies, ensuring seamless connectivity and actual-time interplay for customers throughout the globe.

5.3.2 Immersive Experiences in the Metaverse

The metaverse gives a massive immersive experience for the enjoyment of its users. The metaverse opens up a huge variety of potential monetary opportunities and applications across diverse fields. With the combining of VR and AR, the metaverse creates a surrounding in which customers can engage in reviews that combine a whole lot of audiovisual stimuli and special capabilities to create a 3D immersive international experience. The AR and VR devices use the interface through which the users engage with the virtual international environment and get output from the metaverse's surroundings [13].

In the metaverse, the customers aren't passive spectators but energetic members in the virtual international environment. Users can create personalized avatars that may serve as digital personas that represent them and can interact with different users around the world. The customers of the metaverse interact with the interfaces of the AR and VR devices, giving input such as actions, with the digital camera focus interacting with objects and taking in output from the VR devices. Thus, VR technology creates new opportunities in the metaverse inclusive of digital travel, virtual tours, and digital occasions. The metaverse can facilitate social interaction on a scale previously impossible and unimaginable. The scale of social interaction and its volume is global within the metaverse environment. Within virtual environments, users can connect with friends, family, colleagues, and strangers from around the globe, transcending geographical boundaries and time zones. Whether attending virtual concerts, exploring virtual museums, or simply hanging out in virtual cafes, users can share meaningful experiences and forge connections in ways that feel remarkably real. The metaverse offers users the opportunity to create, customize, and share their content and environment. Some examples include building virtual homes and businesses, designing clothing and accessories, and creating artwork. Cloud storage allows users to create, work with, and store their virtual creations, such as artwork, multimedia, 3D models, and textures, without the need for local storage, thus enabling users to access all this content from any device at any time. All the user-created objects are stored in the cloud object storage along with their digital fingerprint. Blockchain technology, NFTs, and the metaverse's object storage play a crucial role in storing and assigning ownership to digital assets and creations. To render complex 3D environments, objects, and animations, a lot of graphics processing power is required. With regard to this, the cloud can provide the computing resources required for this in the form of shared and virtualized resources. Additionally, cloud computing enables metaverse applications to scale both horizontally and vertically, allowing a wide user base to access the metaverse and build more diverse applications. In addition to supporting social and creative hobbies, the metaverse holds enormous potential for education and mastering the education. Educational institutions and groups may additionally appoint virtual worlds to create immersive mastering stories that engage college students in ways that conventional strategies can't. From digital school rooms and schooling simulations to interactive academic video games and historical reenactments, the metaverse offers a dynamic and engaging method of learning that caters to a wide variety of teaching patterns and hobbies.

Another area where the metaverse indicates notable ability is entertainment, with users able to participate in several quite immersive and attractive events. From multiplayer online games and digital subject matter parks to host occasions and virtual artwork exhibitions, the metaverse gives a huge variety of entertainment alternatives to suit each taste or interest. Users can take part in digital occasions, live concert events, gaming, and many other activities. All the packages and regions of hobby in the metaverse are built on the pinnacle of scaling cloud infrastructure.

5.3.3 Use Cases of the Metaverse

The metaverse has a wide range of applications for different industries and spheres. In the sphere of entertainment, such applications enable users to play games in the considered worlds, watch different films and live events, and become engaged in various storytelling and interactive experiences. As for the educational sector, special apps for personalized and lifelong learning, virtual classes, and various simulations can be created. The metaverse can make corporate meetings, virtual offices, and showrooms run more smoothly. Healthcare implications are also intriguing, and dedicated applications and places may be created to improve virtual consultations, medical training simulations, and rehabilitation [14].

The metaverse may be used to socialize, network, connect, and interact with extraordinary communities for the duration of the sector. As new developments within the metaverse emerge, new use instances in the metaverse might be identified and greater programs and capabilities could be built for the metaverse. The metaverse opens a wide variety of multifaceted and nuanced monetary opportunities throughout distinct industries and sectors. The metaverse offers an upward push to an increasing virtual financial system wherein virtual items, services, and reports keep tangible fees and economic importance. The metaverse offers a big gambling field for innovation, entrepreneurship, and financial growth.

The metaverse can revolutionize healthcare by providing immersive and personalized experiences for patients and healthcare experts alike. Telemedicine systems inside the metaverse help join the patients to the doctors and medical service providers and allow sufferers to acquire digital consultations, diagnostic offerings, and remedy alternatives from the comfort of their own homes. Medical consultations, therapy sessions, and group counseling may be conducted with the assistance of the metaverse, allowing faraway services and increasing accessibility. Metaverse programs can also be leveraged to offer informative educational resources to patients and assist them in recognizing their conditions and treatment plans interactively. The metaverse permits scientific experts to build 3D interactive models to have a look at, teach, and make use of simulations for training and schooling. Healthcare experts can also gain from virtual schooling simulations, surgical rehearsals, and clinical conferences held inside the metaverse, enhancing their capabilities and information in safe and managed surroundings.

Entertainment inside the metaverse has a huge potential to impart to users various interesting stories inclusive of virtual concerts, immersive films, video games, virtual artwork exhibitions, and interactive environments. The metaverse also permits customers to express their creativity and create virtual art, sculpture, and content. All the content made with the aid of the customers is recognized with a unique identifier and saved inside the blockchain and the cloud object garage. There is also an extended record of the development of VR games, providing customers with immersive first man or woman games. The video games also can be mixed with motion factors and surround audio, developing even extra engaging gaming stories. Further possibilities encompass virtual massive multiplayer games and decorated immersion games in the metaverse. Therefore, the economic opportunities of the metaverse are considerable and may be multiplied similarly as increasingly more customers utilize and apply the metaverse to their desires.

5.4 Benefits of Cloud Computing in the Metaverse

Cloud computing has transformed the way we think, store, and get the right of entry to facts. The implementation of cloud computing structure has spread out for several opportunities such as immersive mastering stories, customized healthcare, virtual event management, and increased revenue streams. In this section, we spotlight a number of the benefits of cloud computing in the metaverse and its elements [15].

5.4.1 Scalability

Cloud computing offers scaling of metaverse programs, each horizontally and vertically. Cloud computing offers on-call resource provisioning with its pay-as-you-pass model, which is important for the metaverse due to its dynamic nature. With cloud computing, resources can be easily scaled up or down based on demand, ensuring that clients remain seamlessly connected to the metaverse and access its services without any lag or downtime. Distributed processing may be made feasible with cloud computing, making managing complex tasks in the metaverse less tough. Distributed processing includes breaking down large duties into smaller tasks and dispensing them across a couple of servers, taking into account quicker execution time and multiplied performance. This factor of allotted computing is particularly vital for rendering excellent pics, simulating physics, and processing user interactions in real time. With Cloud Garage, the statistics of the users is long lasting, and the records may be replicated and saved in unique disks, ensuring that information is usually available and may be recovered fast in case of any failure or loss, through the technique known as redundancy. This is vital for the metaverse, as users count on their statistics to be on hand continually, irrespective of any technical problems. Cloud-based tools permit seamless sharing of sources and synchronization of efforts, streamlining workflows, and accelerating challenge timelines. Consequently, businesses stand to benefit from extensive productivity gains and cost efficiencies by harnessing the collaborative power of the metaverse intertwined with cloud computing technology.

5.4.2 Cost Effective

Cloud computing offers pay-as-you-go pricing models, which permit metaverse builders and users to pay for the sources they truly use instead of investing in highly priced hardware and infrastructure in advance, reducing the barrier to entry for developing and web hosting metaverse applications. Metaverse builders can leverage the cloud to construct complex virtual environments without being stressed about the upfront prices of purchasing and preserving their hardware. Load-balancing algorithms utilized in cloud computing and their autoscaling nature are vital for dealing with the unpredictable and relatively diverse utilization styles of the metaverse. A load balancer can routinely distribute incoming traffic throughout a couple of times, making sure that users always have a seamless experience, even during top usage times. Hence, cloud computing gives value savings through aid optimization and efficient utilization. Moreover, metaverse programs regularly require massive quantities of garage and processing energy to deliver awesome photographs, physics simulations, and actual-time user interactions. Cloud computing offerings can optimize the usage of these assets with the aid of imparting functions like car-scaling, spot times, and serverless computing. Cloud computing services can optimize using those assets by offering capabilities like automobile scaling, spot times, and serverless computing. Metaverse applications regularly require high availability and records sturdiness to make sure that customers always have access to their virtual belongings and reports. Cloud computing offerings offer more than one replica of statistics across specific areas and availability zones via the computing technique referred to as redundancy, making sure that statistics are constantly available in case of any failure or loss. Cloud computing gives price savings via redundancy and restoration after a catastrophe. Hence, cloud computing facilitates metaverse builders to build fault-proof, exceedingly available, and scalable packages.

5.4.3 Reliability

Cloud computing offers redundancy through multiple data centers and availability zones, ensuring that metaverse applications are always available even in cases of hardware failures, natural disasters, or any unforeseen circumstances. With cloud computing, real-time monitoring and automatic failover are possible, which allows metaverse developers to quickly identify and resolve any issues before they impact the users. Failover is the ability of a system to switch seamlessly to a different backup system. The load balancer in the cloud architecture ensures that the resources are always allocated optimally, removing possibilities of bottlenecking and lags and ensuring seamless connectivity to all users. Hence, with distributed computing, metaverse engineers can develop scalable and reliable metaverse applications for the users. Encryption, access control, and multifactor authentication can be integrated with the metaverse, user data from unauthorized access is blocked, and losses of user data are prevented.

5.4.4 Accessibility

Metaverse applications require actual-time character interactions and amazing pictures to deliver immersive evaluations, which may be tough to reap over lengthy distances or unreliable net connections. This is addressed using edge cloud computing locations and content delivery networks (CDNs). Metaverse carrier companies can offer multidevice resources permitting customers entry to metaverse applications on numerous devices, such as smartphones, tablets, laptops, and virtual truth headsets. Cloud computing gives scalability and flexibility in terms of aid allocation and cost management, permitting users to get proper access to metaverse applications primarily based on their desires and budgets. The good security options, including encryption, access control, and multi-factor authentication, aid to protect metaverse application servers and client data from unauthorized uses or loss.

5.4.5 Collaboration

Cloud-based tools enable easy sharing of content and efforts, streamline workflows, and accelerate project timelines. Through a virtual environment, individuals from diverse backgrounds can participate in cultural, educational, and social activities without physical barriers. Additionally, cloud-based analytics and data insights derived from virtual event interactions enable organizers to better understand attendee behavior and preferences, leading to more personalized and enjoyable experiences at events in the future. Hence cloud computing leads driving technology to improve performance.

5.4.6 AI Usage

Cloud computing supports the integration of AI and ML in metaverse applications. The usage of AI to create a more interactive and responsive environment that adapts to different users' behavior and changes randomly is being explored. Cloud computing is central in data analytics and the processing of large amounts of data generated by users. Building recommendation systems and user behavior analytics is being done with AI and cloud computing. Scalable and shared relational and nonrelational cloud databases are crucial to store user data and manage authentication and user preferences. Cloud data analysis tools and ML model building can be used to analyze and predict user behavior and trends, and this offers valuable insights to metaverse application developers and service providers.

5.5 Cloud Architecture of a Metaverse Application

The metaverse and its surrounding applications have millions of users around the world, hence there is a need for accessible and reliable metaverse applications

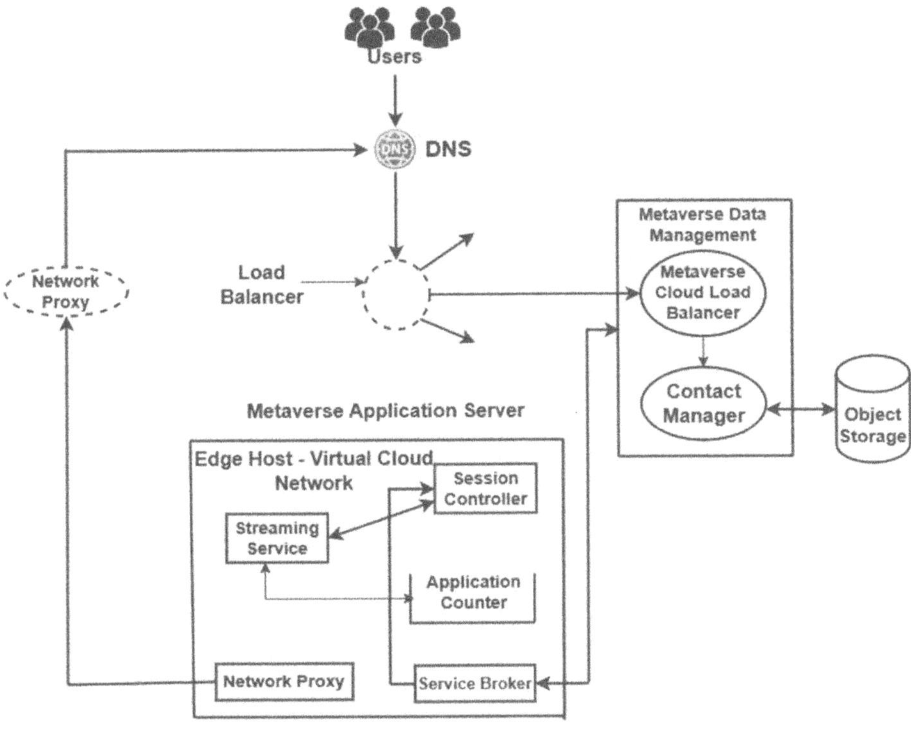

Figure 5.1 Cloud architecture of a metaverse application.

that are available to a wide range of users. The application of cloud infrastructures is of utmost importance in metaverse applications. A metaverse application hosted in the cloud can show good performance accessibility and reliability to a wide range of users from around the world. A robust cloud architecture that is scalable and one that can efficiently manage and allocate resources is of importance here.

Figure 5.1 illustrates the cloud architecture of a metaverse application. This cloud infrastructure makes use of multiple availability domains to ensure the uptime of the server in different regions. Additionally, multiple availability domains can be used to serve the same application to web1, web2, and web3 users. The metaverse cloud application is encompassed by Edge Virtual Cloud Network (VCN). The metaverse application server exists within the VCN. A VCN is a system of devices, virtual machines, servers, and data centers that are connected through a software known as a "virtual switch," or "switch," instead of the traditional physical switch. The application server has four major components, namely a session controller, a streaming service, an application container, and a service broker.

5.5.1 Load Balancer

A metaverse application needs to process the requests of hundreds of millions of users at a time and serve the users different multimedia such as texts, images, audio, and video. The users in turn need to be able to stream their media to other users, and all of this has to occur simultaneously and with good performance and low latency. This is only possible via a distribution of tasks and resources. A load balancer is used to distribute the user requests to different virtual computing instances and to allocate the resources in the virtual network. The process by which a load balancer distributes network traffic over a set of computing resources (computing units) is known as load balancing. The purpose of using load balancing is to make efficient use of the computing units and to reduce the overall time taken to process the requests.

5.5.2 Network Proxy

The users of the metaverse are connected to the metaverse software servers via a network proxy. A network proxy is a middleman server that offers a gateway between customers and the hosted utility or Internet site, which can be a software program or hardware that is placed between the purchaser and the provider's server. The intermediary position of the community proxy is critical in making sure seamless connectivity and data exchange in the metaverse ecosystem. It is responsible for routing visitors, as site visitor actions move through the proxy along its way to the software server. It manages the communication between the customer (the consumer) and the metaverse utility server, and all the requests are made by using the purchaser bypass through the community proxy in order to attain the metaverse utility server. It is a vital a part of a strong network infrastructure and guarantees privacy and safety for customers having access to the metaverse. By acting as a buffer between the patron's tool and the Internet, it can filter and block unauthorized admission to tries, malicious content material, and capability cyber threats, safeguarding touchy data and private statistics. Additionally, encryption techniques can be used to shield information transmission, as an end result similarly improving the confidentiality of personal interactions inside the metaverse.

5.5.3 Session Controller

A session controller, also known as a session border controller (SBC), is a devoted hardware device or software program that regulates and secures IP communications and data flow. Session controllers are a vital part of the shape of the metaverse due to the fact the metaverse entails numerous nonpublic interactions and multi-individual environments. An SBC acts as the regulator of the metaverse provider, allowing best-authorized classes created via authentic customers to bypass the connection factor and avail the provider of the metaverse. Hence, it acts as the gatekeeper to the metaverse application, dealing with access permissions and ensuring compliance with privacy regulations. An SBC carries out the functions of regulating the QoS of the metaverse utility by implementing the call administration control (CAC) regulations, the rate proscribing the metaverse carrier, and the terms of carrier marking. It may additionally dynamically regulate session parameters based on consumer options, environmental factors, or actual-time activities to tailor studies. SBCs reveal community site visitors and preserve the security of the device and may guard the system from distributed denial of service (DDoS) attacks. SBCs also can act as a firewall for session site visitors, enforcing the platform's defined QoS guidelines and identifying capability incoming threats to the infrastructure of the server. Additionally, a consultation controller optimizes the resource allocation, prioritizes person actions, and implements access controls for improved performance and security.

5.5.4 Service Broker

A service broker is a cloud entity that manages the usage, performance, and delivery of a cloud service. It is the link between the users and the cloud service provider, it has the details of the catalogue of the services provided, and it is responsible for carrying out the provisioning of the resources and connecting the users to the application. It acts as the middleman, communicating the needs and requests of the client to the server and the server's responses.

5.5.5 Streaming Service

Streaming is the procedure of continuous transmission of virtual media files, generally audio and video, from one factor to every other. A streaming provider is a platform that promises and serves multimedia content of diverse paperwork, which includes audio, films, textual content, and live publicity to users in real time. It operates by storing the content material at the streaming carrier, which is responsible for delivering multimedia content seamlessly to users in the virtual surroundings. It serves as the spine for transmitting stay events, interactive reports, and on-demand media to members in real time. Seamless collaboration and interplay among users of the metaverse in actual time is made possible by using the streaming carrier as it handles the statistics dispatched to the server by using all the concurrent customers concurrently and sends the digital global surroundings dynamically to the users. A streaming provider consists of the media being sent to the purchaser in a nonstop movement and the client using the client-side utility to display it. This calls for storing the content within the content material supervisor that is a part of metaverse data management and efficiently distributing it to the users' gadgets. The streaming service plays a pivotal role in making sure that clean and uninterrupted person studies result, facilitating engagement and immersion within the metaverse. Leveraging the cloud infrastructure, the service could dynamically scale to house fluctuations in calls for guaranteeing first-rate shipping of multimedia content to a large audience. Additionally, the streaming service frequently carries advanced capabilities inclusive of adaptive bit-rate streaming and content caching to optimize performance and reduce latency, enhancing the user's pleasure.

5.5.6 Metaverse Applications

The metaverse application box includes numerous critical additives that work together to create immersive experiences for the users. The pictures inside the metaverse are the primary aspect of the immersive visuals of the metaverse. The metaverse software field consists of the portrait-rendering engine at the core, also known as photosynthesis, which is the method of producing a complex and distinctive photo from a 2D or a 3D version. The software that performs the rendering is referred to as a photo-rendering engine or a renderer. Rendering in a provider issuer that includes the metaverse is made feasible via cloud technologies. By cleverly managing assets inside the cloud, the metaverse can provide the best graphics for the customers. With the renderer, the digital environment of the metaverse is populated with interactive objects and properties such as digital homes, automobiles, and customers' avatars. All these objects are stored in object storage, where each item is given a unique identifier or ID and the map of the item's identification along with its place is created. Cloud infrastructure plays a vital function in presenting scalable resources for website hosting and managing the software, ensuring seamless overall performance and accessibility across diverse gadgets and platforms.

5.5.7 Content Manager

As part of metaverse information management, the content material supervisor or the content material management machine (CMS) serves as the imperative hub for organizing, storing, coping with, and getting access to various types of virtual content material in the metaverse. The CMS is included with the cloud item records storage for successfully retrieving content properties inclusive of 3D fashions, textures, audio documents, and movies. The content manager interfaces with Object Garage to upload, organize, and retrieve content material assets, leveraging its skills for green data management. The CMS has two additives, a content material management application (CMA), which is the front-stop application for handling the content material, that allows you to be used by the metaverse provider directors. The metadata control equipment of the CMA allows tagging and categorization of content for clean looking and organization. The different element of the CMS is the content material transport software (CDA), which is answerable for compiling and handing over the content material to the users. By offering sturdy content material management talents, a content material supervisor allows developers and creators of the metaverse to create diverse types of content material and broaden new material for the users to interact with.

5.5.8 Object Storage

Cloud object storage is an important component of metaverse data management, as it handles a vast amount of digital content efficiently. In a traditional fire storage system, all the files are organized in a file tree, wherein the storage contains folders that in turn contain subfolders and files. Block storage is a storage system where the data are broken up into blocks and then stored in storage area networks (SAN) as individual pieces, and each block is given its unique identifier or ID, as shown in Figure 5.2.

The SAN management software constantly collects metadata from all the storage devices that are part of the storage system. The metadata includes read-and-write information such as the time of the last write and reads, read-write failures, and faults in the storage devices. The SAN places each data block in a location that is optimal for future access. The data are separate from the user environments, which allows the data to be accessed efficiently across different environments.

Metaverse data management makes use of object storage to store the different forms of multimedia within the metaverse. Unlike traditional file systems, object storage manages data as discrete objects or "blobs" with their associated metadata, enabling seamless scalability and accessibility across distributed environments. The objects in the object storage are stored and managed in sectors and tracks within the data storage system. Object storage allows for large-scale storage of unstructured data in which the data are written and read numerous times. This aspect of object storage is very important because most of the data that users engage with on the metaverse are unstructured. Every digital asset in the metaverse, all the users' avatars, digital belongings, and objects in the environment are stored in the object storage. Object storage abstracts lower-level storage functions, allowing

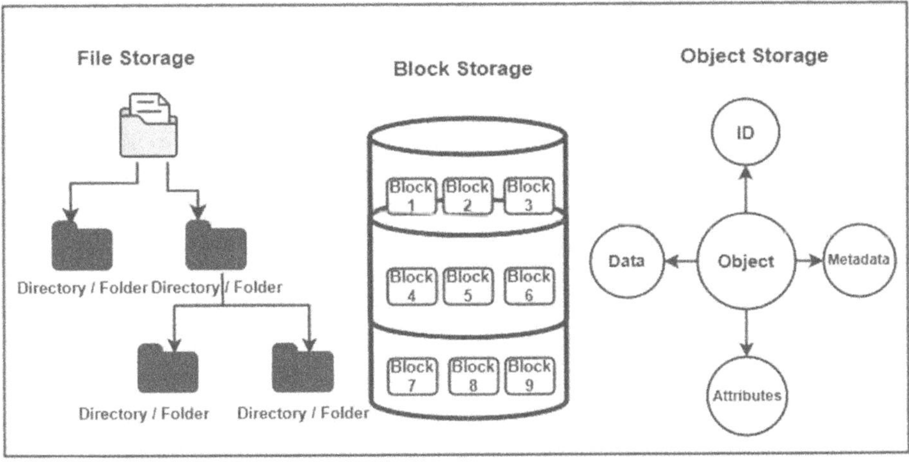

Figure 5.2 Different data storage methods.

the administrators of the object database to focus their attention on managing the content rather than spending their time configuring the storage. This abstraction facilitates simplified data access and identification, enhancing the scalability and usability of the metaverse data infrastructure. By enabling direct programmability and offering expansive namespaces, object storage enhances the flexibility and functionality of metaverse applications, supporting diverse use cases ranging from virtual collaboration to immersive experiences.

5.6 Challenges of Cloud Computing in the Metaverse

Integrating cloud computing with the metaverse offers several advantages, yet it also brings forth several challenges that require attention [16].

5.6.1 Technical Complexity

Metaverse packages require high computational electricity, garage capacity, and network bandwidth to help a big consumer base. Minimizing the latency among the customers and ensuring excessive availability of the server as well as between servers are crucial and call for the setup of disbursed computing architectures. Integrating metaverse packages across one-of-a-kind structures is hard because of the varied technologies involved. Achieving a continuing integration of metaverse software requires overcoming great challenges, consisting of ensuring uniformity in user experience across exceptional gadgets and systems. Some of the other demanding situations faced in this effort are community latency, records synchronization, and computational asset allocation. Developers who can resolve the issues in this domain can supply a cohesive metaverse that is available to users throughout various devices and structures.

5.6.2 Privacy Concerns

As the customers of the metaverse have interacted in various activities, they are at risk of leaking private records, and there are privacy concerns. To ensure the safety and confidentiality of the users' sensitive statistics, there is a need to set up robust protocols. The utilization of facts to get entry to manage methods, encryption standards, and steady authentication mechanisms is crucial in this aspect. Moreover, the metaverse provider carriers want to comply with the statistics protection rules of the governing bodies, including the General Data Protection Regulation (GDPR). Taking safety features and enhancing the device's resilience decreases the danger of malicious attacks being a hit and builds consideration with the customers. Hence, developers must put in force complete privacy measures to mitigate risks and uphold personal privacy, fostering a stable and honest environment within the metaverse [17].

5.6.3 Cybersecurity Risks

As the metaverse ends up increasingly more integrated into the digital panorama, the risks of cyberattacks and threats increase. Cyber threats can vary from direct assaults such as efforts to inject malware and viruses, phishing assaults, data breaches, and social engineering assaults. Hence, there's an absolute necessity for proactive defense mechanisms for the metaverse. In the metaverse, there is excessive opportunity for capability perpetrators to launch malware and malicious software that can exploit vulnerabilities inside client-facet applications. Virtual identities and virtual assets of customers are vulnerable objects for identification theft and users' records, login credentials, or avatars and impersonation. Implementing thorough, rigorous safety features is of utmost significance in protecting consumer records against unauthorized admission and malicious exploitation. Cybersecurity engineers of the metaverse can put into effect encryption protocols, multi-aspect authentication, and intrusion detection structures, which play a pivotal role in securing consumer information. Ensuring secure communication between customers and the servers, encrypting facts at rest and in transit, and enforcing right of entry to control rules are large undertakings. Moreover, steady vigilance and timely response to rising threats are vital. Hence, developers must adopt a proactive stance toward cybersecurity to uphold consumer acceptance and shield the integrity of the metaverse atmosphere [18].

5.6.4 Intellectual Property Issues

In a dynamically developing environment such as the metaverse, the reality of intellectual property disputes may be due to customer makeup or percentage of content that may violate design rights. The creation, sale, or distribution of digital content without proper licensing is a serious concern in the metaverse. This situation creates uncertainty regarding ownership and user rights, and emphasizes the importance of distinct standards for content development and distribution. To avoid legal troubles and guard highbrow property, builders need to deal with those complexities with warning by establishing explicit rules for copyright safety, license agreements, and truthful use provisions. Additionally, approaches for content material attribution and dispute resolution are required to support a creative environment while protecting intellectual assets and rights inside the metaverse.

5.6.5 Regulatory Frameworks

The regulatory framework surrounding the metaverse may be very complicated and evolving with numerous legal guidelines, rules, and regulations on information privateness, protection, and intellectual belongings. Hence, it's of high importance to stick and comply with the rules, policies, recommendations, and legal guidelines of the neighborhood governments in order to function as a metaverse service. Since the rules are constantly changing, there may be a desire to be proactive and adjust the operations of the platform to conform with the policies. Being informed and knowledgeable about the rules is crucial for developers and bosses, with the purpose to navigate the complex criminal landscape and taking preventive measures. Adhering to regulations and requirements together with the GDPR and Central Consumer Protection Authority (CCPA) is of utmost importance, considering the legitimate concerns and user consent views. Therefore, builders should stay informed of the regulatory traits to implement the vital measures and uphold prison and ethical requirements within the metaverse. Robust deep learning fashions may be carried out for content material moderation inside the metaverse. Since the metaverse's contents are considerable, growing, and varied, it also poses the task of creating this sort of system to discover malicious content material being circulated in the platform. Additionally, user-driven rules and content balance must be implemented to complement AI principles and enhance the regulatory system.

5.6.6 Interoperability

The interoperability of the metaverse with existing systems and applications is a challenge to be addressed. There is a lack of universal standards in the metaverse that affects the interoperability with existing websites, apps, and other software. There need to be ways to communicate between different platforms along with collaborative development of the applications and software that can enable a better, interoperable ecosystem. A detailed and well-defined standard can ensure that assets, identities, and functionality can be exchanged between different platforms and also can be integrated with each platform. There is also a challenge of fragmentation between AR and VR components that use different propriety technologies and standards and lead to compatibility issues. Additionally, challenges related to the portability of content, such as 3D models, textures, and virtual assets, between different virtual environments and platforms, can limit user freedom and creativity. The interoperability issues aren't limited to software issues; there can be hardware compatibility issues as well. There may be variations in hardware specifications and capabilities across VR headsets, AR glasses, and other devices that may result in discrepancies in rendering, performance, and user experience.

5.7 Conclusion

The metaverse is a leading and emerging technology in the field of cloud computing and has massive prospects for research and innovation. Some of the important avenues for future research and development include prioritizing the development of an interoperable metaverse, giving rise to seamless interconnectivity across different platforms and devices. Hence, developing application programming interfaces

(APIs) and integration methods that use cloud computing technologies to achieve interoperability and real-time data synchronization is the topmost priority. The usage of AI and ML algorithms and models is promising in improving the user experience in the metaverse. The integration of recommendation systems, task automation, and enhanced communication interfaces can enrich the immersive environment and create more possibilities for collaboration and monetization. The advancements of VR technology open up new possibilities in a wide range of sectors spanning healthcare, education, and entertainment. Real-time rendering is being made possible by cloud computing and gives more high-quality and immersive experiences to the users. Using cloud resources to process and render complex 3D graphics, metaverse applications can deliver higher-quality and more engaging experiences. This is an area of continuing research as we look for more ways to deepen and extend the immersion in VR experiences. The areas of advancement in VR include developing non-audio-visual outputs and improving the way we interact in a virtual environment, in other words, creating a better interface between the user and the virtual environment. This will be an area of longstanding interest and research as more users adopt VR devices and applications. Adopting a decentralized architecture is important for the security and privacy of users of the metaverse. Using decentralized frameworks such as blockchain and NFTs boosts user engagement and confidence in data security and privacy measures. As the metaverse grows, the management of massively scaled data will be done through cloud computing and blockchain. As new trends and technologies in the metaverse emerge, it is important to deliver a user-centric experience and drive research and expansion in that direction.

References

1. Cai, Yang, et al. (2022). Decentralized control of distributed cloud networks with generalized network flows. *IEEE Transactions on Communications 71*(1), 256–268.
2. Cai, Yang, et al. (2023). Joint compute-caching-communication control for online data-intensive service delivery. *IEEE Transactions on Mobile Computing. 23*(5), 4617–4633.
3. Cai, Yang, et al. (2022). Compute-and data-intensive networks: The key to the metaverse. 2022 1st International Conference on 6G Networking (6GNet). IEEE.
4. Shokrnezhad, Masoud, et al. (2024). Towards a dynamic future with adaptable computing and network convergence (ACNC). arXiv preprint arXiv:2403.07573.
5. Chen, Ruxiao, & Guo, Shuaishuai. (2023). Look-ahead task offloading for multi-user mobile augmented reality in edge-cloud computing. arXiv preprint arXiv:2305.19558.
6. Chang, Luyi, et al. (2022). 6G-enabled edge AI for metaverse: Challenges, methods, and future research directions. *Journal of Communications and Information Networks 7*(2), 107–121.
7. Farhoudi, Mohammad, Shokrnezhad, Masoud, & Taleb, Tarik. (2023). QOS-aware service prediction and orchestration in cloud-network integrated beyond 5G. GLOBECOM 2023–2023 IEEE Global Communications Conference. IEEE.
8. Yang, Liang, et al. (2024). Interoperability of the metaverse: A digital ecosystem perspective review. arXiv preprint arXiv:2403.05205.

9. Qian, Liangxin, Liu, Chang, & Zhao, Jun. (2024). User connection and resource allocation optimization in blockchain empowered metaverse over 6G wireless communications. arXiv preprint arXiv:2403.05116.

10. Ismail, Leila, & Buyya, Rajkumar. (2023). Metaverse: A vision, architectural elements, and future directions for scalable and realtime virtual worlds. arXiv preprint arXiv:2308.10559.

11. Balasubramaniam, S, & Kumar, K. S (2022). Fractional feedback political optimizer with prioritization-based charge scheduling in cloud-assisted electric vehicular network. *Ad Hoc & Sensor Wireless Networks*, *52*(3–4), 173–198.

12. Wang, Yitong, & Zhao, Jun. (2022). Mobile edge computing, metaverse, 6G wireless communications, artificial intelligence, and blockchain: Survey and their convergence. 2022 IEEE 8th World Forum on Internet of Things (WF-IoT). IEEE.

13. Balasubramaniam, S, Syed, M. H., More, N. S., & Polepally, V. (2023). Deep learning-based power prediction aware charge scheduling approach in cloud based electric vehicular network. *Engineering Applications of Artificial Intelligence*, *121*, 105869.

14. Choudhury, A., Balasubramaniam, S, Kumar, A. P., & Kumar, S. N. P. (2023). PSSO: Political squirrel search optimizer-driven deep learning for severity level detection and classification of lung cancer. *International Journal of Information Technology & Decision Making*, 1–34. https://doi.org/10.1142/S0219622023500189

15. Subhadra Sarngadharan, A., Narasimhamurthy, R., Sankaramoorthy, B., Singh, S. P., & Singh, C (2022). Hybrid optimization model for design and optimization of microstrip patch antenna. *Transactions on Emerging Telecommunications Technologies*, *33*(12), e4640.

16. Balasubramaniam, S, & Kavitha, V (2013). A survey on data retrieval techniques in cloud computing. *Journal of Convergence Information Technology*, *8*(16), 15.

17. Hariharan, B, Siva, R, Kaliraj, S, Kamaraj, K, & Dinesh, E (2022). Improved beetle swarm optimization algorithm for energy efficient virtual machine consolidation on cloud environment. *Concurrency and Computation: Practice and Experience*, *34*(10), e6828.

18. Paul Raj, D., & Hariharan, B. (2019). WBAT job scheduler: A multi-objective approach for job scheduling problem on cloud computing. *Journal of Circuits, Systems and Computers*, *29*(12), 2050089.

Chapter 6

Blockchain for Healthcare Data Security in the Metaverse: A Comprehensive Study

Rishi Kumar and Hariharasitaraman S

6.1 Introduction

The metaverse, a technological advancement that provides immersive experiences and seamless interactions, is the most sought-after advancement in the healthcare sector. By combining AI and blockchain, we can create a secure and efficient ecosystem that benefits both patients and medical professionals. The integration of artificial intelligence (AI) algorithms and blockchain mechanisms ensures the protection of the medical data generated in the metaverse environment. In the realm of the metaverse, the authors conducted a study of ensuring data protection by integrating such technologies. A metaverse experience is visualized into three verticals, and each vertical can be considered an environment. These verticals include the doctor's arena, the patient's, and the metaverse environment. Doctors or healthcare professionals can access the metaverse through blockchain mode only. The doctors can do online consultations inside the environment as a virtual avatar. The consultation activity involves the generation of data in the form of images, speech, text, videos, and clinical data, which are recorded inside the environment and will be stored on the blockchain. The second component is called the patient's environment, where patients interact with doctors and nurses within the metaverse. The doctor and healthcare professional data are secured in the blockchain; then comes the patients' arena, the patients' data such as consultation, prescriptions, diagnosis data, and follow-up. These all happen in the metaverse and are also stored in a separate entity and stored in the blockchain, which results in privacy and transparency of the data. The data generated in the environment as electronic health records (EHRs) are stored online, which makes the data available and accessible all the time. In addition, the maintenance of EHRs in blockchain mode promises data integrity, immutability, and traceability. The EHR datasets can be used by explainable AI (XAI) models (such as GradCAM and LIME) to analyze data for disease prediction and diagnosis. AI advancements like XAI assist medical professionals with logical reasoning, which ensures trust and transparency in medical decisions and can be used as decision support systems.

The authors' research is concerned with the significance of blockchain in healthcare within the metaverse: Blockchain technology has various benefits in the healthcare industry, especially in the metaverse. With blockchain, patient records remain confidential and tamper-proof, and once stored on the blockchain, data cannot be altered or discarded. This provides enhanced security for sensitive medical information. Additionally, the blockchain ensures transparency in data exchange, allowing patients to track their medical history and treatment journey. The patient data stored in the blockchain can be retrievable and verifiable by the patients, and they can grant or revoke permission for who can access and control their health records from time to time. In the metaverse environment, numerous use cases detail securely maintaining EHR, right from pharmaceutical supplies right from the medicine supplier to patient, to the sharing of data for clinical trials. Despite data maintenance and securing data in blockchain mode, there are shortfalls in such technology, like the scalability of chains for medical records, integration, and coherence with the existing digital data maintenance system and adherence to geographical legal and regulatory guidelines, which vary across the globe in terms of data privacy and data transparency. To mitigate the risks, the healthcare industry has to harden its environment with security protocols, such as data encryption, multifactor authentication (MFA), and firewalls. It is essential to sensitize the cybersecurity measures and various cybersecurity audits and assessments for their frontline staff, who are the primary source of data updating in the environment. In conclusion, while adopting digitalized healthcare has brought immense benefits to the healthcare industry, it has also created new risks. The healthcare industry needs innovations and the adoption of new technologies, such as blockchain, to improve patient care and outcomes, which ensures the privacy and security of patient data.

6.1.1 The Challenge: Data Breaches in Healthcare

IBM's 2023 Data Breach report flagged the healthcare sector, which incurred the highest expenses in data breaches of healthcare records. Any medical data are said to be sensitive data because they contain all information related to patients and doctors, such as personal details and treatment histories, which makes such data the most sought-after data targeted by cybercriminals. The leakage compromises patient privacy but also disrupts healthcare procedures and grinds down public trust. The healthcare sector requires a resilient, robust, and secure system to protect against data breaches and maintain patient privacy.

6.1.2 Blockchain Technology

An exemplar shift called blockchain technology, which is known to the common public through cryptocurrencies like Bitcoin, has exceeded its origins and found applications in cross-domains. Its decentralized storage of data property and data availability make it a suitable choice for securing sensitive data, including healthcare records. The data are stored across a distributed network of nodes where no single entity controls the entire system. Every node maintains a copy of the digital ledger of data storage, which is resilient against attacks or system failures. The data storage in the blockchain is referred to as a transaction, where the users request transactions for data storage or retrieval. The request is logged into the node digital ledger and distributed ledger, which are connected to the distributed nodes. The transaction request is validated using various cryptographic algorithms to ensure the confidentiality, integrity, and authorization of the user, node, and transaction request. Once the verification is done, a new block or storage is created for the user and appended to the distributed network. The process flow is illustrated as a flow chart in Figure 6.1.

6.1.3 Immutability

The blocks listed inside the blockchain hold the transaction of medical data. After the verification of the authenticity of the transaction, the data are appended into the chain of secured blocks, which cannot be deleted or altered by anyone, as they are part of a distributed chain. This immutability property ensures medical data integrity, which prevents unauthorized or accidental alterations of medical records. This property supports the EHR in a tamper-proof system, which ensures that data remain secure and unaltered.

6.1.4 Verifiability and Traceability

All the transactions are verifiable by the user and third-party auditors, which ensures blockchain transparency. All the medical care participants like patients, doctors, other healthcare providers, and regulatory agencies can verify the authenticity of data entries. For example, a patient can verify their treatment history back to its source, which gives them the satisfaction of ensuring accuracy and accountability. The transparency and audibility feature of blockchain technology provides the healthcare sector with a more reliable system to track medical records.

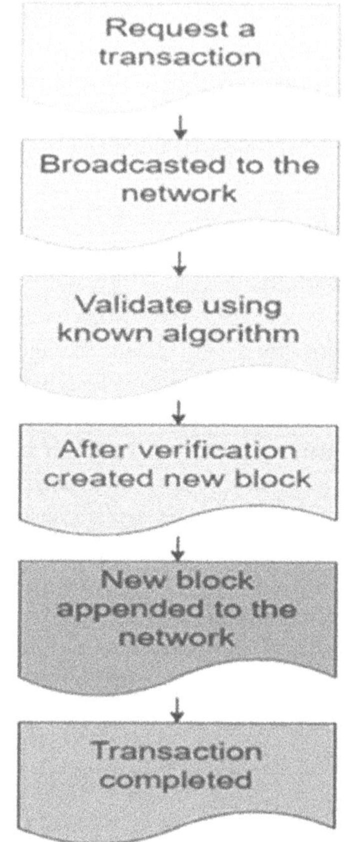

Figure 6.1   Workflow of the blockchain.

6.1.5 Smart Contracts

Blockchain is equipped with a digital ledger for maintaining client data through smart contracts that are self-executing agreements prompted by predefined conditions. In the healthcare sector, such smart contracts can assist in automating processes across allied domains like insurance claims and payments and eliminate administrative overhead and personnel costs. The authors recommend a new advancement called hyper ledger that brings less latency in transacting the data. This advancement is discussed at the end of the chapter as a future avenue.

6.1.6 Compliance and Operational Excellence

To ensure regulatory provider guidelines, healthcare industry providers comply with the standards such as the Health Insurance Portability and Accountability

Act (HIPAA) and Service Organization Control (SOC) version 2. Blockchain supports these regulatory requirements and ensures robust security controls, aligns with audit trails, and delivers data privacy. The presence of such compliance and operational excellence features provides the healthcare industry with a further reliable system to preserve industry standards and regulations.

6.1.7 Case Study: HCA Healthcare Data Breach

The data breach reported by HCA Healthcare, a notable US provider, emphasizes the requirement of data security in the healthcare industry. If there are systems designed with blockchain-based storage, HCA possibly will have minimized the effect of the breach, protecting patient information, and sustained public trust. The case study highlights the need for a secure and robust system to prevent data breaches and maintain public trust. In conclusion, blockchain-based data storage is critical in safeguarding sensitive medical information, emphasizing the need for proactive cybersecurity measures within the healthcare sector. The healthcare sector needs a secure system to protect patient privacy and maintain public trust. Blockchain technology provides a more secure and efficient system that aligns with industry standards and regulations. The chapter is organized into the following sections that describe the rationality of metaverse and blockchain in the context of anticipating security threats in healthcare data. Following this introduction that describes the need for a blockchain with its merits and demerits, in the next section detailed study of the bibliography is conducted to support the chapter's objective and the proposed design of blockchain-enabled healthcare system and future technological avenues in which the system can be improved.

6.2 Related Works

In recent years, the number of ransomware attacks and alternatives has grown extensively. Healthcare facilities have become an important objective for these attacks. Thamer et al. [1] gave a broad overview of ransomware attacks in the healthcare sector, as well as the weaknesses and solutions. Thamer et al. [1] also discussed the classification of cyberattacks in the health sector. The solutions are based on blockchain technology, software-designed networks (SDNs), and machine learning (ML) techniques. Along with this, challenges faced have been highlighted to avoid ransomware attacks. According to Thamer et al. [1], blockchain technology is the best technology to counter ransomware attacks in the healthcare sector. Magnusson et al. [2] described the most common and impactful attack in cybersecurity on healthcare systems. In this paper, all the attacks are mapped according to the CIA triad security principles. Along with this, the authors also suggested mitigation techniques against these attacks. Magnusson et al. [2] note that the most common and impactful attack is a ransomware attack. Such attacks have the capability of stopping the functioning of medical devices, leading to the death of patients. When the CIA mapped these attacks, it concluded that availability is the most important healthcare security goal. Magnusson et al. [2] also suggested some solutions to ransomware attacks. They include investment in security and cybersecurity awareness. Sardi et al. [3] gave an in-depth review of cybersecurity in healthcare organizations. The main theme of the paper was cyber risk. Sardi et al. [3] showed that scientific communities have paid insufficient attention to this topic. The authors highlighted that further studies are needed to investigate the cyber risk, especially in the healthcare sector. Sardi et al. [3] discussed the gaps in the current literature that need to be filled by future research. The authors suggested that scholars may do research on cybersecurity practices in other sectors and apply the same to the healthcare sector.

Safavi et al. [4] discussed how smart homes that aid with smart devices are susceptible to vulnerabilities easily by the hackers. After reviewing this paper, it's very clear that security is a very important aspect of our life as well as new technologies in this modern era. As new technologies are coming daily, there is greater need to secure and protect the privacy of users. Safavi et al. [4] also highlighted the common attacks and threats that healthcare devices and smart homes face. Safavi et al. [4] found that blockchain technology could best mitigate these attacks. Newaz et al. [5] provides an overview of existing security and privacy research in healthcare organizations. The most common trends observed in healthcare device applications are software programmability and wireless network connectivity. These technologies make the applications more vulnerable to cyber threats and attacks. Newaz et al. [5] analyzed different aspects of threats and showed how current solutions can overcome them. These issues should be addressed proactively by the community. This survey had a positive impact on the medical community by highlighting recent attacks and defenses and making the healthcare system more secure and private. The development of networked medical devices in this modern era has transformed healthcare organizations. In the last few years, several networked medical devices have been invented. Along with this, security issues in these devices have also gained the attention of researchers because of the increase in vulnerabilities and cyberattacks. Yaqoob et al. [6] studied more than 100 devices to learn about their security issues leading to cyberattacks. Yaqoob et al. [6] discussed security issues of medical devices along with available solutions for these issues.

Choi et al. [7] showed that hospitals affected by data breaches had significantly higher advertising expenditures. Hospitals affected by data breaches, say 72, were large. The affected hospitals were mostly urban, large, teaching hospitals. This is because large hospitals have multiple entry points through which attackers can attack. The data breach was associated with a 64% increase in annual advertising expenditures. Choi et al. [7] described that breached hospitals had spent more than unbreached hospitals. Choi et al. [7] studied the data breaches that were reported from 2011 to 2014. At that time, ransomware attacks were rare. Choi et al. [7] were the first to study the relationship between hospital expenditures and data breaches. Gabriel et al. [6] said that almost all hospitals are victims of data breaches. The most frequent mode or place of breaches were paper and films. Gabriel et al. [8] used descriptive analysis to characterize the hospitals whether breached or not, to know their breach type and mode of breach. Multivariate logistic regression was then used to analyze the explored hospitals. Results showed a relationship between the data breaches and characteristics of affected hospitals like type and size. There is a need to implement information security systems in this healthcare system. Gabriel et al. [8] also suggested that routine audits by cyber specialists may help healthcare organizations recognize and repair their threats before the breach. The important steps to avoid data breaches are improving access control and securing patient privacy. Pool et al. [9] reviewed and studied the articles on data breaches published between 2009 and 2018. The analysis depicted several direct and indirect causes of protected health information (PHI) breaches. These were mainly unauthorized access, hacking/IT incident, improper disposal, loss, theft, noncompliance, ineffective use, third-party applications, and so on. Pool et al. [9] also discussed the behavioral and operational impacts of PHI breaches. They included privacy concerns, health information sharing, system use, trust, system success, and so on. Most of these causes were not highlighted in any theoretical model of the sample in this paper. The causes and impacts discussed by Pool et al. [9] can help healthcare organizations to make their system more secure.

Smart healthcare systems based on the Internet of Things (IoT) have increased the use of wearable and mobile devices. Modern-day smart healthcare systems based on IoT are vulnerable to security threats. This has increased health data sharing for accurate and improved diagnosis. To overcome these security issues, it is important to know security requirements. IoT-based smart healthcare devices cannot be secured with traditional security methods. Tariq et al. [10] discussed the requirements to make IoT-based healthcare systems more secure. They showed how the blockchain can solve security issues in a scalable, efficient manner. Along with this, Tariq et al. [10] also discussed the challenges faced by blockchain implementation in healthcare infrastructure. H¨olbl et al. [11] described the current trends and research of blockchain technology in the health sector. H¨olbl et al. [11] studied 33 publications, then analyzed them and also searched nine databases for papers published between 2008 and 2019. H¨olbl et al. [11] discussed three questions related to the blockchain in healthcare. Firstly, to what extent the blockchain is established in healthcare and its future. Second, what the current research trends or areas are for the use of blockchain in healthcare. Third, what are the elements of blockchain that are currently in use in healthcare systems? H¨olbl et al. [11] showed that the most common platforms were Ethereum and Hyperledger Fabric (both support smart contracts). They also indicated that the implementation of the blockchain is increasing in the health sector. Currently, it is used for mostly data sharing, access control, and health records. Antwi et al. [12] identified a lot of problems or threats have been faced in the health sector. They discussed how the blockchain can be a solution to these threats. Antwi et al. [12] proposed a solution based on Hyperledger Fabric along with its use case in healthcare domain. They created testing scenarios of Hyperledger Fabric to understand its use case for implementation in healthcare systems. They showed how the blockchain is better than cloud computing. The blockchain-based solution follows the security criteria of privacy, data confidentiality, and access control. Antwi et al. [12] contributed to defining the criteria for implementing secure blockchain-based health applications. Mayer et al. [13] discussed the challenges, issues, and benefits of applying blockchain technology in the healthcare sector. They also highlighted the challenges, current data types, open questions, objectives, related standards, and architectures of blockchain and EHR. After the study of the paper, it can be said that blockchain can be the solution for most security threats in the healthcare sector. Although the blockchain seems to be promising, more research and experiments are needed to ensure that a secure system is implemented before using the blockchain on a large scale, because of the value of patient data. The research questions answered by Mayer et al. [13] may help the future researcher while exploring this topic.

The healthcare sector must invest in cybersecurity response plans for the provision of safe, reliable, and secure operations. Jalali et al. [14] reviewed 13 articles on the topic "Cybersecurity responses recommendations." Then they collected information such as research methodologies, their findings, and implications. Lastly, they combined the recommendations into a framework of "Eight Aggregated Response Strategies" called EARS that come under managerial and technological categories. Jalali et al. [14] also compared their EARS model to the preexisting model for cybersecurity responses. By viewing their comparison, it can be said that the EARS model is better than the preexisting models. Argaw et al. [15] used the PRISMA methodology for writing the paper. The paper was mapped using the six important domains of research. They described all of these in depth. These domains are also an important basis for research in the future. The paper highlights that a total of 97 articles were studied over the past two years and concluded that there are not enough papers. Argaw et al. [15] showed that there was an increase in interest in the research field and the production of articles. Argaw et al. [15] highlighted the areas of research in cybersecurity of medical systems that have been neglected, like cloud storage security, usage of USB ports, and identity and access management. Tervoort et al. [16] found 18 studies describing the risks due to legacy software in healthcare devices. Tervoort et al. [16] discussed solutions that were mainly based on intrusion detection and encrypted communication tunnels. They highlighted different application areas and attack models. Solutions to be used depend upon the type of device to be protected. Technical comprehensive analysis of different solutions is not provided in the paper. The intrusion detection solutions have not been experimentally tested independently. Future research is needed to study the effectiveness of these solutions. The security solution discussed by Tervoort et al. [16] in this paper will help the healthcare organization improve its security.

Razaque et al. [17] collected and analyzed several articles and summarized the solutions of different attacks along with their advantages and disadvantages. For example, cross-site scripting (XSS) attacks can be solved by mathematical methods. More importantly, for data storage assurance, the authors discuss some cybersecurity architectures in the medical field from the existing papers. Razaque et al. [17] also discussed the benefits and deficiencies of cybersecurity architectures in terms of factors like information confidentiality, large scale, low cost, system generality, and transmission efficiency to perform an in-depth analysis of different architectures and find the best architecture. The best architectures for health information system (HIS), cross site scripting (XXS), and analog front end (AFE) have been presented. The COVID-19 period has been very challenging for healthcare information systems. As discussed in the paper, there were multiple attacks on the health sector. He et al. [18] reviewed the security issues and their solutions in the healthcare sector. He et al. [18] also highlighted cybersecurity areas for improvement in the health sector. They identified the main causes of security attacks that have impacted the healthcare sector. They were mainly phishing, distributed denial of service (DDoS), ransomware, and malware. Inadequate endpoint devices, lack of security awareness, and investment in security were the main challenges for cybersecurity in the healthcare sector. He et al. [18] suggested that organizations should plan for long-term cybersecurity resources to deal with this fast-changing situation. Gioulekas et al. [19] showed that healthcare organizations should have security awareness programs along with training procedures. When the findings were presented to the institution's management, reactive and proactive measures for cybersecurity were taken. A certain budget was decided to upgrade or procure cybersecurity systems and software for health institutions. Special workshops were conducted with the support of the European Union Agency for Cybersecurity (ENISA) for information and communications technology (ICT) staff. Along with this awareness, campaigns about antisocial engineering and antiphishing were regularly held for non-ICT employees. In the future, Gioulekas et al. [19] aim to research this topic again for updated cybersecurity strategies and measures and reperform evaluation. The Indian healthcare sector is growing slowly because of increasing expenditure by private and public investors and less usage of capital. Churi et al. [20] discussed various technologies in the healthcare system in India. Along with this, they also described the privacy issues in India. The major causes of these security issues in the healthcare sector are the doctor–patient relationship, improper security policies, constitutional and political issues, and lack of investment in the health sector in India. In the coming times, more attention is needed to understand the privacy issues for healthcare professionals and the government. Churi et al. [20] listed all the major causes of security issues that need to be solved as fast as possible. Hariharasitaraman et al. [21] examined the topic of a Smart Framework for Smart Services based on the blockchain. They investigated the integration of cyber-physical systems (CPS) in the tourism and travel industry. CPSs are capable of self-organizing and reconfiguring systems and devices in real time to respond to changing environments. The study proposes a new blockchain-based framework that aims to create a smart tourism ecosystem designed to meet the changing preferences and needs of tourists. The proposed framework's key idea is to improve the data security of smart tourism services by implementing blockchain-based data security mechanisms.

6.3 Methodology

6.3.1 Background

Khalid et al. [22] designed an access and control mechanism in heterogeneous environment using lightweight IoT devices, which is designed by taking the merits of fog computing and public blockchain technology for demonstrating its usage.

6.3.1.1 Definition and Types of Blockchain

Peer-to-peer decentralized distributed ledger technology that makes immutable and transparent records is blockchain. It can bring down fraud and cybercrimes in a ductile way. It creates a chain of content, i.e., timestamped and unchangeable, using public key cryptography. It can make the system more secure and private by making patients stand at the center of the healthcare system. Types of blockchain depend upon managing data, availability, and actions to be performed. They are public permission less, consortium, and private [23].

6.3.1.2 Working Mechanism and Flowchart of Blockchain

The transaction is requested by a node that wants to place a record in the network. In the next stage, the request is broadcast to the network. Then validation is done using the predefined algorithm of the network. If the validation is successful, the new block is permanently appended to the network. Transaction is then completed, and this record can never be deleted since it's immutable. The diagrammatic representation is shown in Figure 6.1.

6.3.1.3 Software and Tools Available to Implement

Ethereum
Hyperledger Fabric
Solidity
R3 Corda
Multichain
Ripple
Open chain

6.3.1.4 Role of Blockchain in the Healthcare Sector

Healthcare is one of the domains where the blockchain is very important. Safe and secure storage of the records of patients is very necessary. Since the data are very sensitive, attackers keep an eye on it. Currently, these records depend on third-party sources. Although they are trusted, it is important to have a more secure way to store the data. The blockchain benefits the industry in many ways, for example, medical billing, transferring medical records, supporting medicine prescriptions, supply chain management, and interoperability. It makes the data more secure by giving control to patients. Implementing blockchain technology enables patients and medical officers to connect and share data over the Internet safely without any privacy concerns [24].

6.3.2 Problem Statement

Cyberattacks frequently happen in healthcare organizations. Most of these attacks or breaches are because of phishing, ransomware, malware viruses, etc. Currently, blockchain is said to be the most promising technique to make the system secure. Many researchers have proved with their research that blockchain is far better than other traditional techniques. Most of the healthcare system is dependent upon one party for managing the information that is vulnerable to a single point of failure. Since the nature of blockchain is distributive, it can vanquish the attacks. It provides the record of ownership of data and its authenticity [25]. Forty percent of healthcare executives see blockchain as one of the top priorities in the healthcare sector. The use of blockchain in the healthcare sector will save $100−150 billion per year by 2025 by cutting down breach-related costs, IT costs, and operational costs and limiting fraud [26]. A detailed study on different cyberattacks and their solutions was conducted and presented in Table 6.1. Researchers in [22, 24] presented a piece of detailed information about the types of cyberattacks in healthcare and preexisting techniques to mitigate them. The researchers in [21–23] proposed blockchain-based techniques to mitigate these cyberattacks in the healthcare sector. In [25, 26], researchers identified major solutions for these attacks. In [14], researchers proposed an EARS framework for incident response. They compared and proved their framework to be better than the other existing ones. Many researchers have touched upon this issue with different solutions but haven't offered a precise one. Hence, there is scope for improvement. The main contribution of this survey is to (i) identify the current models and approaches of blockchain in healthcare; (ii) identify the extent to which these techniques are successful; (iii) propose the Hyperledger technology; and (iv) identify the advantages of Hyperledger technology over other methods.

Table 6.1 Comparison Table of Various Blockchain Parameters for the Use Case Block with Healthcare, Metaverse Security

Author, Year	Key Contribution	P1	P2	P3	P4	P5	P6	P7	P8
Noor, Thamer et al. 2021	Pointed out that blockchain can be the best technique to protect health data	Yes	No	No	Yes	No	No	Yes	No
Jalali et al. 2019	Proposed EARS framework for cybersecurity response	No	Yes	No	No	No	No	No	No
Safavi et al. 2018	Proposed blockchain-based solutions for future homes and healthcare based on an ideal framework	No	No	No	No	No	No	Yes	Yes
Razaque et al. 2019	Presented the vulnerabilities, attacks, and solutions of healthcare cybersecurity	No	No	No	Yes	No	No	Yes	No
Newaz et al. 2021	Pointed out existing attacks, impacts, and existing solutions in the healthcare industry	No	No	No	Yes	No	No	No	Yes
Yaqoob et al. 2019	Presented policy weaknesses and existing solutions to mitigate attacks on healthcare	No	No	No	Yes	Yes	No	No	No
He et al. 2021	Identified 9 major challenges and 11 solutions in healthcare cybersecurity	Yes	Yes	Yes	No	Yes	No	No	Yes

(Continued)

Table 6.1 (Continued) **Comparison Table of Various Blockchain Parameters for the Use Case Block with Healthcare, Metaverse Security**

Author, Year	Key Contribution	P1	P2	P3	P4	P5	P6	P7	P8
Gioulekas et al. 2022	Assisted in understanding the countermeasures already applied in healthcare, enhancing cybersecurity defense	Yes	No	Yes	No	No	No	No	No
Tariq et al. 2020	Analyzed smart healthcare systems security requirements and proposed blockchain as a solution	No	No	No	Yes	No	No	Yes	Yes
Churi et al. 2021	Listed 14 main privacy issues of the Indian healthcare system	No	No	Yes	No	Yes	Yes	Yes	No
Choi et al. 2019	Depicts the relationship between data breaches and hospital advertising expenditures	No	No	No	No	No	Yes	No	No
Gabriel et al. 2018	Hospitals accounted for approximately 1/3 of all data breaches. Paper and films were the most frequent mode of data breaches	No	No	Yes	No	No	Yes	No	No
Magnusson et al. 2019	Identified the most common cyberattacks, solutions in healthcare	No	No	No	Yes	No	No	No	Yes
Pool et al. 2019	Pointed out the causes and impacts of PHI breaches	Yes	No	No	No	No	Yes	No	No

(Continued)

Table 6.1 *(Continued)* **Comparison Table of Various Blockchain Parameters for the Use Case Block with Healthcare, Metaverse Security**

Author, Year	Key Contribution	P1	P2	P3	P4	P5	P6	P7	P8
Hölbl et al. 2018	Blockchain elements can be implemented for securing EHRs	No	No	No	No	No	No	Yes	No
Antwi et al. 2021	Design and implementation of Hyperledger Fabric to secure healthcare systems	No	No	No	No	No	No	Yes	No
Sardi et al. 2020	Identified knowledge gaps in existing literature for studying cyber risks	Yes	Yes	Yes	No	No	No	No	No
Argaw et al. 2019	Pointed out 6 main research domains in healthcare cybersecurity	Yes	No	Yes	Yes	No	No	Yes	No
Tervoort et al. 2020	Provided solutions based on intrusion detection systems (IDS) and tunneling insecure wireless communications	No	No	No	Yes	No	No	No	No
Mayer et al. 2020	Pointed existing blockchain-based solutions for securing EHRs	No	No	No	Yes	No	No	Yes	Yes

(Continued)

Table 6.1 *(Continued)* Comparison Table of Various Blockchain Parameters for the Use Case Block with Healthcare, Metaverse Security

Author, Year	Key Contribution	P1	P2	P3	P4	P5	P6	P7	P8
Mehdi Letafati et al. 2023	– Digital healthcare in the metaverse demands a thorough study of privacy and security aspects, including data collection and communication security, privacy threats related to AI/ML algorithms, human-centric privacy during social interactions among patients, and distributed differential privacy systems for metaverse healthcare	Yes	No	Yes	Yes	No	No	Yes	No
Hulsen et al. 2023	– Use cases for metaverse in healthcare, including virtual scanning, data sharing, regulatory science, and medical intervention – Discussion of ecosystem issues, including privacy, security, and disparity	Yes	No	Yes	Yes	No	No	Yes	No

Notes: P1 = Lack of security awareness, P2 = lack of coordinated incident response strategy, P3 = lack of budget, technology, infrastructure, P4 = security attacks, P5 = legal policy weakness, P6 = data breaches, P7 = hospital information systems (EHR), P8 = security and privacy goals.

6.3.3 Discussion of Existing Solutions

6.3.3.1 Threats to the Healthcare System

Before moving to the solutions, we need to see the attacks on the healthcare system. In this section, we summarize the most common vulnerabilities and attacks on healthcare.

Ransomware: In ransomware attacks [1, 5], an encrypted file is deleted or stored by already keeping the key to decrypt that file. When victims run this program, it locks all their files and data, and then they are asked to pay a huge amount of money to decrypt those files. The most common forms of ransomware attacks are email phishing, remote desktop protocol, water hole attacks, exploit kits, removable media and USB, installation of pirated software, and botnets.

Malware [6–8]: Malware-infected medical equipment might deviate from its intended functions and slow down or shut down. Patients could not obtain any medical treatments from the attacked facility as a result. X-ray machines and lab equipment made by trusted firms have been among the impacted products. *Passive attacks* [9, 10]: In these attacks, the attackers observe or monitor the contents of messages, but they don't alter them or impact the system resources. This attack is mostly targeted at the privacy of smart homes. Some common passive attacks on the healthcare system are eavesdropping attacks and traffic analysis.

Active attacks [14, 16, 18, 23]: In this attack, the attacker alters the data in the smart home's network. Among such attacks, the most common are masquerade attacks, interception attacks, replay attacks, message modification attacks, malicious codes, denial-of-service attacks, and session-stealing attacks. *Hardware attacks* [16]: An attacker may be aware of or get access to the device's internal hardware architecture and install hardware Trojans (HTs) during chip production, which might seriously impair medical equipment by causing data corruption. *Data breaches* [4–6]: Data breaches in healthcare systems reveal patients' confidential data for public use. They include hacking protected healthcare information, improper disposal, unauthorized access/disclosure, and theft loss.

6.3.3.2 Blockchain as a Solution

Blockchain has led to the development of the healthcare sector. It's reformulating data modeling in healthcare applications. Blockchain gathers data from different sources and keeps their records in a transaction audit log, which ensures data accountability, availability, and transparency. Maintenance of medical records has become easier because of the chain-like structure of blockchain. They are stored in the form of a linked list where each node stores the timestamp and links to the previous one. The general architecture used for integrating blockchain in the healthcare systems to make them secure is represented in Figure 6.2.

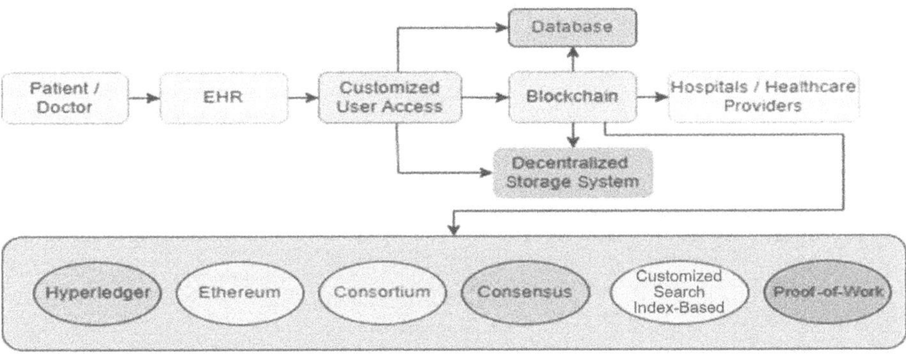

Figure 6.2   Architecture of the blockchain.

The steps include the following. (1) In hospitals, when a patient comes they are registered on the counter. Their details, like name, age sex, and previous medical issues, are fed into the local database. The data also include medical tests, medicines prescribed, nursing care, etc. (2) From the given data, an EHR is generated. (3) The owner of the EHR is the patient. The patient has full control over with whom the patient wants to share the data. (4) Now blockchain comes into process. It stores all the data securely in a decentralized storage system using different algorithms, technology, and platforms. Data are also stored in the local database to ensure that records can be updated whenever required before pushing to decentralized storage. (5) Healthcare practitioners have access to the distributed ledger to provide medical aid to patients by accessing their data. EHR can be safely and securely transferred to anyone using blockchain technology. Different blockchain technologies have been used to date for securing EHRs. Each has merits and demerits. Important ones are listed in Table 6.1.

The relationship between medical practitioner–patient and EHR has been represented through the unified modeling language (UML) diagram shown in Figure 6.3. Data can be accessed only by specific persons, and others will not have any access. Persons who can access the data include the admin, patient, member, and doctor. The admin is the one who has full access to the data stored in the blockchain for all the patients. EHR is generated for the patient, and the doctor is assigned to him for medical treatment. Now the patient and the doctor have access to the data, but another person, Member, cannot view the data. Even the doctor cannot view the data of another patient if assigned to that patient.

6.3.3.3 Evaluation Metrics

The most commonly used evaluation criteria are discussed in the following list. The researchers evaluated the blockchain-based solution for cyberattacks based on these

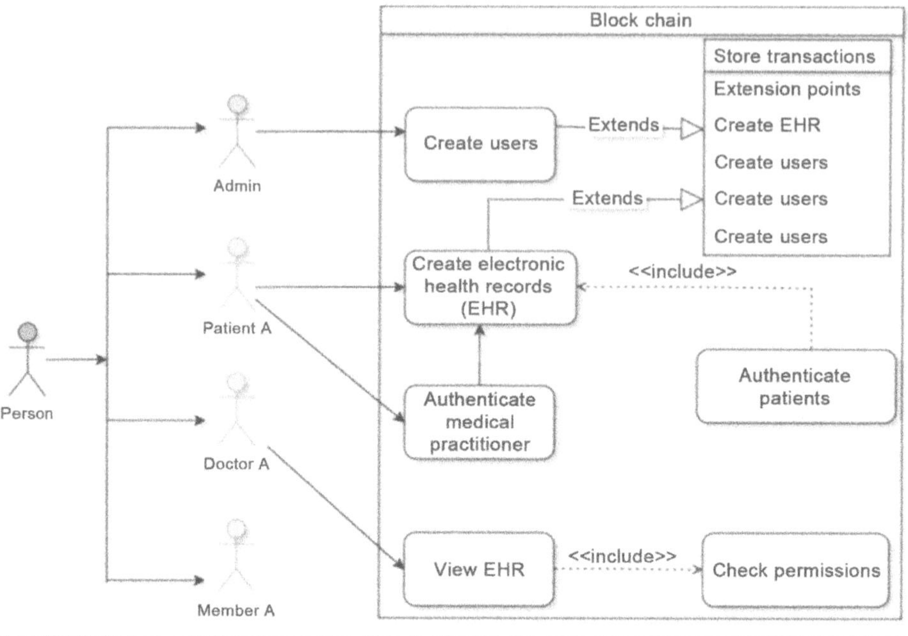

Figure 6.3   UML diagram showing the basic scenario of the connection.

criteria. These criteria help us to decide whether a solution should be implemented or not. They include the following:

Confidentiality: Healthcare data are safely stored, and unauthorized users cannot access that data. In the current era of technology, all the devices are connected, so it is necessary to ensure that the data cannot be altered by any unauthorized users.

Integrity: Healthcare data gathered from different sources or distributed to different sources cannot be changed by anyone, and the data transfer should be correct.

Availability: Ensure that the patient/doctor does not wait for healthcare data to do the treatment.

Ownership: It is important that the patient has the authority to decide with whom to share their data.

Secure data transit: This ensures that the records in transit cannot be accessed or altered by the nemesis.

Anonymity: This ensures secrecy of identification details of patients from unauthorized people.

Auditing: A log of all the modifications or additions in healthcare data should be maintained.

Performance: The volume of data moving from one point to another should always be as fast as possible.

Scalability: Healthcare records should be able to respond quickly in case of periodic fluctuations.

6.4 Hyperledger Fabric–Based Blockchain Solutions

We can look forward to a platform called Hyperledger Fabric. The features of this platform are privacy, scalability, efficient transaction, easy and secure access to data, less turnaround time for storing and sharing EHR over the network, better decision-making, and less capital required to implement. To create a peer-to-peer consortium network, multiple hospitals are connected. Based on agreement among the involved stakeholders, authorization to join the fabric network is decided. The byzantine fault-tolerant consensus protocol is used by the fabric for ordering and execution of transactions to the ledger.

6.4.1 Architecture Diagram

Figure 6.4 represents the architecture of the Hyperledger Fabric–based blockchain solution. Choosing a private permissioned consortium blockchain that is Hyperledger enabled and runs on the Hyperledger Fabric platform. The health authority uses the membership service (MSP) component of the Fabric and certificate issuing authorities (CAs) to identify and register each of the participating healthcare stakeholders and their end users. A membership service that establishes rules and regulations by which various stakeholders (identities) are governed, authenticated, validated, and verified to be part of the network and allowed to access the EHR systems is provided by the fabric to establish a trusted environment

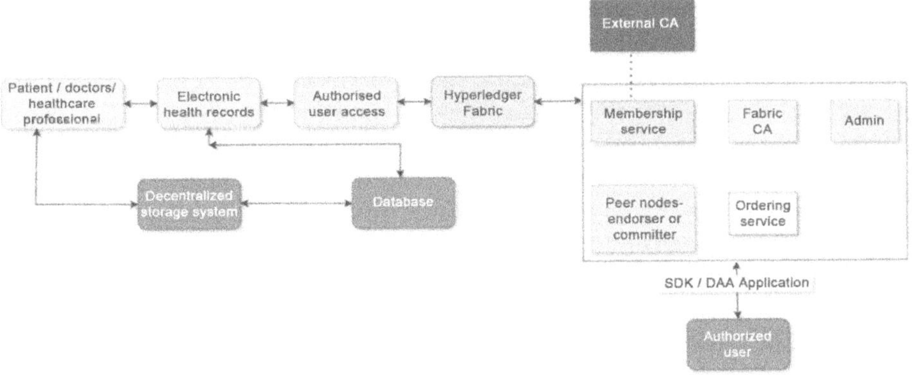

Figure 6.4   Hyperledger Fabric–based blockchain solution.

between untrusted participants. Each peer node in the fabric network has the potential to be an endorser or committer. Additionally, it has a part known as Borderers that provides an ordering service. This service collects endorsed transactions from the patient, arranges them into blocks with the ordering peers' cryptographic signatures, and then broadcasts these blocks to the committed peers on the blockchain network for endorsement policy validation [7].

6.4.2 How It Will Be Better than Other Platforms

The uniqueness of the Hyperledger Fabric compares favorably to other distributed ledger-based technologies:

- Blockchain networks offer a privately permissioned and modular architecture for carrying out various transactions.
- Consensus can be achieved among the stakeholders because of flexibility and a pluggable support model.
- While performing transactions, the latency is less in comparison to other platforms.
- By employing channels, it offers a method that enables transaction integrity and privacy.
- Privacy and secrecy are more important because different member organizations can communicate through channels created.
- Smart contracts can be created using various programming frameworks like JS, Java, and Go.

6.5 Conclusion

The authors did a comprehensive study on various cybersecurity parameters. They recommend blockchain technology–enabled software systems for the healthcare industry with the case study of healthcare data generated through a metaverse environment. Additionally, the cryptographic algorithms inherent in the blockchain ensure data security through verifiability, traceability, and immutability of records. The chapter summarizes the current solutions available to mitigate these attacks. Through the in-depth analysis done in this chapter, we can see that blockchain technology is most capable of making systems secure from these attacks. To achieve this result, 20 survey papers based on "cyberattacks on healthcare" or "solutions for healthcare cyberattacks" were studied in detail as presented in Table 6.1. The blockchain can process and manage sensitive data securely. Since blockchain is a new technology, we need more research work on blockchain technology. By exploring this technology more, we can unlock the abilities of blockchain to make the healthcare system more secure.

References

1. Thamer, N., & Alubady, R. (2021). A survey of ransomware attacks for healthcare systems: Risks, challenges, solutions, and opportunity of research. In *2021 1st Babylon International Conference on Information Technology and Science (BICITS)*, pp. 210–216. IEEE.
2. Magnusson, J., & Sloof, J. (n.d.). A literature survey on cyber attacks in healthcare. Retrieved from https://hex.cse.kau.se/~jonamagn102/DVAD03_Sloof_Magnusson.pdf.
3. Sardi, A., Rizzi, A., Sorano, E., & Guerrieri, A. (2020). Cyber risk in health facilities: A systematic literature review. *Sustainability*, 12, 7002, 1–17.
4. Safavi, S., Meer, A. M., Melanie, E. K. J., & Shukur, Z. (2018). Cyber vulnerabilities on smart healthcare, review and solutions. In *2018 Cyber Resilience Conference (CRC)*, pp. 1–5. IEEE.
5. Newaz, A. I., Sikder, A. K., Rahman, M. A., & Uluagac, A. S. (2021). A survey on security and privacy issues in modern healthcare systems: Attacks and defenses. *ACM Transactions on Computing for Healthcare*, 2(3), 1–44.
6. Yaqoob, T., Abbas, H., & Atiquzzaman, M. (2019). Security vulnerabilities, attacks, countermeasures, and regulations of networked medical devices – a review. *IEEE Communications Surveys & Tutorials*, 21(4), 3723–3768.
7. Choi, S. J., & Johnson, M. E. (2019). Understanding the relationship between data breaches and hospital advertising expenditures. *American Journal of Managed Care*, 25(1), e14–e20.
8. Gabriel, M. H., Noblin, A., Rutherford, A., Walden, A., & Cortelyou-Ward, K. (2018). Data breach locations, types, and associated characteristics among US hospitals. *American Journal of Managed Care*, 24(2), 78–84.
9. Pool, J. K., Akhlaghpour, S., Fatehi, F., & Burton-Jones, A. (2019). Causes and impacts of personal health information (PHI) breaches: A scoping review and thematic analysis. In *Twenty-Third Pacific Asia Conference on Information Systems, China, July 2019*, Available at SSRN: https://ssrn.com/abstract=3584865 or http://dx.doi.org/10.2139/ssrn.3584865.
10. Tariq, N., Qamar, A., Asim, M., & Khan, F. A. (2020). Blockchain and smart healthcare security: A survey. *Procedia Computer Science*, 175, 615–620.
11. Hölbl, M., Kompara, M., Kamišalić, A., & Nemec Zlatolas, L. (2018). A systematic review of the use of blockchain in healthcare. *Symmetry*, 10(10), 470.
12. Antwi, M., Adnane, A., Ahmad, F., Hussain, R., ur Rehman, M. H., & Kerrache, C. A. (2021). The case of Hyperledger Fabric as a blockchain solution for healthcare applications. *Blockchain: Research and Applications*, 2(1), 100012.
13. Mayer, A. H., da Costa, C. A., & Righi, R. D. R. (2020). Electronic health records in a blockchain: A systematic review. *Health Informatics Journal*, 26(2), 1273–1288.
14. Jalali, M. S., Russell, B., Razak, S., & Gordon, W. J. (2019). Ears to cyber incidents in health care. *Journal of the American Medical Informatics Association*, 26(1), 81–90.
15. Argaw, S. T., Bempong, N.-E., Eshaya-Chauvin, B., & Flahault, A. (2019). The state of research on cyberattacks against hospitals and available best practice recommendations: A scoping review. *BMC Medical Informatics and Decision Making*, 19(1), 1–11.
16. Tervoort, J. K., De Oliveira, M. T., Pieters, W., Van Gelder, P., Olabarriaga, S. D., & Marquering, H. (2020). Solutions for mitigating cybersecurity risks caused by legacy software in medical devices: A scoping review. *IEEE Access*, 8, 84352–84361.

17. Razaque, A., Amsaad, F., Khan, M. J., Hariri, S., Chen, S., Siting, C., & Ji, X. (2019). Survey: Cybersecurity vulnerabilities, attacks and solutions in the medical domain. *IEEE Access, 7,* 168774–168797.

18. He, Y., Aliyu, A., Evans, M., & Luo, C., et al. (2021). Health care cybersecurity challenges and solutions under the climate of COVID-19: Scoping review. *Journal of Medical Internet Research,* 23(4), e21747.

19. Gioulekas, F., Stamatiadis, E., Tzikas, A., Gounaris, K., Georgiadou, A., Michalitsi-Psarrou, A., & Marin, S. (2022). A cybersecurity culture survey targeting healthcare critical infrastructures. *Healthcare, 10,* 327.

20. Churi, P., Pawar, A., & Moreno-Guerrero, A.-J. (2021). A comprehensive survey on data utility and privacy: Taking Indian healthcare system as a potential case study. *Inventions,* 6(3), 45.

21. Hariharasitaraman, S., Yadav, R., & Agrawal, P. (2023). Some insights of cyber-physical systems in the context of the tourism and travel industry: A blockchain-based smart framework for smart services. In Thangavel Murugan and Nirmala E. (eds.), *Handbook of Research on Data Science and Cybersecurity Innovations in Industry 4.0 Technologies.* 620. Hershey, PA: IGI Global.

22. Khalid, U., Asim, M., Baker, T., Hung, P. C., Tariq, M. A., & Rafferty, L. (2020). A decentralized lightweight blockchain-based authentication mechanism for IoT systems. *Cluster Computing, 23*(3), 2067–2087.

23. Arsene, C. (2021). The global blockchain in healthcare report: The 2021 ultimate guide for every executive. healthcareweekly.com, https://healthcareweekly.com/blockchain-in-healthcare-guide/ Accessed 10 Nov 2023.

24. Liang, X., Shetty, S. S., Tosh, D., Njilla, L., Kamhoua, C. A., & Kwiat, K. (2019). Provchain: Blockchain-based cloud data provenance. In S. Shetty, C. Kamhoua, and L. Njilla (eds.), *Blockchain for Distributed Systems Security,* 69. *Wiley-IEEE Press* https://doi.org/10.1002/9781119519621.ch4

25. Letafati, M., & Otoum, S. (2023). Digital healthcare in the metaverse: Insights into privacy and security. *IEEE Consumer Electronics Magazine.* http://dx.doi.org/10.48550/arXiv.2308.04438

26. Hulsen, T. (2023). Applications of the metaverse in medicine and healthcare. *Advances in Laboratory Medicine/Avances en Medicina de Laboratorio,* 5(2), 159–165. https://doi.org/10.1515/almed-2023-0124

Chapter 7

MetaHealth: Transforming Healthcare through AI Integration

Ashwini A, Kavitha V, Balasubramaniam S, and Seifedine Kadry

7.1 Introduction to MetaHealth

Amid a period that includes swift technology progress and the growing complication of healthcare specifications, MetaHealth rises as a ray of hope and inspiration. By redefining the surroundings of medical services through the broad possibilities of the metaverse and the revolutionary potential of artificial intelligence (AI), MetaHealth offers an abrupt shift in the method of delivery of healthcare. Fundamentally, MetaHealth promises to surpass the constraints of conventional healthcare systems by integrating AI-driven solutions with virtual environments in a seamless manner, so offering consumers global access to individualized, cost-effective, and customized treatment [1]. To provide greater insights on the large quantities of the patient data, MetaHealth with the AI algorithm can be used effectively. MetaHealth helps nurses and doctors in providing efficient chances for effective diagnosis. Thus the modes of continuous tracking and remote counseling with virtual effect helps in utilization of immersive qualities in virtual reality for the user experience. This helps in providing assistance in executing healthcare professionals. The virtual environment combined with the intelligence tracking provides medical diagnosis. This helps in treating the diagnosed condition efficiently with high accuracy, supporting an approach that focuses on the individual patient for healthcare applications.

DOI: 10.1201/9781003491668-7

Furthermore, inclusion and equality provide accurate healthcare detection. This helps in overcoming obstacles geographically thus providing a guaranteed option to everyone for high-quality healthcare. MetaHealth democratizes virtual healthcare, providing unprecedented control in creating wellness through health monitoring through the amalgamation of AI and a virtual interface. This transformational potential of MetaHealth gives the prominent transformation on healthcare globally, from its traditional technological framework [2]. Figure 7.1 shows various roles in the MetaHealth framework. The MetaHealth structure helps identify rare ailments. By using the infinite possibilities of the virtual world to deliver top-notch healthcare to a wide spectrum of global populations, MetaHealth transcends territorial boundaries. Machine learning (ML) and deep learning (DL), two subfields of AI, have become the de facto norm in identifying medical conditions and are used in schools, agriculture, robotics, transportation, and other industries.

MetaHealth has, however, attracted little study up to this point, and it remains difficult to identify and foresee unusual illnesses simply because of the lack of data. There are several uses for the metaverse in therapeutic settings. Through MetaHealth's AI integrating, which leverages ML techniques to generate accurate forecasts and useful information, large-scale patient data may be merged. Through immersive virtual environments that allow for remote discussions, continuous tracking, and comprehensive simulations for procedural assistance and medical

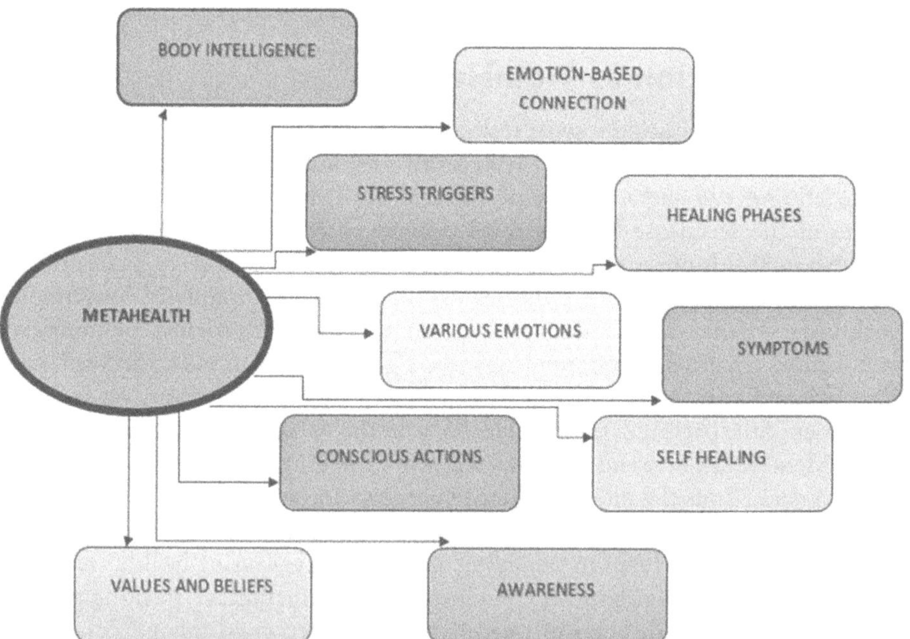

Figure 7.1 MetaHealth roles in healthcare applications.

training, patients as well as healthcare providers engage in previously unheard-of ways. As such, researchers, scholars, and medical professionals need to give serious thought to this important topic. Interoperability in digital healthcare is necessary. The use of blockchain technology and token economies will enable the safe and profitable sharing of intellectual property and data. By allowing medical personnel to display medical pictures, such as CT (digitized scanner) scans, immediately from patients, coordinating with their physical characteristics even while they are moving, augmented reality (AR) when used alongside radiography can provide better insights into interior anatomy. With the use of AR, physicians may interact internationally and take advantage of possibilities to alleviate the shortage of health personnel. In order to pay the society as a whole and specialists for their work to promote health, MetaHealth establishes a completely new economy and source of revenue.

7.2 AI in Healthcare

In the healthcare sector, AI has fixed an important place in growing as most prominent force to all healthcare providers, enabling determination of proper cures. This method of embedding AI with healthcare helps in providing proper care for the customers, maximizing the range of productivity, and increasing patient outcome ranges. Different volumes of volumetric data, pattern identification, and predictions are made possible with the help of AI [3]. AI is accurate in analyzing patterns, like MRI, CT, and X-rays. Doctors can easily identify various anomalies, making diagnosis easier. The number of mistakes related to the missing diagnosis ranges is reduced, thus accelerating the diagnosis process.

AI-driven forecasting systems provide a broader way in identifying healthcare conditions. They help in recognizing people a risk of ailments and giving proper treatment suggestions for the entire treatment. This provides precise management and treatment, thus evaluating the patient data, including health history, lifestyle variables, and gene information [4]. This is a long-term approach that may yield better results for the patients with the lowest possible cost relating to their healthcare conditions. AI is also used in providing facilities for medical services, particularly for the diagnosis and predictive-based modeling. This reduces stress, thus minimizing the management responsibilities and improving productivity [5]. Robots are made to act as automated assistants for conducting meetings, delivering patients with individual database health records, and freeing up the medical staff to concentrate mainly on the medical-based services. Figure 7.2 shows the basic block diagram of MetaHealth as DL exploration.

The application of AI in healthcare has evolved crossing many difficulties despite its immense promise. The algorithmic bias, complying with effective regulations and proper data security, provides a moral and ethical guarantee of data that is to be addressed thoroughly. In order to maintain AI fully utilized with

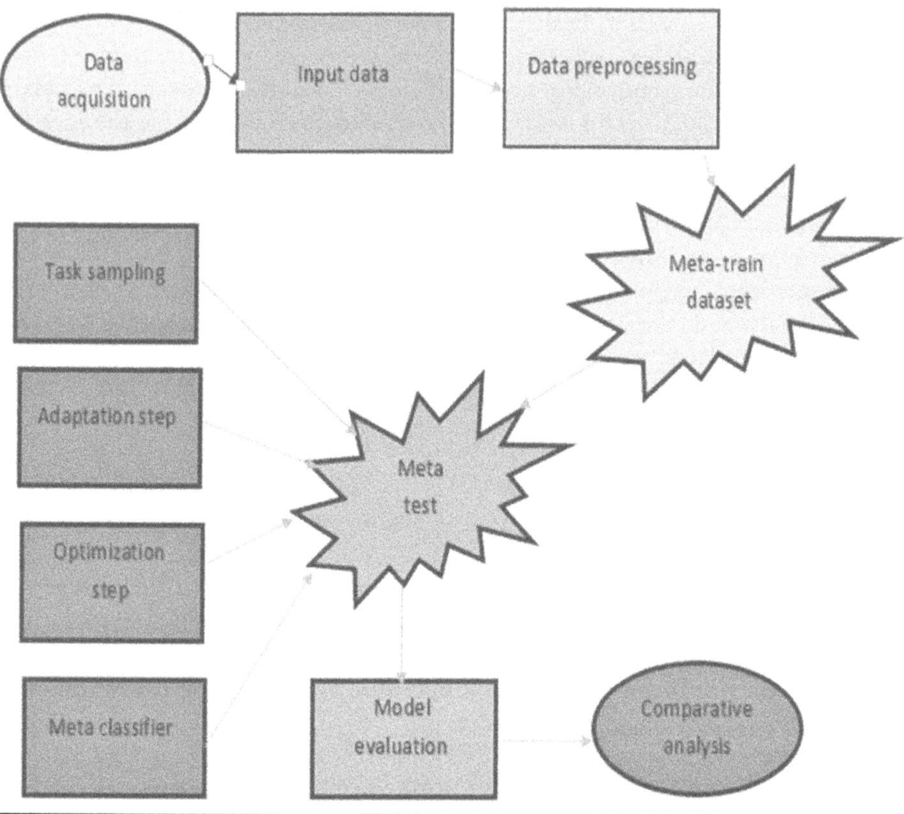

Figure 7.2   Basic block diagram of MetaHealth in DL exploration.

the society and patient, research cooperation among technologies, doctors, nurses, and politicians is required [6]. AI has greater potential in changing the healthcare field from increasing productivity and cost required for diagnosis, concentrating on the satisfaction of the patients and enabling forward thinking with intelligent individual treatment.

7.3 Metaverse in Healthcare

The integration of the virtual world in healthcare has brought forth significant shifts to the delivery, usage, and availability of medicine. The multiverse presents a unique opportunity to revolutionize healthcare, academic study, and development, among other facets of healthcare, with its interactive simulated environments and linked digital spaces. Two significant applications of AR in the field of medicine are electronic health records and web-based therapy. Patients may speak to doctors from any part of the globe via the Internet, reducing geographical restrictions and strengthening the accessibility of medical information. Internet healthcare systems in the virtual realm enable asynchronous inquiry, assessment, and therapies, as well as everyday problems with connections between doctors and their clients. Additionally, the virtual world offers novel approaches to medical education and instruction. Healthcare professionals can practice medicinal skills, operations, and response to disasters by performing active modeling and realistic situations in an atmosphere that is secure and monitored. Effective exercises in such potential situations maximize learning outcomes, reduce demands for resources, and boost patient safety by ensuring that healthcare employees feel educated and proficient in their roles [7].

With technological developments and new approaches of individualized attitudes and learning, virtual reality (VR) has an opportunity to alter the field of medicine. Experts can team up, immediately impart ideas and knowledge, while carrying out studies and cases in virtual laboratories. The collaborative method encourages inventiveness, speeds the pace of medical investigation, and opens novel chances for breakthroughs in areas such as accurate healthcare, disease modeling, and developing medicines.

7.4 AI Diagnostic Solutions with MetaHealth

There are many AI tools for diagnosing that may be used in the framework of MetaHealth, which combines AI and other dimensions for applications in healthcare that will enhance diagnosis and treatment of illness. This section provides a few examples.

7.4.1 AI-Powered Medical Imaging Analysis

ML algorithms may be used by MetaHealth to evaluate information gathered from diagnostic tests, including CAT, MRI, and an X-ray. Algorithms like these can help medical practitioners find trends, assess patients accurately, and spot problems. Guided by AI, medical imaging evaluation has the possibility to greatly improve the availability, efficacy, and reliability of hospital imaging reading. It is a breakthrough development in healthcare research. The use of this method gives healthcare practitioners the ability to interpret complicated medical pictures, such X-rays, MRIs, and scans using CT, with previously unheard-of quickness and accuracy by utilizing advanced intelligent algorithms [8]. AI systems can recognize patterns, spot small anomalies, and help clinicians diagnose patients quickly and accurately. This helps to improve patient outcomes and lowers the possibility of diagnostic mistakes.

Furthermore, doctors may concentrate their skills upon more difficult cases and supervisors' managerial tasks by using AI-powered analyses of medical images to improve their workflows, shorten translation occasions, and ease the pressure on them. AI's incorporation into medical image analysis has enormous potential to improve the process of diagnosis for individualized, data-driven medicine as it develops and matures.

7.4.2 Natural Language Processing (NLP) for Medical Records

To get useful data from medical papers and medical records, NLP algorithms may be linked into MetaHealth. The result makes it possible for medical professionals to swiftly obtain test findings, histories of individuals, and other pertinent information to support diagnostic and therapy choices. Healthcare records, such as doctor notes, summary discharges, and laboratory reports, include unstructured text information that may be extracted, analyzed, and interpreted with the use of NLP methods [9]. NLP raises the velocity of finding knowledge for healthcare workers, optimizes documents procedures, and optimizes the precision of data by digitally analyzing and organizing this enormous volume of textual information.

7.4.3 Predictive Analytics for Disease Risk Assessment

MetaHealth uses an array of mathematical techniques to help determine a patient's mean chance of infection. This keenly helps in the genetic ranges with the use of pertinent information. Predictive analytics of data also serves in developing risk mitigation that is tailored to the profile of each specific affected person. This acts as a screen for preventing disease with quicker treatments.

7.4.4 Clinical Decision Support Systems (CDSS)

MetaHealth with AI CDSS helps in giving the suggestions to the research professionals for an effective diagnosis process. The suggestions are mainly based on the excellence standards adopting keen medical advice to evaluate the information of the patients in real-time scenarios and taking up a multiple range of suggestions with relevant medication and test values [10].

7.4.5 Virtual Symptom Checker and Triage Systems

The individual candidates can use the AI virtual condition tools for checking and getting suggestions and care from MetaHealth. By the use of such structures, better medical resource allocations are made possible that are based entirely on the intensity of the ailments for medical prescription.

7.4.6 Genomic Analysis for Personalized Medicine

Genetic analysis for individualized treatment is a creative approach to healthcare that customizes medical care to an individual's unique personality traits based on

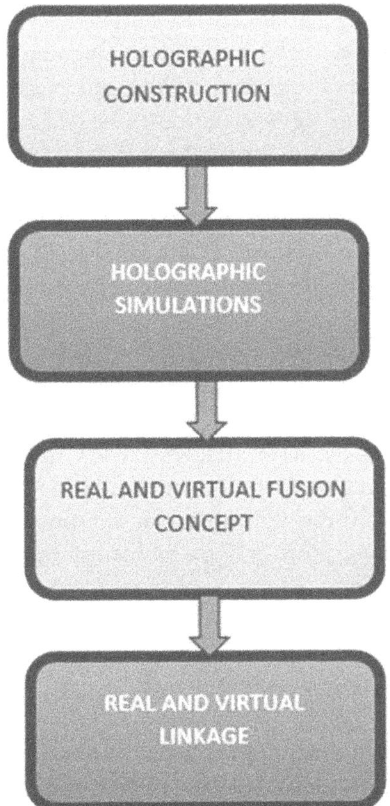

Figure 7.3   Metaverse in digitalized medicine.

genetic information. Genomic sequencing examines a person's genomes, containing variations in chromosomes and genes, in order to identify inherited sensitivity to a specific sickness, determine possible treatments, and direct personalized therapeutic methods.

In general, the use of genetics for individual therapy has enormous potential to revolutionize society by facilitating more accurate, proactive, and customized methods of medical diagnosis, therapy, and prevention, which will ultimately enhance patient outcomes as well as quality of life [11]. Figure 7.3 shows the metaverse in developing digital medicine.

7.4.7 Remote Patient Monitoring and Early Warning Systems

Real-time ongoing tracking of client health data, including indicators of health and level of activity, is possible by artificially intelligent algorithms embedded into MetaHealth. These algorithms allow for swift action and the avoidance of complications by detecting variations from initial results and notifying physicians. Using wearable technology, instruments, and apps for mobile health, RPM gives medical professionals the ability to keep an eye on patients' bodily functions, indications, and vital signs instantaneously. These machines can identify minute variations or departures from the normal range that might point to a decline in overall wellness or the beginning of difficulties by gathering and evaluating data on heartbeat, blood pressure, sugar levels, and movements. Predictive analytical methods are used by alert systems connected with remote patient monitoring (RPM) platforms to identify patients who are in danger of adverse reactions or serious illness.

7.4.8 Statistical Analyses for Psychology Evaluation

MetaHealth may employ methods that utilize AI to assess people's verbal and nonverbal patterns with the objective of testing for mental illnesses such as mood disorders and stress [12]. These algorithms for computers recognize little changes that might be indicators of more serious problems, allowing for prompt aid and rehabilitation.

7.5 Metaverse in Healthcare Disorders

In the subject of metaverse-driven medication, a variety of conditions and illnesses are explicitly addressed via innovative use of VR and technology advancements. But in the other reality, novel approaches to diagnosis, treatment, and recovery hold promise. The following are among these circumstances.

7.5.1 Social Anxiety Disorder (SAD)

Under supervision provided by a psychotherapist, individuals can steadily face social events they are afraid of, such as speeches or having conversations with others in an online environment. Because VR is vivid, people can witness similar circumstances in a secure environment. This helps them acquire coping techniques and progressively lessen their anxious reactions [13]. A belief in belonging and mutual assistance may also be fostered through electronic assistance networks and conversations inside the realm of illusion, so this is advantageous for those who may might feel alone or misjudged in actual life.

7.5.2 Post-Traumatic Stress Disorder (PTSD)

PTSD may significantly hinder a person's ability to operate each day and their standard of living. It is typically the outcome of encounters with stressful experiences. Some individuals may find it difficult to engage in standard therapeutic procedures like cognitive behavioral therapy (CBT) and exposure counseling since they involve reliving unpleasant experiences. Through exposure exercises, counselors can help individuals reframe their perception of the upsetting incident and gradually become less sensitive to recollections [14]. VR and mindfulness exercises can also aid with controlling stress and mood regulation, providing people who have PTSD with additional support.

7.5.3 Chronic Pain Disorders

Prolonged pain syndromes such as neurological pain and fibromyalgia present challenging issues for both patients and healthcare providers. Patients receiving AR distraction therapies are absorbed into immersive virtual worlds that stimulate all of their senses, taking their attention away from their pain.

7.5.4 Autism Spectrum Disorder (ASD)

Autism is considered a neurodevelopmental disorder that is typified by limited and recurrent behaviors in addition to challenges with social interactions and involvement. In the metaverse, virtually reality-based social ability education is presented as a possibly effective solution.

7.6 VR in MetaHealth

With the use of interactive digital spaces, a revolutionary method of delivering healthcare is offered by virtual reality (VR) in Meta Health. Now the several facets and uses of VR in Meta Health are presented.

7.6.1 Immersive Patient Care

This care enables professionals to customize the care of the clients based on their need for smooth visualization. This helps in redirecting and focusing the patient awaiting surgery, using VR in MetaHealth to eliminate the tediousness of the wait [15–17]. VR can also be employed to replicate medical procedures, operations, and rehabilitation activities.

7.6.2 Virtual Consultations and Telemedicine

Through remote visits and conferencing with MetaHealth, patients may engage with doctors anywhere in the world thanks to the usage of AR. Through VR-enabled online workplaces, patients may interact with physicians and other specialists in immersive virtual worlds, eliminating geographical obstacles and improving getting treatment.

7.6.3 Medical Education and Training

VR-based anatomy lessons offer participatory depiction of intricate neural networks, improving comprehension and memory of important ideas. Furthermore, individualized discussions and simulated reality big circles encourage peer learning and cooperation of medical experts, supporting ongoing career advancement and information sharing.

7.6.4 Therapeutic Interventions and Rehabilitation

VR is a medical technology that MetaHealth uses for physical rehab and treatment. VR-based services for rehabilitation provide individuals suffering from operations, accidents, or neurological ailments with stimulating and inspiring encounters. VR settings provide patients possibilities for ongoing training and growth in function by simulating real-life tasks and exercises [18]. Additionally, by encouraging flexibility and cognition recovery, VR-based cognitive rehab therapies can target cognitive deficits linked to neurological illnesses, including Alzheimer's disease and brain trauma.

7.6.5 Pain Management and Distraction Therapy

VR equipment is used by MetaHealth as a distraction treatment to reduce distress and suffering. Clients may successfully distract themselves from suffering by immersing themselves in multisensory, intense virtual realities through realistic VR sessions.

7.7 Workflow on Diagnosis of Various Diseases

MetaHealthcare technology employs a mixed approach to therapy to optimize the efficacy of the illness identification procedures for various illnesses [19–23]. The following elements are often included in the process of evaluating different diseases under MetaHealthcare systems.

7.7.1 Patient Intake and Assessment

Online surveys, online counseling, or the addition of an electronic health record (EHR) may all be used to collect these data. Sophisticated AI computers examine the data provided by the patient to find pertinent multiple illnesses, medical conditions, and any warning signs that might direct to a diagnostic test.

7.7.2 Multimodal Data Collection

Multidisciplinary data collecting technologies are utilized by MetaHealthcare systems to get comprehensive data on the well-being of the individual who is being treated. This might involve physiological parameters (like vital signs or physiological data), testing at the laboratory (like blood tests or genomic screenings), clinical investigations (like X-rays or MRIs), and subjective evaluations (like the results reported by patients or severity of symptoms ratings). The real-time interpretation and analysis of diverse information is made easier by the implementation of AI computational methods, which also helps to identify diagnostics trends and abnormalities.

7.7.3 AI-Powered Differential Diagnosis

In order to provide an appropriate diagnosis, AI algorithms inside MetaHealthcare systems evaluate the client's clinical history. They then rank possible illnesses according to the individual's presentations and chance of occurrence. Refinement of diagnostics theories and recommendation of suitable steps to take for additional examination and care are facilitated by AI algorithms that have been trained on large-scale datasets of medical tracks, medical recommendations, and expert knowledge.

7.7.4 VR Simulation and Visualization

VR simulation and technology for visualization are used by MetaHealthcare technologies to improve planning of treatment and correctness of diagnosis for diseases that need visual evaluation or procedures planning. VR settings can mimic physiology, pathological alterations, and anatomical structures. This makes it possible for medical professionals to connect with and examine 3D models in a natural and engaging way. Thus medical professionals can see intricate processes associated with diseases, spot minute anomalies, and practice treatments before implementing them in actual situations with patients.

7.7.5 Collaborative Decision-Making

Multidisciplinary teams (MDTs) of healthcare workers, comprising medical specialists, radiographers, and pathologists, in particular, and affiliated healthcare providers, may make decisions more collaboratively with the help of the MetaHealthcare system. Clinicians may collaborate to evaluate complicated cases, debate diagnostic issues, and develop evidence-based treatment recommendations through remote transdisciplinary group discussions.

7.7.6 Patient Education and Engagement

With the use of the MetaHealthcare system, various groups of healthcare professionals — including medical experts, radiographers, and pathology in particular, and linked healthcare providers — may decide more cooperatively. AI-powered decision-support systems offer viewpoints, recommendations, and medical standards in real time to assist in making educated decisions and enhancing outcomes for patients.

7.7.7 Continuous Monitoring and Follow-up

Monitoring remotely tools, patient-reported results, and online follow-up meetings make it more straightforward for both patients and medical professionals to stay in continuous contact, guaranteeing that the client's treatment is proactive, individualized, and receptive to changing standards.

7.8 Treatment Plans in MetaHealth

VR, AI, and information-based knowledge of the meta world are just a few of the cutting-edge technologies that MetaHealth employs to construct customized treatment regimens for a variety of health issues [24]. At MetaHealth, the main goals of treatment programs are to enhance patients' quality of life and optimize therapeutic results. These programs are made specifically to fit each patient's needs, preferences, and physiological traits. This section describes the key elements and methods that MetaHealth uses while developing therapies.

7.8.1 Comprehensive Assessment

Creating a plan of action begins with a detailed review of the patient's medical history, current indicators, diagnostics results, and psychosocial factors. AI algorithms are used to analyze the individual's data and identify relevant clinical findings, risk indicators, and treatment objectives in order to produce a customized medicinal routine.

7.8.2 Evidence-Based Guidelines

MetaHealth integrates medical standards, recommendations, and evidence-based decisions and considerations into the curative scheduling process to ensure that therapies are backed by biomedical research and tailored to the patient's specific condition. With the use of AI-powered decision-support technologies, which provide prompt suggestions and alerts that follow the most recent research and expert opinion, providers may make properly educated treatment decisions.

7.8.3 Multimodal Interventions

Multimodal treatments focus on the complex interconnections between all the factors that contribute to a patient's illness. This may involve nutritional psychotherapy, behavioral therapy, exercise regimens, and pharmaceutical therapies, to name a few. The integration of VR equipment opens up new avenues for treatment in the transportation industry or immersion VR exposure treatments for anxiety disorders [25].

7.8.4 Shared Decision-Making

Through promoting collaborative decision-making between physicians and patients, MetaHealth empowers individuals to take ownership of developing customized treatment plans. The implementation of an interactive strategy has been shown to enhance patient involvement, commitment, and satisfaction, resulting in superior treatment results and higher standards of life.

7.8.5 Remote Monitoring and Telehealth Services

MetaHealth employs virtual channels, online health products and services, and surveillance equipment to provide continuous conditions for a patient's oversight and tracking beyond conventional medical offices. Patients may track their accomplishments, get specific comments on treatment adherence and conclusions, and benefit from timely assistance and direction from healthcare experts through virtual further investigation evaluations, telehealth visits, and online health education programs [26]. The capacity to monitor clients remotely improves continuity of care, encourages early action, and gives patients more control over how their physical well-being is managed.

7.8.6 Outcome Evaluation and Continuous Improvement

MetaHealth uses achievement indicators and data analyses to track adherence among patients to professional recommendations, assess treatment results, and pinpoint areas for improved quality during the course of therapy. Therapy responsiveness with the side effects and the plans required for treatment are powered by means of the system analytics posed with AI. This aids the surgeons or the doctors in determining the patients' health over time period with refined strategies for therapies on changing demands of the patients with the means of continuous survcillance.

7.9 Comparative Analysis of Metaverse-Based Techniques

MetaHealth integrates cutting-edge technology, based on proof protocols and customer-centered concepts to improve patient happiness, maximize treatment results, and modernize medical care in the age of digital devices [27–28]. The comparative assessment of the metaverse is given in Table 7.1.

Table 7.1 Comparative Analysis of VR Chart and the Metaverse

Parameters	VR chart	Metaverse
Use	Gaming and Socialization	Gaming, education, life socialization, medical, etc.
Description	Virtualized social problem	Digital twin of the world
Earning	Premium subscriptions	Each element holds value and gives an opportunity to learn
Scope	Users cannot get digitized land	Users get rented digital land that can be resold
Virtual universe	Mono universe with many virtual worlds	Multiple universes with several worlds in it

7.9.1 VR

Strengths: Delivers accurate simulations for imparting treatment, and diagnosis through deep involvement. Useful for rehabilitation, sensitization medication, and chronic diversion.

Weaknesses: Minimal physical involvement, needs specific gear (VR headsets), and may cause motion nausea in certain people.

Applications: Pain administration, psychotropic drugs, radiation therapy, clinical training, and operation simulators are among the therapies offered.

7.9.2 AR

Strengths: Improves communication and perception by fusing both tangible and digital material. Beneficial for online help, healthcare instruction, and procedural navigation.

Weaknesses: Less immersive than VR, suitable equipment (cell phones, AR specs) is needed, and there is a chance of disruption in healthcare situations.

Applications: Laparoscopic advice, online medical care, online help, education for patients, and healthcare instruction with the human anatomy simulation.

7.9.3 Mixed Reality (MR)

Strengths: Blends combining tangible and digital elements to create engaging and dynamic engagements. Ideal for teaching, product imagining, and group projects.

Weaknesses: Requires sophisticated gear (MR helmets), is more difficult to get than AR and VR equipment, and may have connectivity issues.

Applications: Telecommuting, remote collaboration, participation of patients, and healthcare instruction and training.

7.9.4 AI

Strengths: Permits identification of patterns, analysis of information, and judgment assistance. Improves analytics for prediction, planning of therapy, and diagnosis.

Weaknesses: Possibility for partiality in making computational decisions; reliance on accurate algorithms and reliable information [29–31].

Applications: Clinical decision assistance systems (CDAS), ML for customized medical practice, medical imaging analysis, and digital assistants for medicine.

7.9.5 Telemedicine and Telepresence

Strengths: Enables remote discussions, notifications, and the provision of therapy. Decreases disparities in medicine and increases likelihood of receiving specialist treatment.

Weaknesses: Depends on connectivity to the Internet, might not be able to be examined physically, and raises security and confidentiality concerns.

Applications: Online monitoring of patients, a form of teleeducation, and a program is called online counseling.

7.9.6 Multimodal Interaction

Strengths: mixes speech, motion, and haptic feedback with other input and output technologies to create natural and engaging engagements. Improves access and involvement among users.

Weaknesses: Technology specifications, possibility for overstimulation of the senses, and technological complexity.

Applications: Instruction for patients, surgery instruction, treatments, medical care simulators, and assistance technology.

In conclusion, every metaverse-based approach has advantages and disadvantages of its own, and the best approach relies on the particular use situation and standards in the context of healthcare. Using several treatments to take advantage of their own benefits and successfully serve a range of medical needs may be part of a holistic strategy.

7.10 Impact on Global Healthcare Accessibility

Some of the primary methods that MetaHealth is using to expand access to healthcare internationally are through the use of contemporary instruments throughout the multiverse, as shown in Figure 7.4.

7.10.1 Remote Consultations and Telemedicine

Meta Health makes telemedicine services and remote consultations possible, allowing patients to consult with doctors from any location in the globe [32–34]. Patients who have trouble moving around or getting about, as well as those who live in distant or impoverished areas with little access to healthcare, can all benefit greatly from this method.

7.10.2 Virtual Clinics and Specialty Services

People may obtain information and treatment that may be limited in some places by using MetaHealth, which makes it simpler to establish online medical clinics and specialized facilities in the metaverse. Remote clinics can offer a wide range of medical specialties, including cardiology, oncology, neurology, and mental health. By eliminating long wait times and extensive travel, these clinics can save patients time and money.

7.10.3 Health Education and Awareness

In order to improve the keen understanding of medical datasets and increasing medical preventive care, MetaHealth provides the way for making reality and instructional technologies [35]. Interactive tutorials, immersion tests, and prominent health courses help people to gain better insight on medical topics, which promotes good habits to enable patients to make sensible choices regarding their mental and physical well-being.

7.10.4 Capacity Building and Training

MetaHealth provides courses on educational basics to children, which is the main criterion of instructional simulation facilities, which helps in enhancing the healthcare capacity development in resource-based environments. Furthermore, telementoring systems supply the connection between regional healthcare professionals and global specialists, allowing for the sharing of information, transferring of skills, and joint decision-making aimed at improving the standard medical services provided in underprivileged regions.

7.10.5 Disaster Response and Humanitarian Aid

MetaHealth is essential in enabling quick responses and providing impacted communities with life-saving assistance medical treatment during crises or humanitarian catastrophes. In disaster-affected regions with inadequate facilities or access to healthcare providers, collaborative efforts to assess requirements, distribute resources, and give medical aid are made possible by telehealth triage points,

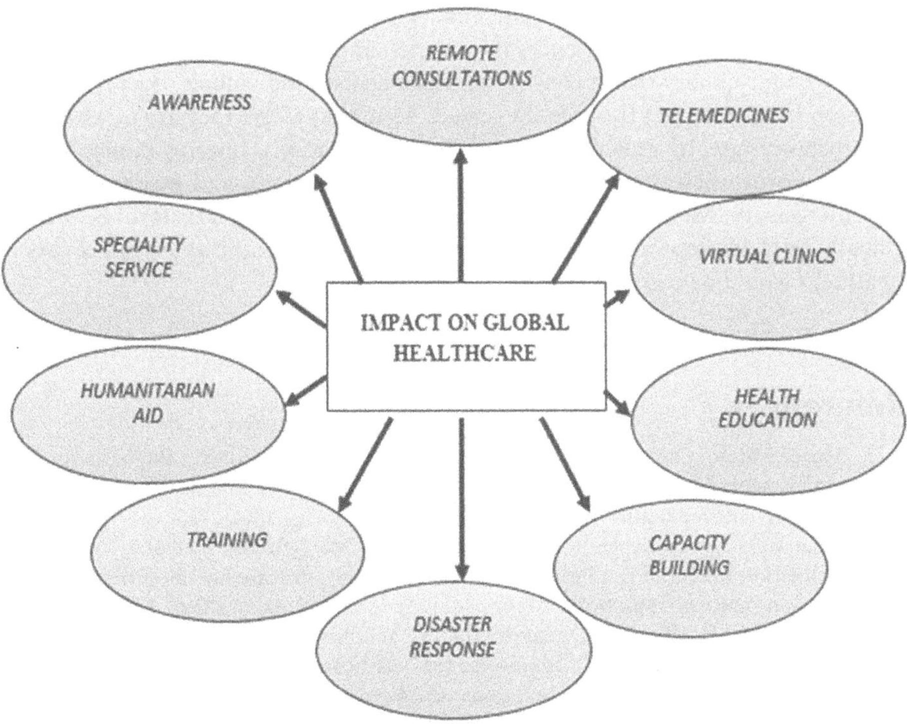

Figure 7.4 Impact on global healthcare.

remote medical professionals, and VR-based catastrophe exercises [36–37]. This makes immediate action possible, lowers rates of morbidity and death, and builds tolerance in populations that are already at risk of health problems.

MetaHealth uses cutting-edge technology and creative solutions to remove obstacles from the delivery of medical treatment, which has a revolutionary effect on the affordability of medical care worldwide. MetaHealth provides more opportunities for telemedicine, such simulated clinics, health-related schooling, and disaster recovery services. These resources enable people, clinicians, and the general public to overcome practical, financial, and geographical obstacles to receive excellent healthcare whenever and wherever it needs to be.

7.11 Conclusion

In summary, MetaHealth is a shining example of creativity and promise for the future of globally accessible treatment. By incorporating cutting-edge technologies like telecommunications- augmented reality and intelligent systems into the wider universe, MetaHealth has the chance to revolutionize the way healthcare is offered, enhance the experiences of patients, and close strong gaps in the availability of high-quality treatment. MetaHealth enables individuals, doctors, nurses, and communities to get the care they need, no matter where they are or what their circumstances are, by providing on-demand consultations, Internet clinics, educational opportunities, professional development applications, and guidance regarding emergencies. MetaHealth has the potential to completely transform healthcare globally as it develops and spreads, paving the way for a time when fair access to treatment would be considered inherent.

References

1. Moztarzadeh, O., Jamshidi, M., Sargolzaei, S., Jamshidi, A., Baghalipour, N., Malekzadeh Moghani, M., & Hauer, L. (2023). Metaverse and healthcare: Machine learning-enabled digital twins of cancer. *Bioengineering, 10*(4), 455.
2. Elhenawy, I., AL-baker, S. F., & Mohamed, M. (2023). Intelligent healthcare: Evaluation potential implications of metaverse in healthcare based on mathematical decision-making framework. *Neutrosophic Systems with Applications, 12*, 9–21.
3. Chengoden, R., Victor, N., Huynh-The, T., Yenduri, G., Jhaveri, R. H., Alazab, M., & Gadekallu, T. R. (2023). Metaverse for healthcare: A survey on potential applications, challenges and future directions. *IEEE Access, 11*, 12765–12795.
4. Yang, Y., Zhou, Z., Li, X., Xue, X., Hung, P. C., & Yangui, S. (2023). Metaverse for healthcare: Technologies, challenges, and vision. *International Journal of Crowd Science, 7*(4), 190–199.
5. Ullah, H., Manickam, S., Obaidat, M., Laghari, S. U. A., & Uddin, M. (2023). Exploring the potential of metaverse technology in healthcare: Applications, challenges, and future directions. *IEEE Access, 11*, 69686–69707.
6. Gupta, O. J., Yadav, S., Srivastava, M. K., Darda, P., & Mishra, V. (2023). Understanding the intention to use metaverse in healthcare utilizing a mix method approach. *International Journal of Healthcare Management, 12*(2), 318–329. https://doi.org/10.1080/20479700.2023.2183579
7. Bashir, A. K., Victor, N., Bhattacharya, S., Huynh-The, T., Chengoden, R., Yenduri, G., ... & Liyanage, M. (2023). Federated learning for the healthcare metaverse: Concepts, applications, challenges, and future directions. *IEEE Internet of Things Journal, 15*, 21873–21891
8. Kumar, V., Joshi, K., Kumar, R., Anandaram, H., Bhagat, V. K., & Baloni, D. (2023). Multi modalities medical image fusion using deep learning and metaverse technology: Healthcare 4.0 a futuristic approach. *Biomedical and Pharmacology Journal, 16*(4), 1949–1959.
9. Athar, A., Ali, S. M., Mozumder, M. A. I., Ali, S., & Kim, H. C. (2023, February). Applications and possible challenges of healthcare metaverse. In *2023 25th International Conference on Advanced Communication Technology (ICACT)* (pp. 328–332). IEEE.
10. Ashwini, A., & Sriram, S. R. (2023). Quadruple spherical tank systems with automatic level control applications using fuzzy deep neural sliding mode FOPID controller. *Journal of Engineering Research*. https://doi.org/10.1016/j.jer.2023.09.022

11. Ashwini, A., Purushothaman, K. E., Rosi, A., & Vaishnavi, T. (2023). Artificial intelligence based real-time automatic detection and classification of skin lesion in dermoscopic samples using DenseNet-169 architecture. *Journal of Intelligent & Fuzzy Systems*, (Preprint), *45*(4), 6943–6958.
12. Zhang, T., Shen, J., Lai, C. F., Ji, S., & Ren, Y. (2023). Multi-server assisted data sharing supporting secure deduplication for metaverse healthcare systems. *Future Generation Computer Systems*, *140*, 299–310.
13. Bang, J., & Kim, J. Y. (2023). Metaverse ethics for healthcare using AI technology: Challenges and risks. In *International Conference on Human-Computer Interaction* (pp. 367–378). Springer Nature Switzerland, Cham.
14. Ashwini, A., & Sangeetha, S. (2024). IoT-based smart sensors: The key to early warning systems and rapid response in natural disasters. In *Predicting Natural Disasters with AI and Machine Learning* (pp. 202–223). IGI Global.
15. Ashwini, A., Sriram, S. R., Manisha, A., & Prabhakar, J. M. (2024). Artificial intelligence's impact on thrust manufacturing with innovations and advancements in aerospace. In *Industry Applications of Thrust Manufacturing: Convergence with Real-Time Data and AI* (pp. 197–220). IGI Global.
16. Letafati, M., & Otoum, S. (2024). Digital healthcare in the metaverse: Insights into privacy and security. *IEEE Consumer Electronics Magazine*, *13*(3), 80–89.
17. Kim, E. J., & Kim, J. Y. (2023). The metaverse for healthcare: Trends, applications, and future directions of digital therapeutics for urology. *International Neurourology Journal*, *27*(Suppl 1), S3.
18. Ashwini, A., & Kavitha, V. (2023). Automatic skin tumor detection using online tiger claw region based segmentation – a novel comparative technique. *IETE Journal of Research*, *69*(6), 3095–3103.
19. Zhang, G., Dai, Y., Wu, J., Zhu, X., & Lu, Y. (2023). Swarm learning-based secure and fair model sharing for metaverse healthcare. *Mobile Networks and Applications*, *28*(4), 1498–1509.
20. Akbari, A. A., & Teymouri, M. (2023). The role and position of metaverse in health care. *Medical Law Journal*, *17*(58), 839–850.
21. Çeçen, Z., & Yüksel, O. (2023). Metaverse and healthcare sector. *International Journal of Engineering and Innovative Research*, *5*(3), 280–290.
22. Ashwini, A., Vaishnavi, T., Rosi, A., Shahila, D. F. D., & Nalini, N. (2023, December). Deep learning based drowsiness detection with alert system using Raspberry Pi Pico. In *2023 International Conference on Data Science, Agents & Artificial Intelligence (ICDSAAI)* (pp. 1–8). IEEE.
23. Al Kuwaiti, A., Nazer, K., Al-Reedy, A., Al-Shehri, S., Al-Muhanna, A., Subbarayalu, A. V., ... & Al-Muhanna, F. A. (2023). A review of the role of artificial intelligence in healthcare. *Journal of Personalized Medicine*, *13*(6), 951.
24. Ashwini, A., & Murugan, S. (2023). Automatic skin tumour segmentation using prioritized patch based region – a novel comparative technique. *IETE Journal of Research*, *69*(1), 137–148.
25. Shahila, D. F. D., Ashwini, A., Vaishnavi, T., Rosi, A., & Evangelin, D. L. (2023, August). IOT based object perception algorithm for Urban Scrutiny System in Digital City. In *2023 International Conference on Circuit Power and Computing Technologies (ICCPCT)* (pp. 1788–1792). IEEE.
26. Stephanie, V., Khalil, I., & Atiquzzaman, M. (2024). DSFL: A decentralized SplitFed learning approach for healthcare consumers in the metaverse. *IEEE Transactions on Consumer Electronics*, *70*(1), 2107–2115.

27. Ashwini, A., Purushothaman, K. E., Prathaban, B. P., Jenath, M., & Prasanna, R. (2023, April). Automatic traffic sign board detection from camera images using deep learning and binarization search algorithm. In *2023 International Conference on Recent Advances in Electrical, Electronics, Ubiquitous Communication, and Computational Intelligence (RAEEUCCI)* (pp. 1–5). IEEE.
28. Balasubramaniam, S, Joe, C. V., Manthiramoorthy, C., & Kumar, K. S. (2024). ReliefF based feature selection and gradient squirrel search algorithm enabled deep maxout network for detection of heart disease. *Biomedical Signal Processing and Control*, *87*, 105446.
29. Wu, T. C., & Ho, C. T. B. (2023). A scoping review of metaverse in emergency medicine. *Australasian Emergency Care*, *26*(1), 75–83.
30. Choudhury, A., Balasubramaniam, S, Kumar, A. P., & Kumar, S. N. P. (2023). PSSO: Political squirrel search optimizer-driven deep learning for severity level detection and classification of lung cancer. *International Journal of Information Technology & Decision Making*, 1–34. https://doi.org/10.1142/S0219622023500189
31. Yang, E. (2023). Implications of immersive technologies in healthcare sector and its built environment. *Frontiers in Medical Technology*, *5*.
32. Li, Y., Gunasekeran, D. V., RaviChandran, N., Tan, T. F., Ong, J. C. L., Thirunavukarasu, A. J., & Ting, D. S. (2023). The next generation of healthcare ecosystem in the metaverse. *Biomedical Journal*, *47*(3), 100679.
33. Huang, H., Zhang, C., Zhao, L., Ding, S., Wang, H., & Wu, H. (2023). Self-supervised medical image denoising based on WISTA-Net for human healthcare in metaverse. *IEEE Journal of Biomedical and Health Informatics*, *28*(11), 6329–6337. https://doi.org/10.1109/JBHI.2023.3278538
34. An, P. H. (2023). Exploring the digital healthcare product's logistics and mental healthcare in the metaverse: Role of technology anxiety and metaverse bandwidth fluctuations. *iRASD Journal of Management*, *5*(4), 223–241.
35. Ramamurthy, S., Yammahi, A. S., & Rahim, A. A. (2023). The role of the metaverse in transforming healthcare. *Research Journal of Pharmacy and Technology*, *16*(11), 5506–5513.
36. Balasubramaniam, S, Kadry, S., & Kumar, K. S. (2024). Osprey Gannet optimization enabled CNN based transfer learning for optic disc detection and cardiovascular risk prediction using retinal fundus images. *Biomedical Signal Processing and Control*, *93*, 106177.
37. Tripathi, A., Chauhan, N., Choudhary, A., & Singh, R. (2023). Augmented reality and its significance in healthcare systems. In *Meta-Learning Frameworks for Imaging Applications* (pp. 103–118). IGI Global.

Chapter 8

Leveraging MIR to Metaverse: Immersive Exploration with HCI

Banu Priya Prathaban, R. Subash, Ashwini A, and B. Sundaravadivazhagan

8.1 Background

Computer-aided diagnosis (CAD) has advanced as one of the precise and substantial probe domes in medical imaging. Cutting-edge technologies in CAD are the machine learning (ML) and deep learning (DL) algorithms, which are commonly utilized to examine medical images via sequential patient data trials and to generate a classifier model for assessing the current physical state of patients [1]. The established classifier model helps clinicians make rapid verdicts in case of any medical emergencies. The field of study under computer vision (CV) involving the popular techniques like ML and DL for analyzing and interpreting the medical images is popularly termed as medical image recognition (MIR) [2]. Those medical images are mostly like X-rays for imaging the internal organs, bones, and tissues; a computed tomography (CT) scan for imaging the internal injuries and tumors in the body; magnetic resonance imaging (MRI) for viewing the soft tissue parts of brain and its disorders; positron emission tomography (PET), used for viewing the malignant tumor cells; and ultrasound for viewing the internal organs [3]. MIR is used for distinguishing the different objects in the medical images. From these, interpretation can be done very easily for diagnosing the diseases in the body. It is more favorable for detecting, distinguishing, and localizing the objects in medical

DOI: 10.1201/9781003491668-8

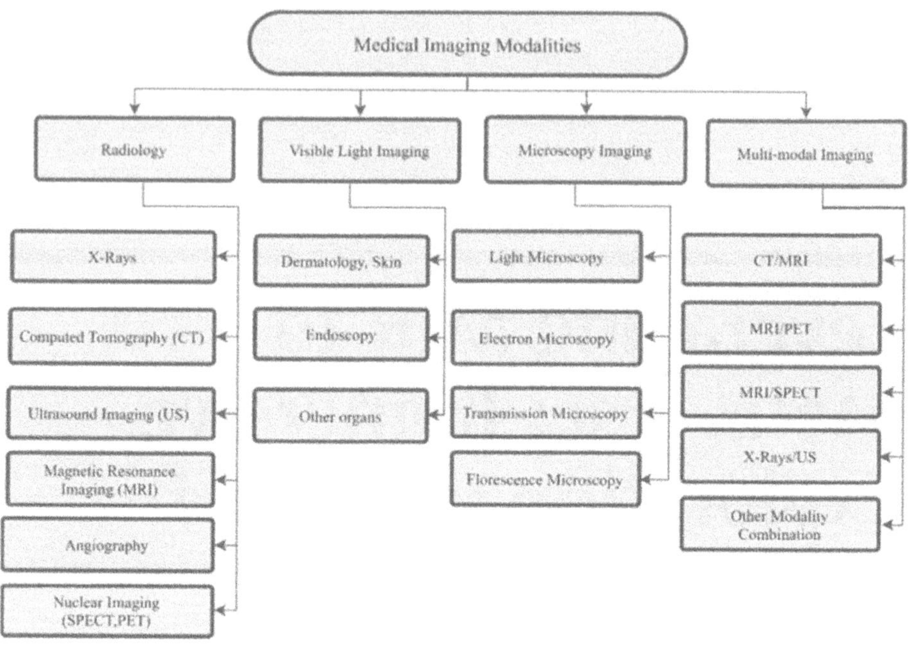

Figure 8.1   MIR modalities.

images. Such a technology is better suited to revolutionize this medical era by disease diagnosis, early disease prediction, and even in the therapy and assistive planning of treatment procedures [4]. Figure 8.1 depicts the various modalities of MIR.

MIR is used extensively for locating the internal organs from the digital images for therapeutic dedications like determining or otherwise reviewing different syndromes in our body. The key goal of MIR is to increase the effectiveness of medical research and disease management opportunities [5]. The major needs for which MIR is utilized are the following: image segmentation, augmentation, localization, disease diagnosis, early disease prediction, classification, or sorting different types/stages of a disease [6]. In the past, low-level techniques like thresholding, region expanding, and edge tracing were used to process medical images [4]. MIR is utilized for the automation of detecting the anomalies found in the input digitalized medical images, like in detecting breast tumors from mammogram images, lung nodules from chest X-rays, fractures from bone X-rays, etc. Medical image segmentation, which entails determining the borders of various tissues and organs, can be accomplished with MIR [7]. Surgical operations or radiation therapy treatments can be planned using this imaging data. Medical images are segmented using MIR, which requires localizing the boundaries of numerous tissues and organs. Strategies for radiation therapy management or surgical trials are accomplished exhausting this medical image information. Also, MIR can be utilized for discovering the potential novel drug objects by examining the input medical image information [8].

In recent times, the metaverse has drawn out abundant attractiveness and responsiveness everywhere. Currently this generation is flowing on the way to the metaverse, which empowers users to maintain a relation between the physical and the virtual world in the way of immersiveness. Through the usage of metaverse technology, individuals are able to form an enhanced reality world even though it is just digitalized [9]. MIR in the metaverse offers an exciting frontier for healthcare, blending powerful AI analysis with immersive virtual environments for diagnosis, treatment, and education. Moreover, MIR also can be used toward advancing the reality of metaverse medical simulations and virtual healthcare settings in a more professional manner [10]. Figure 8.2 depicts the healthcare applications of the metaverse.

Human–computer interaction (HCI) in the metaverse involves the use of interfaces, devices, and technologies to facilitate communication and interaction between users and the virtual environment. Medical image recognition enhances the visualization of medical data within the metaverse [11]. Users can navigate and interact with 3D representations of medical images. Metaverse HCI facilitates remote consultations where medical professionals collaborate and discuss cases using virtual representations of medical images. The integration of medical image recognition in the metaverse's HCI holds the potential to revolutionize medical visualization, training, and collaboration in virtual environments. MIR and its potential usages in the metaverse are significantly reliant on HCI [12]. Interfaces

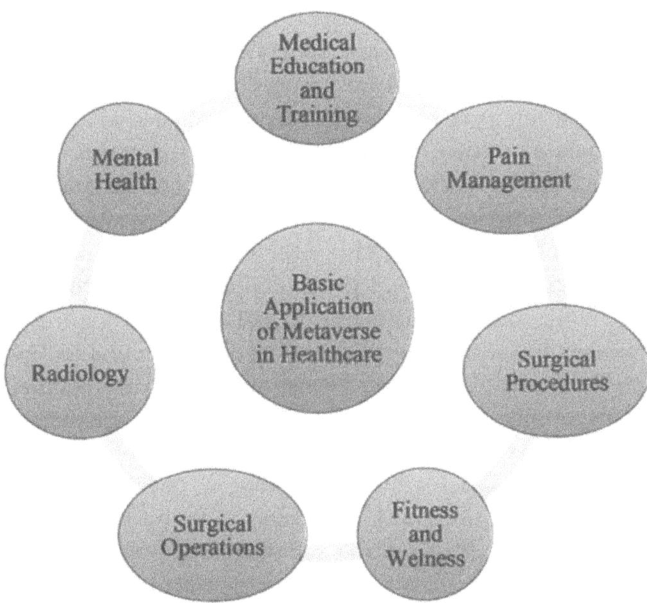

Figure 8.2 Healthcare applications of metaverse.

are very simple to practice and are essential for radiologists and other medical practitioners to connect with MIR coordination. On the road to appropriately assess medical images, the rudiments like user-friendly navigation tools, coherent visualization tools, and adaptable procedures are needed [13]. Smart neural networks can be built into the virtual world to give medical practitioners on-the-spot medical assistance. Through extensive analysis of client information, encompassing imaging scans, testing outcomes, and patient records, systems based on AI are able to provide recommendations, highlight pertinent discoveries, and spot possible error in diagnosis. When clients interact with the user interface, they ought to get prompt, unambiguous input that validates the information they provide and indicates system replies. This consists of sense, aural, and optical signals to recognize behaviors and smoothly navigate users around the metaverse.

8.2 Metaverse and HCI in the Field of Radiology

The metaverse is a cutting-edge technology in the field of radiology that leverages medical image analysis to the next arena, integrating the augmented reality (AR) and virtual reality (VR) in MIR powered with AI for disease detection, diagnosis, and treatment planning. The notion of the metaverse is an extensive, unified digital world with combinational components of AR, VR, and the Internet. Within the perspective of radiology, this technology will possibly transfigure the way clinical images are inferred, united, and exploited. The amalgamation of the metaverse along with HCI unwraps a domain of opportunities aimed at making individuals and digital environs much more interactive [14]. Radiologists might practice their imaging by the use of VR headsets for immersing their mind inside a virtual setting where they can interpret and handle medical images as 3D models, possibly refining their capability to detect multifaceted medical diseases. VR environments enable doctors and nurses to participate in extremely lifelike simulation of patient visits. These risk-free simulations emulate a wide range of medical scenarios, giving medical professionals a chance to hone their diagnostic competencies, improve their decision-making methods, and get acquainted with uncommon or complicated ailments. Clinicians can become more proficient and confident in their ability to diagnose a variety of medical problems through holographic encounters [15].

Radiologists from all over the world may possibly work together in real time inside a common computer-generated, virtual environment, deliberating any medical circumstances and providing their vision, irrespective of their current physical localities. This might be particularly advantageous for physically isolated healthcare groups, consultants, authorities, and counselors required for exceptional medical emergency circumstances. Medical and radiology students may very well utilize this technology for immersiveness and convincing training imitations for practicing, inferring medical images, and accomplishing medical trials. Such a virtual environment might develop their knowledge and advance their preparation for practical medical situations. Such an immersive technology might empower the imagining of enormous datasets, like inhabitants' well-being statistics and medical imaginary collections, as a more instinctive and enlightening learning method than outmoded two-dimensional presentations [16].

Patients in distant or unallocated regions might contact skilled radiologists over simulated cybernetic sessions, refining admittance to dedicated attention. HCI provides gesture acknowledgment, speech instructions, and eye stalking, which all might permit radiologists to work together with medical descriptions in an extra innate and effectual way of utilizing the metaverse. HCI expertise such as haptic response and three-dimensional audio might augment the immersiveness of inspecting and inferring medical imaginings in any simulated setting, offering an added convincing and appealing involvement. HCI progressions might make the situation much relaxed for patients with infirmities to intermingle with medical imagining statistics operating under the metaverse by refining approachability to healthcare evidence and amenities [17].

Planning consumer interfaces in the metaverse requires a profound knowledge of HCI principles that will guarantee the continuous, instinctual, and entertaining utilization for radiologists and patients. Better knowledge of HCI along with ergonomics might keep the customization of the virtual immersive experience grounded on distinct inclinations and desires, permitting radiologists to adapt their workstation and apparatuses, better suiting them for their own environment and working style. HCI progressions confirm that the metaverse is available to individuals with debilities, permitting them a comprehensive computer-generated world. Employment of such a metaverse with HCI expertise will resolve the practical issues in the usage of three-dimensional imagining and simulated direction-finding for practical design; however, these technologies can certainly not imitate the profundity of human association along with lushness of real-life involvements and genuineness of living [18].

Advancement in the metaverse is the digital twin comprising of the creation and cyber-simulated illustration of any physical entities. In the case of healthcare, this technology is quite useful for modeling the distinct human parts or entirely as a generic model, which in turn is useful for surgical procedures [19, 20]. Surgeons may customize this technology to organize and mimic multifaceted surgical techniques formerly accomplished on real subjects, which in turn moderates the jeopardies, increases results, and improves surgical preparation. Figure 8.3 depicts the elements of the digital twin. Merging digital twin technology with HCI can augment the approach of healthcare specialists and patient interaction by leveraging the cybernetic demonstrations.

HCI procedures along with AR and VR will generate immersive atmosphere for digital twin interaction by delivering larger convincing, pleasing imitation of familiarity aimed at preparation and surgical arrangement [21]. HCI is utilized to distinguish the communication by means of the digital twins grounded on the favorites and requirements of specific healthcare specialists, permitting additional

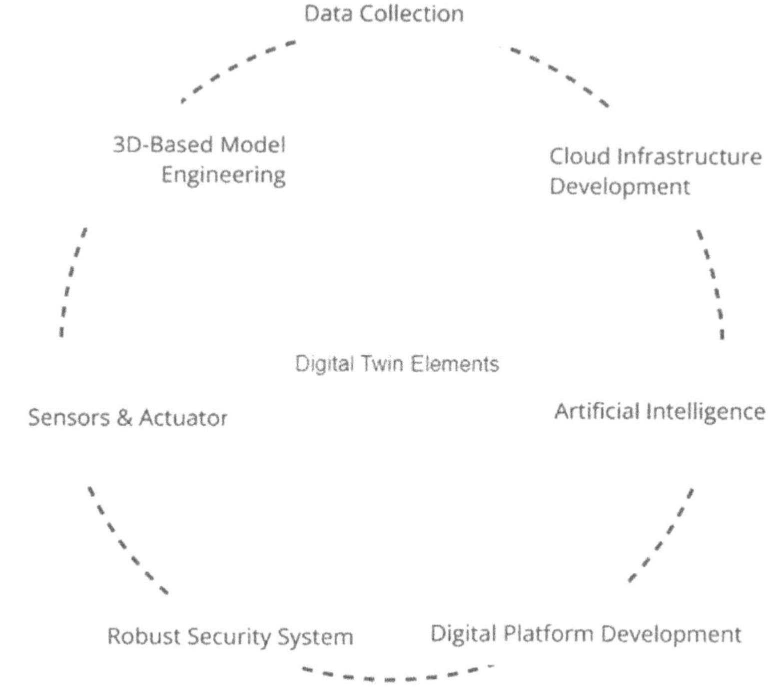

Figure 8.3 Elements of a digital twin.

personalized and well-organized functioning. HCI procedures can augment the imagining of information contained in the digital twins, building it as a healthier approach for healthcare specialists to infer multifaceted medical evidence and to sort conversant assessments. Figure 8.4 depicts the concept of the digital twin along with its determinants. This technology will aid healthcare specialists professionally to observe the conditions of a patient distantly, which is predominantly advantageous for telehealth scenarios [22].

In addition to medical imaging being performed distantly, elderly patients often have difficulty accessing the amenities of this technology. In these cases, such remote observing helps doctors obtain immediate updated information about the status of their patient. Likewise, if there exists an uncertainty in medical data, showing some inconsistencies, then doctors can easily contact the patients to obtain immediate updated information about the status of their patient by planning their regular medical inspections before the condition worsens [23]. Figure 8.4 depicts the concept of the digital twin for healthcare applications in the physical and cyber worlds. This technology practices and understands input information via sensors, which permits it to track the body in real time, forecast its activities, and accomplish numerous investigations through the virtual environment [24]. Imaging specialists and other experts can modify and understand medical photos, such as MRI, CT,

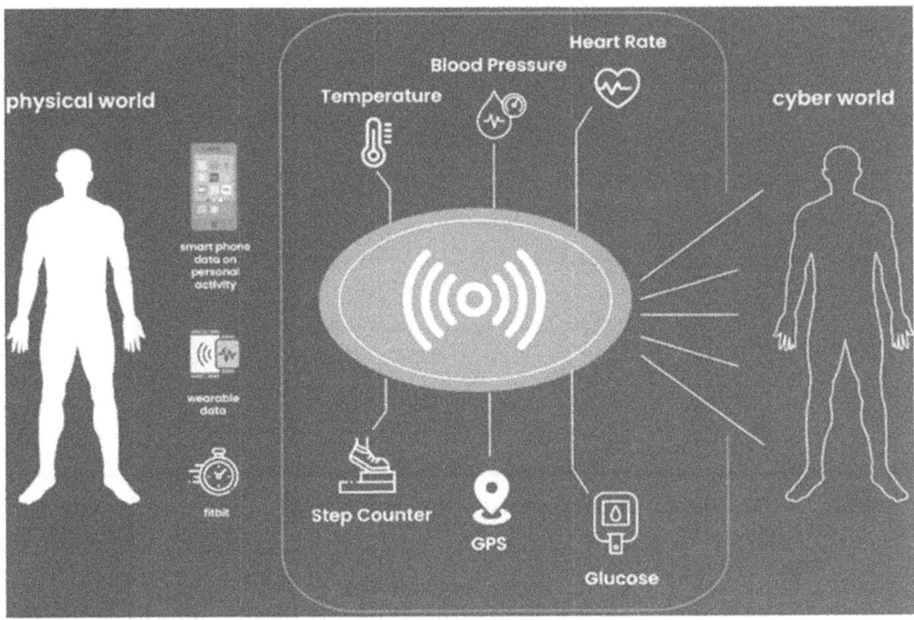

Figure 8.4 **Digital twin for healthcare applications.**

and X-ray scans in 3D by using AR and VR interfaces. Professionals may study anatomical features, collaborate more effectively with colleagues, and identify issues throughout the diagnostic process by using speech, gesture recognition, and touch-based instructions. By employing VR simulations that replicate the environment of a surgical procedure, for example, surgeons may practice challenging procedures and view the anatomy for patients before they even arrive at the surgery center [25]. The established classifier model helps in helping clinicians to make rapid verdicts in case of any medical emergencies. The popular technologies like ML and DL are used for the analysis and interpretation of CT scan and MRI images for visualizing the internal parts of the body [26, 27].

Distant located patients can easily contact the radiologists by means of telemedicine along with HCI [28]. Figure 8.5 depicts the healthcare determinants of digital twin technology. Healthcare professionals may explore cells, tissues, and biological functions in extraordinary depth by immersing the user in highly detailed models of human tissue into this virtual space. They may see data about patients immediately in these simulated images with AR overlays, which enable greater understanding of intricate healthcare issues [29].

These modern AI algorithms help common physicians to evaluate the accuracy in biological irregularities and imagery forecasting the key ailments. Practitioners in the medical field may receive immediate feedback and make more timely interventions with the help of these AI-driven tools for diagnosis

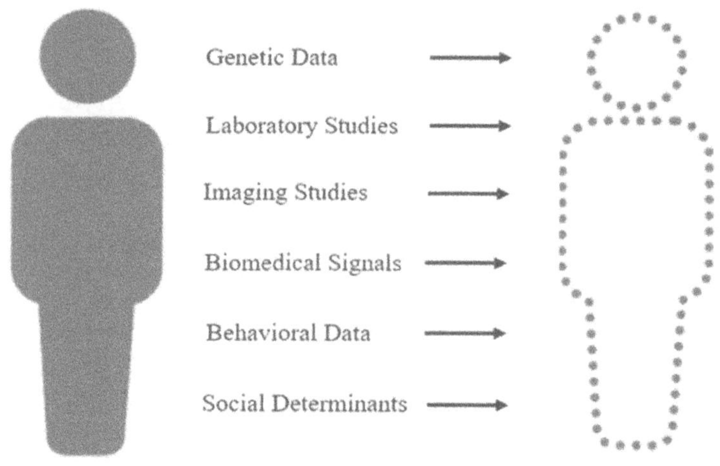

Figure 8.5   Healthcare determinants of the digital twin.

that can quickly assess imaging scans, pathological slides, and other types of diagnostic procedures [30]. This metaverse-based diagnostic paradigm not only aids physicians but also enables people to take greater responsibility in regard to their wellness treatment. Complex clinical information may be actively seen in the metaverse with the help of multifunctional systems. Healthcare professionals may see data related to patients in realistic three-dimensional locations using VR and AR tools, encompassing genetic data, laboratory findings, and digital health records. Therapists can search through databases, collect important information, and obtain deeper insights into their patients' health state to aid in diagnostic selections by combining spoken words, gestures of the hands, and eyes tracking [31].

8.3 Metaverse and HCI in Brain Tumor Detection

The usage of cutting edge technologies leverages HCI, extraordinary VR controllers are capable of manipulating and exploring three-dimensional brain tumor simulations in very immersive surroundings. Customized diagnostic and treatment regimens are made achievable by the integration of multiple modes of interaction and personalized medical care. However, difficulties regarding security of data, moral issues, and technical advancements remain crucial areas of concentration for enhancing the confidence and wide adoption of Multimodal Diagnosis [32]. The growth of the metaverse will enable novel ways for offering healthcare and lead to significant improvements in the treatment of long-lasting problems. Such immersiveness will expand the profundity of insight toward the disease when compared to conventional two-dimensional inspection of medical images, which is possibly superior to previous and extra-precise recognition of a tumor in a brain. The metaverse technology when combined with HCI will be able to incorporate ML and DL algorithms for the real-time detection and prediction of brain tumors via MRIs or any kind of brain scans inside the virtual immersive environment by emphasizing doubtful regions, releasing distinctive identification. All these will prominently increase the indicative efficacy and accurateness of the entire AI model [33].

Currently, multimodal datasets are used for brain tumor detection. Collaboration of different modal medical input data is meant to provide minimized operations with enhanced communication, transforming the means of providing proper healthcare advice. This can help in meeting the specific unique demands of both the workers and the patients with the prominent means of gesture, sound, reach, and graphical interfacing tasks. Additionally, it offers a new range of engaging the patients with the medical educational content and home-based medical providers, thus enabling multimodal interfaces to bring about active participation in a medical journey [34]. Furthermore, irrespective of physical distance, multimodal contact in telemedicine promotes confidence and connection among patients and clinicians by enabling online meetings that resemble in-person conversations. Healthcare institutions may improve patient engagement, optimize treatment delivery, and ultimately improve individual and community health effects by employing a variety of technological advances [35].

Multimodal involvement performs a substantial part in healthcare, delivering a range of strengths and uses that increase patient care, streamline clinical procedures, and encourage interaction between providers and patients. The main intention for multimodal detection of a brain tumor is concentrated on providing the diagnosis experience on a comprehensive scale to providers' own clients, taking only the list of the passive consumers on the prominent medical evaluation. These clients are enabled to develop the active participation of the passive consumers having an online meeting with the medical specialist on such medical evaluations. This helps in determination of high degree of realistic participation to the virtual world. More significant connections between customers and healthcare practitioners are made possible by these realistic and interactive surroundings, which encourage participation and working together.

Figure 8.6 depicts the steps in an ML-based brain tumor diagnosis system. In order encourage deeper comprehension and analysis, dynamic visualization enables users examine data from different perspectives, explore into specific factors, and modify graphics elements in real time. Managers of healthcare may use visualizations for tracking important measures of performance, consumption of resources, and public health trends, while healthcare providers can use these to follow illness development over time or discover irregularities in medical imaging data [36]. Graphical medical information visualization also improves interprofessional teams' interactions and collaboration, facilitating more effective transfer of information, analysis, and decisions.

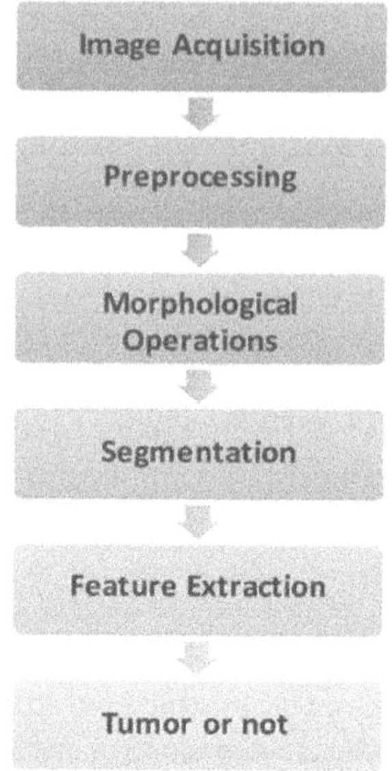

Figure 8.6   General flow brain tumor detection.

8.4 Optimized Decision Tree Algorithm (ODTA) for Brain Tumor Detection along with Immersiveness

The ODTA is a fine-tuned decision tree involving adjusting various parameters to achieve a better model performance. This includes changing the splitting criteria, such as selecting either information gain or Gini impurity as the criterion for choosing the best split at each node, or changing the maximum depth of the tree. Other parameters that can be modified include the minimum number of samples in a leaf node or the minimum number of samples required to split a node. Additionally, different pruning techniques can be used to reduce overfitting and improve generalization. Finally, ensembling techniques such as bagging and boosting can also be applied to further improve accuracy.

All these will prominently increase the indicative efficacy and accurateness of the entire AI model. We utilized two different MRI datasets such as Harvard medical dataset [29] and Figshare dataset [30].

Figures 8.7 and 8.8 depict the types of brain tumor, such as meningiomia, glioma, and pituitary, and the stages of brain tumor such as grade 1, 2, 3, and 4 under the glioma-type benign (cancerous) brain tumor. Fundamentally, brain tumor detection along with the metaverse and HCI helps utilization in a wide range of sensory inputs and highly immersive virtual environments in order to offer

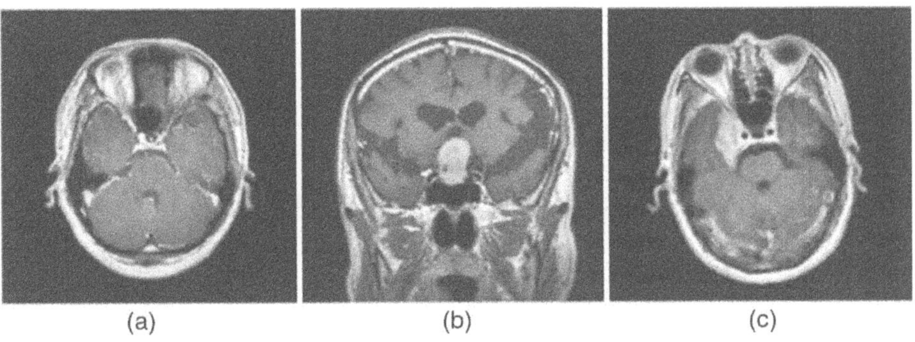

Figure 8.7   Types of brain tumor: (a) meningiomia, (b) glioma, and (c) pitutiary.

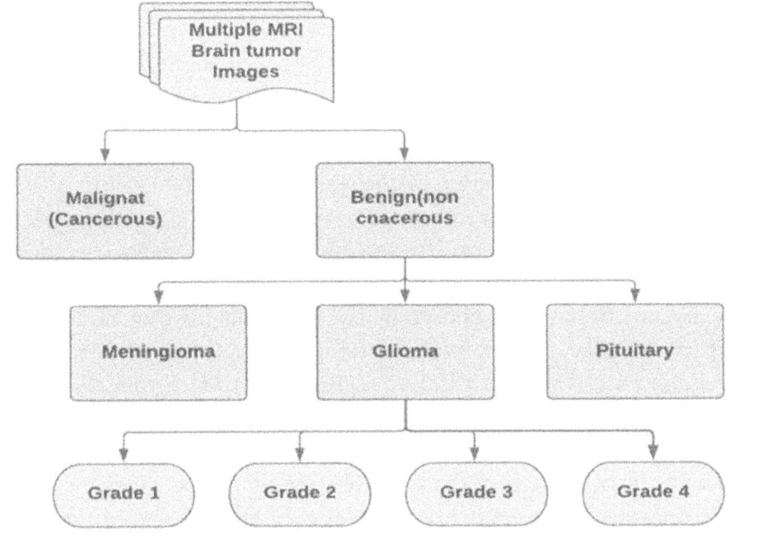

Figure 8.8   Stages of brain tumor detection using MRI.

an enjoyable and dynamic diagnosis procedure. Figure 8.9 depicts the steps in brain tumor detection using the random forest classifier.

Gini impurity is used to evaluate candidate splits at each node when building the tree. Gini impurity, denoted as Gini (D), for a dataset D with multiple classes is calculated by Equation 8.1, where D is the number of distinct classes in the dataset and dp is the proportion of data points belonging to class k in the dataset DS.

$$Gini\ (DS) = 1 - \sum_{k=1}^{D} dp_k^2 \qquad (8.1)$$

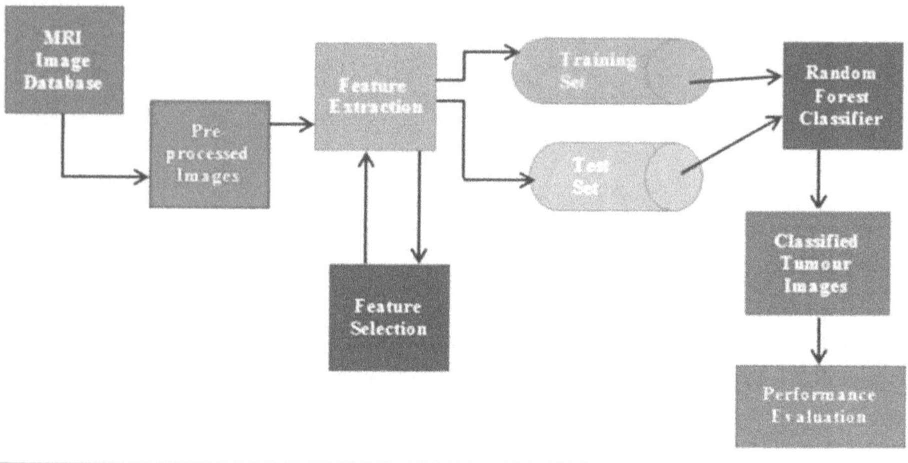

Figure 8.9   Steps in brain tumor detection.

The Gini impurity of a node is calculated as a weighted average of the Gini impurity of its child nodes. Then the Gini impurity of each child node is calculated. Weight each child's Gini impurity by the proportion of data points that belong to that child node. Subtract the weighted Gini impurities of the child nodes from the Gini impurity of the parent node. This results in the Gini impurity reduction (also known as the Gini gain) achieved by the split. The split that achieves the greatest reduction in Gini impurity is chosen as the best split for that node. This process is repeated recursively for each internal node in the tree until a stopping condition (e.g., maximum depth, minimum samples per leaf) is met. Gini impurity is a critical metric used in decision tree algorithms to assess the quality of attribute splits. It is used to select the most informative features for splitting and, as a result, is instrumental in constructing the decision tree that maximizes the separation of classes or categories in a classification problem. Table 8.1 shows the pseudo code for ODTA. Healthcare professionals may explore cells, tissues, and biological functions in extraordinary depth by becoming immersed in highly detailed models of human tissue into this virtual space. They may see data about patients immediately into these simulated images with AR overlays, which enable more understanding of intricate healthcare issues. These modern AI algorithms help common physicians to evaluate the accuracy in biological irregularities and imagery forecasting the key ailments. Practitioners in the medical field may receive immediate feedback and make more timely interventions with the help of these AI-driven tools for diagnosis that can quickly assess imaging scans, pathological slides, and other types of diagnostic procedures. People can research alternatives to treatment, learn more concerning their health issues, and establish peer support communities with people going through similar difficulties by using VR interactions. Moreover, the technology framework has made it easier for scholars, developers, and healthcare

Table 8.1　Pseudo Code of ODTA

Input: Trained dataset
Output: Classifier trained accuracy
Step 1: Start with assigning the root node to the entire dataset.
Step 2: Determine the best attribute to split the data for the root node by calculating the entropy and information gain for each attribute.
Step 3: Split the root node into subnodes based on the values of the best attribute.
Step 4: Repeat steps 2 and 3 until all of the data are covered in the leaf nodes.
Step 5: Prune the tree to avoid overfitting.
Step 6: Evaluate the performance of the decision tree using cross-validation or other appropriate methods.

experts from throughout the world working with one another. Experts may work cooperatively on difficult issues, share expertise, and co-design creative approaches to important health-related issues via shared virtual environments [9]. All things thought out, the metaverse's technical foundation for illness identification has enormous potential to transform healthcare delivery, raise the benchmark for clinical precision, and possibly enhance the results for patients in ways that were previously unimaginable. A pruning technique is used to reduce the size and complexity of decision trees. This can improve the generalization performance of the model, which means that it will be more likely to perform well on new data that it has not seen before. There are two main types of decision tree pruning. Prepruning involves stopping the growth of the tree before it reaches its full depth. This can be done by setting a maximum depth for the tree or by using a heuristic to decide when to stop growing the tree. Postpruning involves removing parts of the tree that have already grown. This can be done by removing subtrees that do not contribute significantly to the accuracy of the model or by removing subtrees that are likely to overfit the training data. Table 8.2 shows the MDL pruning algorithm.

Table 8.2　MDL Pruning Algorithm

Step 1: Start with the full decision tree.
Step 2: For each subtree, calculate the MDL of the tree with the subtree removed.
Step 3: Remove the subtree that results in the smallest increase in MDL.
Step 4: Repeat steps 2 and 3 until no further subtrees can be removed without increasing the MDL.

8.5 Experimentation

In this experiment, sample size was calculated for the control group of two using several baseline circumstances. The 3,726 input MRI datasets were considered and categorized into five classes with an accuracy of 92.7%. We utilized a previously preprocessed dataset from the Kaggle source, from two different MRI datasets such as the Harvard medical dataset [29] and the Figshare dataset [30]. Figure 8.10 depicts the proposed model implementation.

The following are the steps to be carried out for the implementation: Collect a dataset of historical accident data. This dataset should include information about vehicle physiognomies. Clean and prepare the data. This may involve removing outliers, converting categorical variables to numerical variables, and scaling the data. Split the data into training and test sets. The training set will be used to train the decision tree model, and the test set will be used to evaluate the performance of the model. Train the decision tree model. This involves feeding the training data to the decision tree algorithm. The algorithm will learn to predict whether an accident will occur based on the input data. Evaluate the performance of the model on the test set. Then integrating the model with a software application or a hardware device [37].

For the experiment, all analyses were carried out using statistical software for social sciences (SPSS). For the ODTA and the support vector machine algorithm, descriptive statistics (mean, standard deviation, and standard error) are computed. The independent variables include road type, hidden correlation between weather conditions, time, and vehicle domain, where time frequency comprises

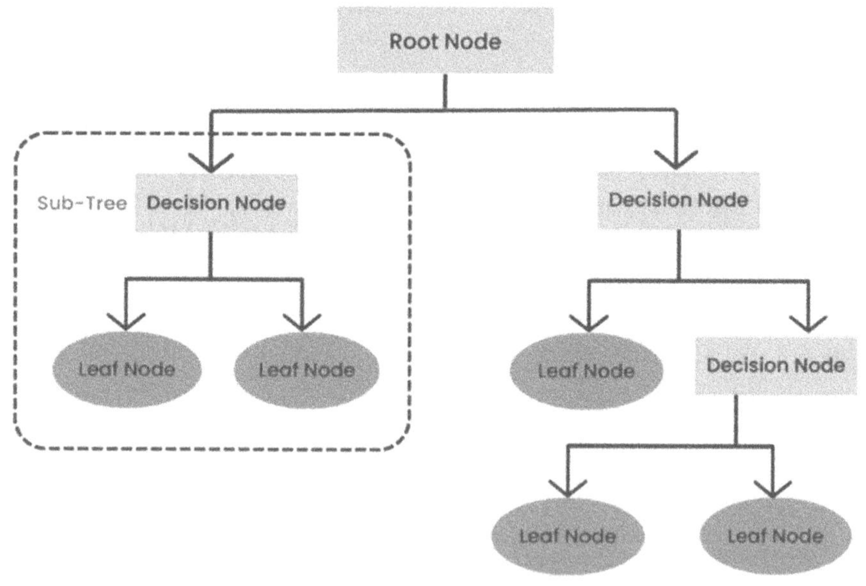

Figure 8.10   Basic structure of the proposed ODTA classifier.

mean, median, and variance and vehicle domain includes wavelet transforms. The dependent variables were the driver's age, the vehicle's age, and the road conditions. To compare the performance of an algorithm, an independent sample t is used. According to the results of the analysis, the accuracy rate has improved. In this comparison, the accuracy of the ODTA method (92.70%) appears to be higher than that of the convolutional neural network (CNN) approach (61.80%).

8.6 Results and Discussions

For forecasting the accuracy, ODTA (N = 10) was used, and other ML algorithms were iterated for various times. Two sample groups are considered and tested, and G-power is calculated, which includes two separate groups, alpha (0.05) and power (80%), and an environment ratio. Our ODTA gained 99.12% precision, 98.26% recall, 98.7% accuracy, and an F1 score of 99.24%. With a p-value of 0.001, the ODTA approach appears to be more significant than the other machine algorithms. In the context of the present subject, the ODTA provides the highest accuracy in detecting the brain tumors from two different MRI datasets, such as the Harvard medical dataset [29] and the Figshare dataset [30]. The CNN gained precision of 80%, recall of 78.09%, the accuracy of 71.80%, and an F1 score of 81.10%. Table 8.3 depicts the predicted efficiency.

Table 8.4 presents the ODTA and CNN classifier mean, standard deviation, and difference. This table summarizes the results based on accident prediction

Table 8.3   Predicted Road Design Efficiency

Algorithm	Accuracy (%)	Precision (%)	Recall (%)	F1-Score (%)
ODTA	98.7	99.12	98.26	99.24
CNN	71.80	80.0	78.09	81.10

Table 8.4   Individual T Test Result Comparison

Metrics		T Test for Equality of Mean		
		Mean Difference	Std, Error Difference	95% Confidence Interval of the Difference
Accuracy	**Anticipated equal variances**	0.62	0.4308	−0.388
	Unanticipated equal variances	0.62	0.4308	−0.3409

```
d on accuracy score
df_acc=pd.DataFrame(list(zip(algo_lst, accuracy_lst)), columns=['Algorithm','Accuracy_Score']).s
ort_values(by=['Accuracy_Score'],ascending = True)

# Export to a file
df_acc.to_csv('./Accuracy_scores_algorithms_{}.csv'.format(state),index=False)

# Make a plot
ax=df_acc.plot.barh('Algorithm', 'Accuracy_Score', align='center',legend=False,color='0.5')

# Add the data label on to the plot
for i in ax.patches:
    # get_width pulls left or right; get_y pushes up or down
    ax.text(i.get_width()+0.02, i.get_y()+0.2, str(round(i.get_width(),2)), fontsize=10)

# Set the limit, lables, ticks and title
plt.xlim(0,1.1)
plt.xlabel('Accuracy Score')
plt.yticks(y_ticks, df_acc['Algorithm'], rotation=0)
plt.title('[{}-{}] Which algorithm is better?'.format(state, county))
```

Figure 8.11   Model implementation of ODTA classifier.

using ODTA and achieves significantly better results, as the difference between the two groups were p = 0.03 using Independent Sample T Test. Figure 8.11 depicts the brain tumor detection using the ODTA approach. Based on the results from Table 8.5, the statistical significance of the ODTA is high. The ODTA approach has an accuracy mean of 92.7%, a standard deviation of 1.09 for the sample size of N = 5, whereas the CNN has an accuracy mean of 71.80% and a standard deviation of 0.875 for the sample size of N = 5.

Figure 8.12 depicts the brain tumor detection using ODTA approach. Medical datasets of Harvard and Figshare are classified as no tumor, tumor, meningiomia, glioma, and pituitary.

Table 8.5 shows group statistics results. A mean of ODTA 92.7 is more compared with the support machine algorithm 61.80, the standard error mean for CNN is 1.09, and OTDA is 0.87. Comparing ODTA and CNN in terms of mean accuracy and precision, the ODTA is better than the support vector machine algorithm. The standard deviation of ODTA is slightly better than CNN. The y-axis shows the mean accuracy of detection is ± 1 SD. Also, along with AI, the metaverse permitted

Table 8.5   Group Statistical Result Comparison

Metrics	Algorithm	N	Mean	Std. Deviation	Std. Error Mean
Accuracy	**ODTA**	5	92.7	1.09	0.3541
	CNN	5	61.8	0.876	0.2769

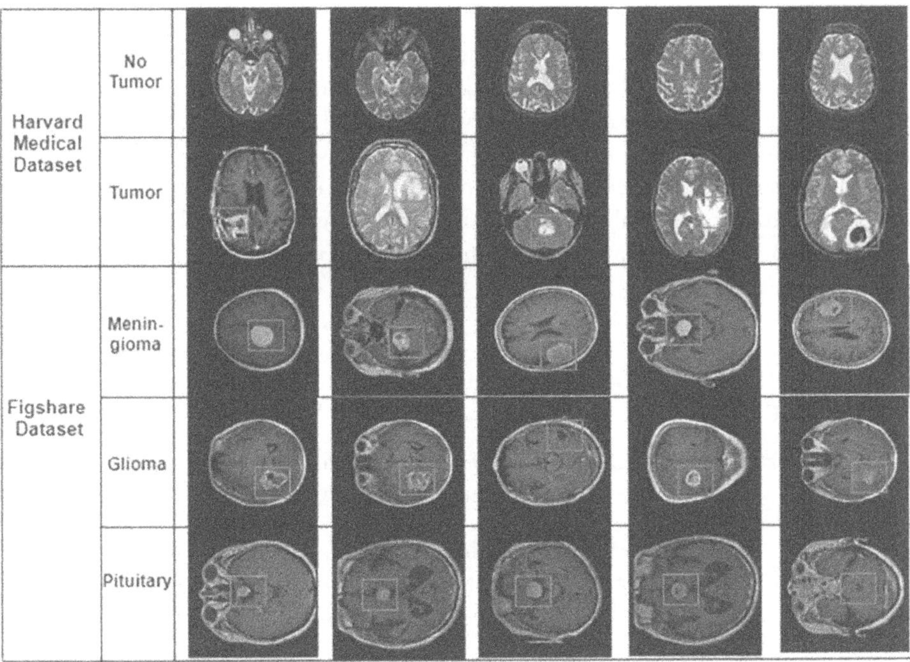

Figure 8.12   Results of the ODTA classifier in brain tumor detection.

the creation of groundbreaking cloud and immediate interaction technologies, which greatly improved the near-term prospects of the medical field. Furthermore, the realm of the metaverse may be able to achieve its maximum potential due to breakthroughs in technology like wearables as well as intelligent machines, which could have a big influence on the field of healthcare.

8.7 Conclusion

MIR is extensively used for locating the internal organs from the digital images for therapeutic dedications like determining otherwise reviewing about different syndromes in our body [38–39]. The key goal of MIR is to increase the effectiveness of medical research and disease management opportunities. The major needs for which MIR is utilized are the following: image segmentation, augmentation, localization, disease diagnosis, early disease prediction, classification, and sorting different types/stages of a disease. In the past, low-level techniques like thresholding, region expanding, and edge tracing were used to process medical images. The metaverse is a cutting-edge technology in the field of radiology that leverages medical image analysis to the next arena, integrating the AR and VR in MIR powered with AI for disease detection, diagnosis, and treatment planning. The notion of the metaverse is an extensive, unified digital world with combinational components of AR, VR, and the Internet. Within the perspective of radiology, this technology will possibly transfigure the way clinical images are inferred, united, and exploited. The amalgamation of the metaverse along with HCI unwraps a domain of opportunities aimed at making individuals and digital environs much more interactive. Radiologists might practice their imaging by the use of VR headsets for immersing their mind inside a virtual setting, where they can interpret and handle the medical images as 3D models, possibly refining their capability to detect multifaceted medical diseases.

References

1. Magadza, T., & Viriri, S. (2021). Deep learning for brain tumor segmentation: A survey of state-of-the-art. Journal of Imaging, 7(2), 19. https://doi.org/10.3390/jimaging7020019
2. Yaqub, M., Feng, J., Zia, M. S., Arshid, K., Jia, K., Rehman, Z. U., & Mehmood, A. (2020). State-of-the-art CNN optimizer for brain tumor segmentation in magnetic resonance images. Brain Sciences, 10(7), 427. https://doi.org/10.3390/brainsci10070427
3. Zhao, Y., Ren, X., Hou, K., & Li, W. (2021). Recurrent multi-fiber network for 3D MRI brain tumor segmentation. Symmetry, 13(2), 320. https://doi.org/10.3390/sym13020320
4. Alam, M. S., Rahman, M. M., Hossain, M. A., Islam, M. K., Ahmed, K. M., Ahmed, K. T., & Miah, M. S. (2019). Automatic human brain tumor detection in MRI image using template-based K means and improved fuzzy C means clustering algorithm. Big Data and Cognitive Computing, 3(2), 27. https://doi.org/10.3390/bdcc3020027
5. Joshi, D., & Channe, H. (2020). A survey on brain tumor detection based on structural MRI using deep learning and machine learning techniques. International Journal of Scientific & Technology Research, 9(4), 17–23. http://www.ijstr.org/final-print/apr2020/A-Survey-On-Brain-Tumor-Detection-Based-On-Structural-Mri-Using-Machine-Learning-And-Deep-Learning-Techniques.pdf
6. Liu, Z., Chen, L., Tong, L., Zhou, F., Jiang, Z., Zhang, Q., & Zhou, H. (2021). Deep learning based brain tumor segmentation: A survey. Journal of Latex Class Files, 14(8), 15460–15476.
7. Suganthe, R. C., Revathi, G., Monisha, S., & Pavithran, R. (2020). Deep learning based brain tumor classification using magnetic resonance imaging. Journal of Critical Reviews, 7(9), 347–350. http://www.jcreview.com/?mno=111627
8. Wu, W., Li, D., Du, J., Gao, X., Gu, W., Zhao, F., & Feng, X. (2020). An intelligent diagnosis method of brain MRI tumor segmentation using deep convolutional neural network and SVM algorithm. Computational and Mathematical Methods in Medicine, 2020, 6789306.
9. Nasor, M., & Obaid, W. (2020). Detection and localization of early-stage multiple brain tumors using a hybrid technique of patch-based processing, k-means clustering and object counting. Hindawi International Journal of Biomedical Imaging, 2020, 9035096. https://doi.org/10.1155/2020/9035096

10. Hasan, A. M., Jalab, H. A., Meziane, F., Kahtan, H., & Ahmad, A. S. (2019). Combine deep and handcrafted image character for MRI brain scan classification. IEEE Access, 7, 79959–79967. https://ieeexplore.ieee.org/stamp/stamp.jsp?arnumber=8736208

11. Zaw, H. T., Maneerat, N., & Win, K. Y. (2019). Detection of brain tumor based on Naïve Bayes classification. International Conference on Engineering, Applied Sciences and Technology, pp. 1–4. https://www.jetir.org/papers/JETIR2104081.pdf

12. Anaraki, A. K., Moosa, A., & Kazemi, F. (2019). MRI-based brain tumor grades classification and grading via convolutional neural networks and genetic algorithms. Biocybernetics and Biomedical Engineering, pp. 63–74. https://www.sciencedirect.com/science/article/abs/pii/S0208521618300676

13. Gupta, N., & Khanna, P. (2017). A non-invasive and adaptive CAD system to detect brain tumor from T2-weighted MRIs using customized Otsu's thresholding with prominent features and supervised learning. Signal Processing Image Communication, pp. 1–9.

14. Deepak, S., & Ameer, P. M. (2019). Brain tumor classification using deep CNN features via transfer learning. Computers in Biology and Medicine, 111, 103345. https://doi.org/10.1016/j.compbiomed.2019.103345

15. Ronneberger, O., Fischer, P., & Brox, T. (2015). U-net: Convolutional networks for biomedical image segmentation. Lecture Notes in Computer Science, Proceedings of the International Conference on Medical Image Computing and Computer-Assisted Intervention, Munich, Germany, 5–9 October 2015, 234–241. https://arxiv.org/abs/1505.04597

16. Heinrich, M. P., Oktay, O., & Bouteldja, N. (2019). Obelisk-net: Fewer layers to solve 3D multi-organ segmentation with sparse deformable convolutions. Medical Image Analysis, 54, 1–9. https://doi.org/10.1016/j.media.2019.02.006

17. Naseera, S., Rajini, G. K., Venkateswarlu, B., & Priyadarisini, J. P. (2017). A review on image processing application in medical field. Research Journal of Pharmacy and Technology, 10(10), 3456–3460. https://doi.org/10.5958/0974-360X.2017.00644.8

18. Muthumeenakshi, M. (2016). An application of pentagonal valued hesitant fuzzy set in medical diagnosis. Research Journal of Pharmacy and Technology, 9(10), 1823–1826.

19. Dange, V. N., Shid, S. J., Magdum, C. S., & Mohite, S. K. (2017). A review on breast cancer: An overview. Asian Journal of Pharmaceutical Research, 7(1), 49–51.

20. Zhao, Y. X., Zhang, Y. M., & Liu, C. L. (2020). Bag of tricks for 3D MRI brain tumor segmentation. In A. Crimi & S. Bakas (Eds.), Brainlesion: Glioma, Multiple Sclerosis, Stroke and Traumatic Brain Injuries (pp. 210–220). Springer International Publishing.

21. Anaraki, A. K., Ayati, M., & Kazemi, F. (2019). Magnetic resonance imaging-based brain tumor grades classification and grading via convolutional neural networks and genetic algorithms. Biocybernetics and Biomedical Engineering, 39(1), 63–74.

22. Ker, J., Wang, L., Rao, J., & Lim, T. (2018). Deep learning applications in medical image analysis. IEEE Access, 6, 9375–9389.

23. Işın, A., Direkoğlu, C., & Şah, M. (2016). Review of MRI-based brain tumor image segmentation using deep learning methods. Procedia Computer Science, 102, 317–324.

24. Dong, H., Yang, G., Liu, F., Mo, Y., & Guo, Y. (2017). Automatic brain tumor detection and segmentation using U-net based fully convolutional networks. Communications in Computer and Information Science, 1, 506–517.

25. Cheng, J., Huang, W., & Cao, S., et al. (2015). Enhanced performance of brain tumor classification via tumor region augmentation and partition. PLoS One, 10(10), e0140381.

26. Kumar, R., & Arthanariee, A. M. (2014). Performance evaluation and comparative analysis of proposed image segmentation algorithm. Indian Journal of Science and Technology, 7(1), 39–47.

27. Liu, J., Li, M., Wang, J., Wu, F., Liu, T., & Pan, Y. (2014). A survey of MRI-based brain tumor segmentation methods. Tsinghua Science and Technology, 19(6), 578–595.

28. Bahadure, N. B., Ray, A. K., & Thethi, H. P. (2017). Image analysis for MRI based brain tumor detection and feature extraction using biologically inspired BWT and SVM. International Journal of Biomedical Imaging, 2017, 9749108.

29. Li, H., Li, A., & Wang, M. (2019). A novel end-to-end brain tumor segmentation method using improved fully convolutional networks. Computer Methods and Programs in Biomedicine, 108, 150–160.

30. Glorot, X., & Bengio, Y. (2010). Understanding the Difficulty of Training Deep Feedforward Neural Networks. In Proceedings of the Thirteenth International Conference on Artificial Intelligence and Statistics (pp. 249–256).

31. Balasubramaniam, S, Kadry, S., & Kumar, K. S. (2024). Osprey Gannet optimization enabled CNN based transfer learning for optic disc detection and cardiovascular risk prediction using retinal fundus images. Biomedical Signal Processing and Control, 93, 106177.

32. Pereira, S., Pinto, A., Alves, V., & Silva, C. A. (2016). Brain tumor segmentation using convolutional neural networks in MRI images. IEEE Transactions on Medical Imaging, 35, 1240–1251.

33. Casamitjana, A., Puch, S., Aduriz, A., Sayrol, E., & Vilaplana, V. (2016). 3D Convolutional Networks for Brain Tumor Segmentation. In Proceedings of the MICCAI Challenge on Multimodal Brain Tumor Image Segmentation (BRATS), 65–68.

34. S, B., Kadry, S., & Dhanaraj, R. K., et al. (2024). Res-Unet based blood vessel segmentation and cardiovascular disease prediction using chronological chef-based optimization algorithm based deep residual network from retinal fundus images. Multimedia Tools and Applications. https://doi.org/10.1007/s11042-024-18810-y

35. Mlynarski, P., Delingette, H., Criminisi, A., & Ayache, N. (2019). Deep learning with mixed supervision for brain tumor segmentation. Journal of Medical Imaging, 6, 034002.

36. Iqbal, S., Ghani Khan, M. U., Saba, T., Mehmood, Z., Javaid, N., Rehman, A., & Abbasi, R. (2019). Deep learning model integrating features and novel classifiers fusion for brain tumor segmentation. Microscopy Research and Technique, 82, 1302–1315.

37. Gollagi, S. G., & Balasubramaniam, S (2023). Hybrid model with optimization tactics for software defect prediction. International Journal of Modeling, Simulation, and Scientific Computing, 14(2), 2350031.

38. Sethy, P. K., & Behera, S. K. (2021). A data constrained approach for brain tumour detection using fused deep features and SVM. Multimedia Tools and Applications, 80, 28745–28760.

39. Lamrani, D., Cherradi, B., El Gannour, O., Bouqentar, M. A., & Bahatti, L. (2022). Brain tumor detection using MRI images and convolutional neural network. International Journal of Advanced Computer Science and Applications, 13, 452–460.

Chapter 9

Brain–Computer Interface of an Immersive Virtual Metaverse for Preventive Brain Healthcare and Neurorehabilitation

Pankaj Rahi, Abolfazl Mehbodniya, Julian L. Webber, Sayed Sayeed Ahmad, and Radha Raman Chandan

9.1 Introduction

The metaverse is an emerging technology concept that seeks to integrate multiple virtual world technologies to enhance the depth and longevity of 3D experiences. The main emphasis is on social aspects and the creation of information, rather than virtual or augmented reality. While virtual reality (VR) and augmented reality (AR) have proven to be effective in addressing mobility and cognitive impairments, they have inherent limitations when it comes to those with neurological disorders [1].

The metaverse is centered on the concept of providing services and is specifically designed to facilitate social interaction and content creation. The progress relies on advancements in virtual experiences and technology, encompassing artificial intelligence (AI), the Internet of Things (IoT), and blockchain. These technologies aim to establish a seamless connection between the virtual and physical realms, mirroring

DOI: 10.1201/9781003491668-9

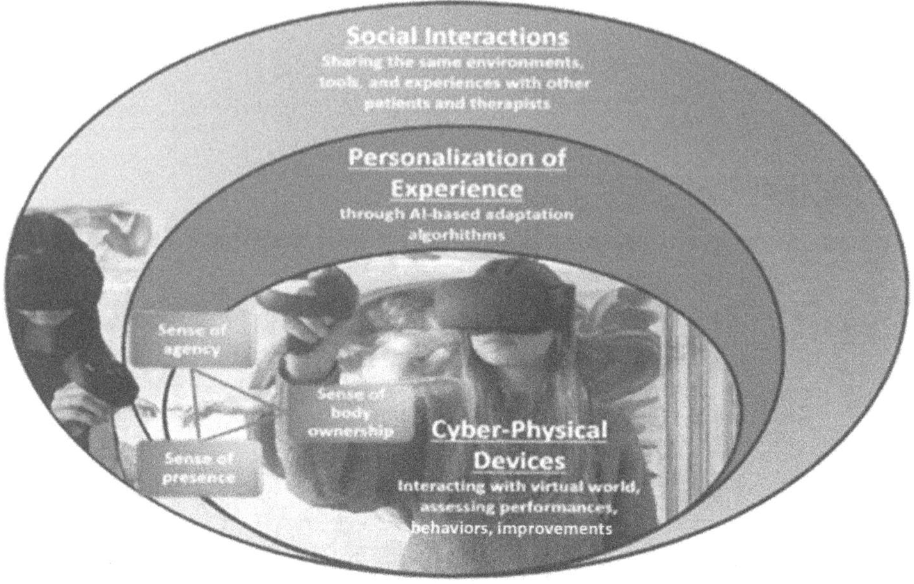

Figure 9.1 Hierarchical framework of application of the metaverse in clinical care.

the functioning of human brains. AI has the capacity to revolutionize customized mental healthcare by enabling the creation of customized treatment alternatives for each person [2]. To incorporate the metaverse into medicine, substantial advancements and the creation of novel technologies are necessary to enhance the level of immersion in virtual encounters (refer to Figure 9.1). The upcoming phase of innovation has the capacity to overcome the current constraints of VR usages in medical procedures, hence enhancing the effectiveness of VR-constructed medications in comparison to traditional methods. According to the most recent research [1], multiple investigations have demonstrated that altering patients' internal body perceptions through the use of virtual bodies can effectively impact specific clinical issues [2]. The topmost layer facilitates social interaction via Internet connections, enabling individuals, therapists, carers, and friends to share their environments, resources, experiences, and data. From this standpoint, the concept of possessing one's own body is connected to the most essential aspect of human identity. The correlation between the sense of organization in one's activities and individual experiences within the virtual realm is evident. The concept of proximity encompasses not only an individual's personal existence but also the existence of others in social environments [1, 2].

The diagram in Figure 9.1 depicts the hierarchical framework for utilizing the metaverse in therapeutic neurorehabilitation. The infrastructure layer consists of a unique array of wearable sensors and devices that offer various physical-digital environments to enhance immersive experiences. To deliver a tailored metaverse therapy session, the customization layer integrates AI services with other distributed web functionalities. This personalized experience is meticulously crafted to align with the patient's distinct characteristics and address their specific clinical requirements. Positioned at the pinnacle is a layer that fosters online social interaction among patients, therapists, caregivers, and family members, facilitating the sharing of settings, resources, knowledge, and information. Autonomy over one's own body is a fundamental aspect of individuality [1, 2].

9.1.1 Explanation of Metaverse

A. The metaverse is a useful grouping of implicit interaction, collaborative gaming, and AR using eyewear that represents the enhancement of all real-world objects in the form of digital elements. Advanced VR reality headsets allow users to interact with others in fully simulated digital worlds, facilitated by digital currencies [3].
B. The metaverse comprises of a complex association of connected simulated domains that aid entities to participate in legitimate societal collaborations, events, function, and spending and buying activities [4].
C. The metaverse is a radiant simulated sphere comprising of persistent digital surroundings. By agreeing to avatars, which behave as digital depictions of themselves, individuals can enter this shared digital space and actively participate in live discussions and interactions [5].
D. The metaverse employs cutting-edge technologies such as AI, AR, VR, telepresence robots, digital twinning, and blockchain-based secure online transaction systems to have a substantial influence on healthcare [6].

Utilizing these technologies allows for the exploration of novel methods for delivering treatment at a substantially reduced expense, hence improving patient outcomes. Using the metaverse, an online platform that simulates a virtual world, users can act and feel as if they are in the real thing. In its whole, the idea incorporates the digital and physical worlds' social and economic structures [7].

9.2 Metaverse in Healthcare Domains

The field of digital health is fundamentally transforming the provision of healthcare and playing a crucial role in driving innovation in the biotechnology and pharmaceutical industries. The COVID-19 pandemic has also spurred innovators and healthcare professionals to devise methods for remotely handling patients and reducing their reliance on hospitals.

The proliferation of smartphones and the growing adoption of wearable gadgets have also played a significant role in facilitating this trend.

As per the prediction in 2021, four major changes in the worldwide medical sector are expected: the entry of major technology corporations into healthcare, the exploitation of consumer data for financial gain, the establishment of health data markets, and the rise of Asia as a prominent player in digital health. The metaverse is commonly linked to games and entertainment, although its underlying technology has practical uses in healthcare at present. AR, VR, and mixed reality (MR), which encompass extended reality (XR); Web3 technology and applications, such as blockchain and virtual assets; and M-worlds, which are interactive virtual environments where users gather and create content. Currently, the majority of healthcare applications are around XR. These technologies are being used in various diagnostic and therapeutic applications, as well as in medical education, meetings, and conferences. Companies are also conducting trials with blockchain technology for other purposes, such as verifying supply chains and managing and storing healthcare data.

Metaverse technology has the potential to enhance the value of organizations through various means, which include:

- Enhancing healthcare accessibility by connecting patients with physicians irrespective of their geographical location.
- Using advanced technologies to enhance the precision of diagnoses and the quality of surgical procedures.
- Minimizing expenses in healthcare provision, medical education, and data management.
- Enabling novel opportunities for storing, sharing, and retrieving data related to patients, claims, and healthcare providers.
- Enhancing the satisfaction of patients and insurance plan members while expanding sources of income through the introduction of new services.
- Optimizing processes such as recruitment, training, and payment, operating expenses can be minimized.

Phase-wise representation of technology mapping with metaverse applications shown in Figure 9.2.

9.3 Metaverse and Brain–Computer Interface

The metaverse is a nascent technological development in the digital realm that holds immense promise in the field of healthcare, facilitating lifelike encounters for both patients and medical professionals. The metaverse is a convergence of several advanced technologies like AI, VR, additive reality, the Internet of medical equipment, robotics, quantum computing, and more. It offers opportunities to explore innovative approaches for delivering high-quality healthcare treatment and services. The combination of all these technologies guarantees a fully immersive, close, and

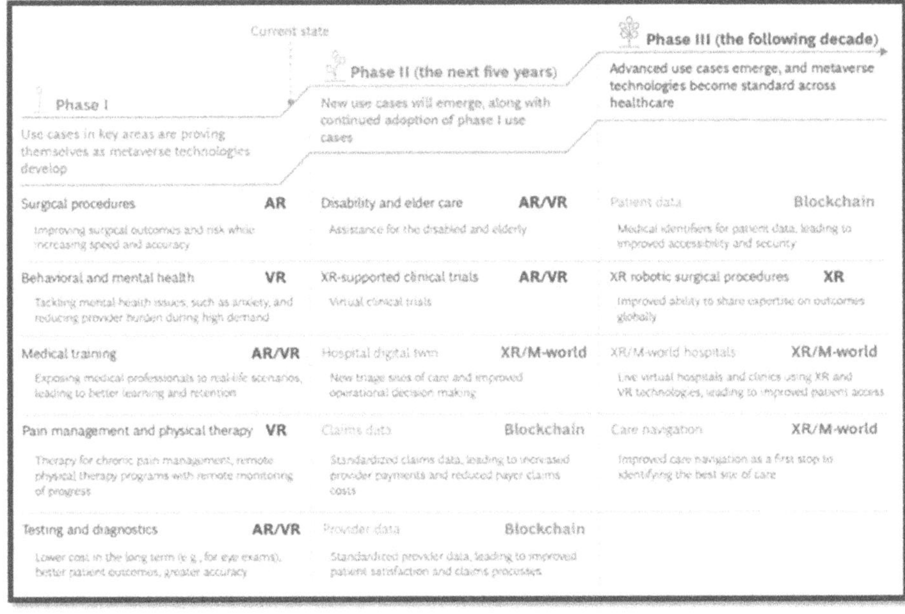

Figure 9.2 Phase-wise representation of technology mapping with metaverse applications.

tailored patient care experience. Additionally, it offers adaptable intelligent solutions that remove the obstacles between healthcare professionals and recipients.

9.3.1 Noninvasive Brain Stimulations

The brain is a highly responsive structure in the body that can detect and adapt to both external and interior environmental stimuli. Neuroscience has made significant progress in understanding the mechanism of neuronal plasticity in the present year [8]. Noninvasive brain stimulation (NIBS) represented in Figure 9.3, describes that NIBS has the ability to enhance the excitability of certain regions of the brain. Combining it with personalized, activity-specific, rigorous therapy can result in more significant enhancements in function compared to rehabilitation alone. NIBS is a painless and safe technique that has been widely employed in thousands of individuals globally, with minimal occurrence of side effects. The objective is to enhance the overall well-being and mitigate the impact of challenges associated with speech, swallowing, mobility, cognition, and other bodily processes [9]. There are two possible techniques to achieve this:

- Applying targeted stimulation to the impaired region of the brain in order to facilitate the recovery of the afflicted function
- Inducing neural activity in an alternative brain region to offset the impairment in functionality

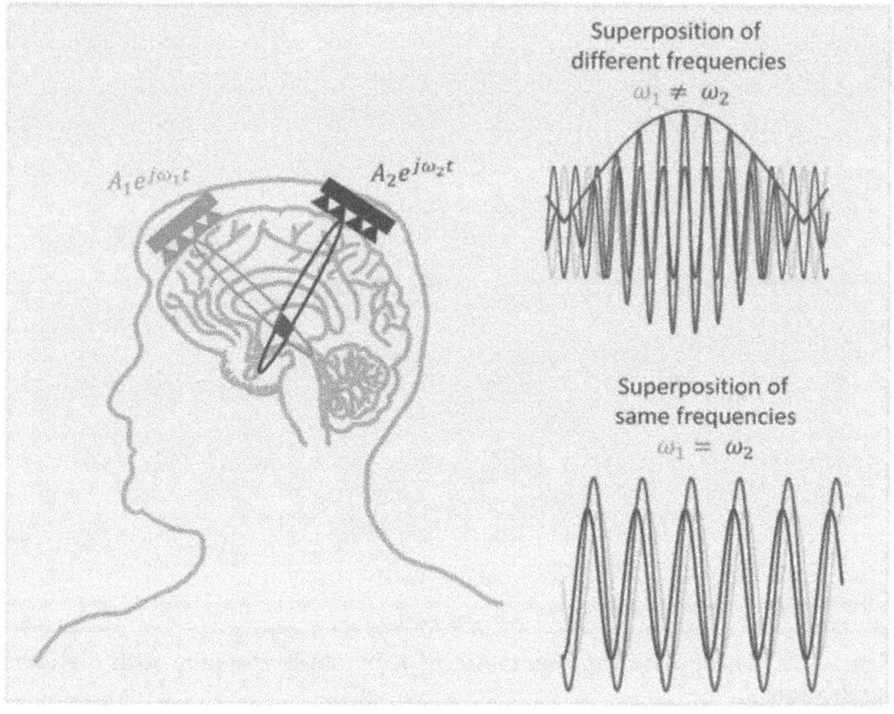

Figure 9.3 Noninvasive stimulation of brain.

9.4 Brain–Computer Interface, Immersive Metaverse, and Neurorehabilitation

Neurotechnology encompasses the utilization of sophisticated methods and approaches within the realm of neuroscience.

Neurotechnology refers to any technologies that have the ability to study the human brain and its activities. Neurotechnology applies countless practices and methodologies for recording brain motion and accelerating numerous chunks of the intellect/brain. Figure 9.4 elucidates an electroencephalogram (EEG) representation which captures the brain's electrical activity via electrodes placed on the scalp. The EEG signal displays wave patterns generated by synchronized neural firing, commonly categorized into different frequency bands, such as delta, theta, alpha, beta, and gamma waves. These patterns offer insight into various brain states, from deep relaxation to intense cognitive processing, and serve as a valuable tool in brain–computer interface (BCI) applications, enabling real-time monitoring and interpretation of brain activity for neurorehabilitation and preventive brain healthcare.

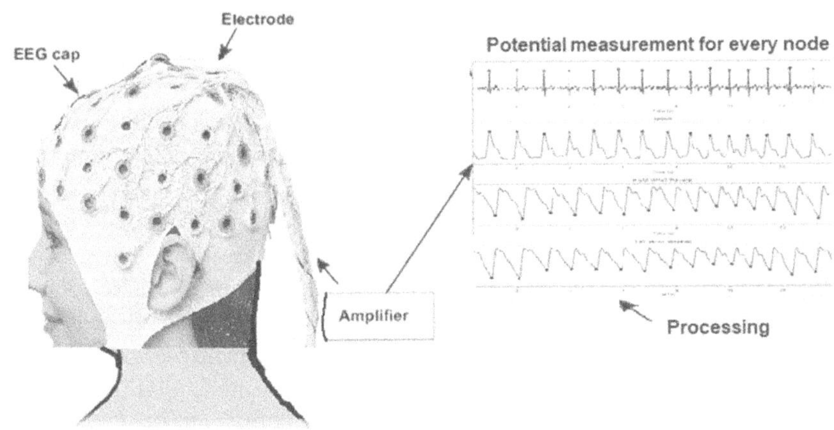

Figure 9.4 Depiction of an electroencephalogram (EEG).

An EEG is a method utilized to record and measure the electrical activity of the brain by situating electrodes on the scalp [10, 11].

Functional near-infrared spectroscopy (fNIRS) is a technique that employs a portable sensor to accurately assess brain activity. fNIRS is a noninvasive method for imaging the brain.

There exist various techniques that can stimulate the brain, including:

a. Deep brain stimulation (DBS) is a clinically invasive method that involves the infusing the placement of an electrode to identify and improve indications and other brain-related troubles. Focused ultrasound (FUS) is a noninvasive device that uses pulsing waves to selectively activate certain areas of the brain [12]. In addition, it can be applied to the nasal and ocular regions, providing cures for ailments and assisting in the patient's expeditious recuperation.
b. Transcranial magnetic stimulation (TMS) is a method that uses a magnetic field to generate electrical currents in the brain. Moreover, it possesses the capacity to increase interneuronal transmission and augment cognitive activities such as learning, perception, and memory.
c. Transcranial electrical stimulation (TES) is a noninvasive technique that entails placing electrodes on the scalp to activate certain brain activities.

9.5 Neurorehabilitation Approach Using Metaverse and VR Technologies

9.5.1 Sleep Management for Preventive Mentacare-Metaverse

A large number of people suffer from sleep disruptions, including insomnia, which have a substantial impact on their daily functioning. Studies have shown that almost a quarter of adults have insomnia [12]. Furthermore, researchers asserted that insomnia has an adverse effect on both physical health and emotional well-being. Sleep disorders, such as disruptions in sleep patterns, have been theorized to be strongly linked to various factors, including psychological stress, lack of acknowledgment, inadequate social support, feelings of danger, emotional strain, and an imbalance between work and personal life [13].

Neurorehabilitation technology, such as robotics, exoskeletons, VR, brain user interfaces, and observation procedures, are improving the advancement of neuro-rehabilitation technology development by tackling different obstacles. The future research tool that employs a brain—machine interface is combined with software specifically tailored to improve neurorehabilitation [14]. Neuro-oncology is a constantly evolving area that seeks to understand the diverse molecular underpinnings of the central nervous system. Novel medications are being employed to investigate the categorization of tumors, specifically those affecting the brain.

EEGs are instruments employed to observe and analyze brain activity by detecting electrical impulses transmitted through the skull. They play a vital role in the detection of several seizure disorders that impact brain functionality. Wearable monitoring technologies play a vital role in evaluating the neurological state of patients and monitoring their activities. Pedometers, accelerometers, and diverse multisensory systems possess the capacity to understand physical capacities and track neurological conditions. The rehabilitation therapy is classified into three main categories: occupational, speech, and physical. This classification is beneficial for treating developmental problems and helping patients achieve a strong and active lifestyle. fMRI is a commonly employed magnetic resonance imaging (MRI) technique that is essential for understanding alterations in brain functions. Nanotechnologies are being employed to augment future healthcare by enabling physicians to identify early indications of cancer, formulate precise treatments, and ensure treatment efficacy. It should be emphasized that these developments do not have any effect on the three primary areas of oncology, specifically radiation oncology, medical oncology, and surgical oncology [15]. The radio frequencies are monitored using diverse GPS devices, which are beneficial for understanding the process of expansion.

Intraoperative computed tomography (ICT) is an advanced medical imaging method that improves the accuracy and safety of electrode implantation in the brain. The patients stay unresponsive during the surgical operation and do not regain consciousness during the medical imaging process.

People who are tetraplegic and use sophisticated prostheses understand the idea of brain plasticity, which is helpful when understanding how brain-controlled limb stimulators work. The electric currents generated by these stimulators help to improve brain activity. Neurorehabilitation is improving as a groundbreaking innovative technique for improving the growth by employing and following the perceptions from neuroscience [16]. MRI is a complicated procedure utilized to analyze the brain and produce complete three-dimensional structural images. The monitoring system has been enhanced by integrating four distinct categories: observation, analysis, storage, and action. These technical advancements are essential for comprehending the complexities of monitoring brain restoration. AI is improving the skill of surgeons by reducing errors in neurosurgery. The discipline of robotics is experiencing substantial expansion, which has the potential to ultimately supplant neurosurgeons in the utilization of numerous minimally invasive procedures for the brain and spine. Modern operations utilize highly efficient technologies such as AI, surgical robots, 3D printing, and imaging systems. Obstacles to overcome in the field of neurorehabilitation technologies include time limits, social influence, low energy levels, and limited skills and resources.

Neurostimulation technologies are assisting paralyzed persons in recovering the capacity to walk, highlighting the importance of different prosthetic technologies in promoting progress in the medical profession [17]. Technological advancements including DBS, visual stimulation, and phytopharmacology procedures are employed to facilitate the growth of neuroscience. Neurogenetic disorders are defined by the presence of specific gene abnormalities, which offer important understanding of the process of social stimulation.

9.6 Radio Frequency and SAR Value Emissions and Effect on Metal Health

9.6.1 Current Research Investigating the Impact of Mobile Phones on Human Health

Numerous global research has been conducted on radio frequency (RF) radiation and its impact on the human body. A significant distinction exists between a biological effect, which refers to an impact on the body, and a health effect [18].

For instance, the RF radiation emitted by a mobile phone causes a localized increase in brain temperature by a small fraction of a degree. This biological phenomenon does not inherently pose any health hazards. The human body possesses the ability to tolerate significant fluctuations in temperature without suffering any detrimental effects.

9.6.2 Mobile Phones and Potential Health Impacts

Current research is examining the possible health impacts of cell phone use beyond cancer, although no harmful health effects have been found up to this point. Mobile phone usage can potentially lead to other indirect health implications. For example:

■ RF radiation can potentially disrupt medical electronic equipment that is susceptible to the electromagnetic field. Mobile devices should be powered off within hospital premises.

■ Empirical evidence suggests that engaging in mobile phone use while driving substantially increases the probability of being engaged in a motor vehicle collision. It is illegal to operate a handheld mobile phone while operating a motor vehicle in any Australian state or territory.

9.6.3 Measures to Minimize Exposure to Mobile Phone Radiation

■ The current evidence indicates that mobile phones do not pose any harm. However, the long-term hazards and repercussions associated with their use still need to be explained.

■ To mitigate your exposure to RF radiation, you can take the following measures: To minimize your exposure to RF radiation, it is recommended to use a mobile phone model that has a low specific absorption rate (SAR). The SAR quantifies the extent to which tissues in your body absorb RF radiation. It is recommended to use a landline telephone if possible. In addition, it is recommended to keep mobile phone talks brief and utilize a hands-free device. Avoid placing the mobile or gadget in closure-proximity of the body once it is gone on. Exercise caution when assessing claims that protective equipment or "shields" can reduce your exposure to RF radiation, as there is no scientifically proven evidence supporting the effectiveness of such devices. The existence of a shield can really enhance RF radiation, as the phone will increase its RF emission to compensate for the shield's effect and achieve the best possible communication efficiency.

9.6.4 Potential Advantages of the Metaverse on Psychological Well-Being

Collaborations and exchanges in the metaverse are expected to be an enhanced iteration of existing VR experiences, characterized by more authentic and realistic interactions. The metaverse has the ability to create a community where people may establish new connections, engage in social activities, and sustain relationships. It can enable effortless relationships between patients and psychological care providers by employing avatars in simulated environments. Considering the boundless potential of virtual simulation, it is expected that the metaverse could provide numerous chances to create innovative methods for addressing various mental health disorders. The metaverse is emerging as a platform for mental health support. It offers dedicated spaces for group therapy, led by professionals or peers [19]. Additionally, immersive environments enhance practices like meditation, mindful breathing, and yoga [19]. Companies are creating virtual clinics staffed by mental health specialists for immediate therapy access [20]. Even governments are getting involved, establishing VR-based psychotherapy services within the metaverse [21].

- Mental health support exists in the metaverse.
- Group therapy (professional or peer-led) and immersive self-care practices are offered.
- Virtual clinics with therapists are available.

Governments are exploring VR therapy in the metaverse, and the clinics have recently started accepting cryptocurrency as a valid payment method for their services. Nonfungible tokens (NFTs) will function as reward tokens that may be granted upon the achievement of predetermined objectives in therapy. NFTs can also be exchanged on the online marketplace. These virtual clinics will specifically assist individuals who face difficulties in obtaining mental healthcare due to disability, geographical limitations, or time restrictions, as well as those who opt to stay unidentified because of the societal stigma associated with mental diseases. Nevertheless, it remains unknown if virtual environments and avatars can serve as substitutes for the genuine human interactions that are crucial in traditional mental therapy.

The most-recent COVID-19 epidemic was characterized by multiple lockdowns and contracts requiring persons to stay at their dwellings. Individuals who contracted COVID-19 were mandated to undergo isolation either in their own residences or in officially designated medical isolation centers. Research has indicated that individuals who are placed under quarantine experience increased levels of isolation, anxiety, and a limited amount of social contact [22]. Even in nonpandemic circumstances, marginalized individuals such as the elderly frequently encounter constraints in their ability to participate in social contacts with loved ones due to a variety of issues. Similarly, individuals with physical limitations may encounter feelings of frustration as a result of their restricted independence [23].

The metaverse also acts as a weapons platform where prenatal females as well as recently wedded pairs can come jointly to share their experiments and capabilities [24].

9.6.5 Possible Unpleasant Impact of NFTs and the Metaverse on Mental Well-Being

The impact of NFTs and the metaverse on mental well-being is a topic that raises concerns about potential adverse effects. The pervasive presence of digital media, including Internet usage, social networking platforms, and electronic games, has brought about a profound shift in societies worldwide [25]. It is noteworthy that around 75% of individuals in developed countries, accounting for approximately 25% of the global population, have Internet access [26]. The rapid and remarkable expansion of the hyperconnected Internet era over the past decade has been an exceptionally accelerated transformation experienced by humanity. The World Health Organization (WHO) has implemented measures to restrict mobile usage in schools due to research findings that have linked excessive digital media use to a decline in working memory capacity and the emergence of negative emotions such as melancholy, anxiety, and sleep disorders [27]. The incidence of attention deficit hyperactivity disorder (ADHD) has been consistently increasing over the previous decade merely by having a smartphone nearby, even while not actively using it, might reduce memory processing capacity and lead to poorer performance in cognitive activities. Furthermore, exercising self-restraint to refrain from using the Internet reduces cognitive resources. Moreover, the effects of these gadgets on unborn fetuses of pregnant users remain uncertain.

Furthermore, prolonged exposure to virtual profiles unintentionally encourages the inclination to make comparisons with others, which can greatly weaken one's mental well-being. For example, widely used social media platforms such as Instagram and Snapchat provide users built-in photo filters that can modify reality, leading to the spread of unattainable standards of beauty and lifestyle. Multiple investigations have irrefutably shown a robust correlation between the emergence of body dysmorphia and an excessive utilization of photography filters [28]. Body dysmorphia can result in negative outcomes, such as a higher vulnerability to mental health conditions like eating disorders, compulsive behaviors, and mood disorders [29]. VR and AR function based on similar concepts, allowing users to modify, improve, or manipulate the visual representation of their virtual character in a three-dimensional immersive environment. Nevertheless, emerging technologies also heighten the probability of adverse effects on mental well-being. Previous research has identified a phenomenon called the "Proteus effect," which suggests that people who invest significant time and effort in shaping their online persona prefer to adopt the characteristics and appearance of their virtual avatar. This can result in noticeable modifications in their behavior [30]. Undoubtedly, this would have great importance inside the three-dimensional virtual world of the metaverse.

Consider the anticipated widespread adoption of NFTs, which operate on digital money and blockchains. NFTs are expected to be used to access metaverse applications [31]. A diverse array of individuals and established content creators/ artists from many regions throughout the world participate in the production, trade, sale, and acquisition of digital art to create their virtual assets. The general public frequently tracks news on forthcoming NFT projects and subsequently engages in competition with others to obtain the new tokens, with the intention of creating virtual assets. This leads to a widely acknowledged psychological and behavioral disorder known as Fear of Missing Out (FOMO). FOMO is a prevalent phenomenon marked by worry arising from the recognition that one would be unable to partake in intellectually stimulating or fulfilling pursuits. Social media users are disproportionately likely to suffer from this condition [32]. FOMO is associated with negative effects on mental health, according to research by Gupta and Sharma et al. [33]. Sleep abnormalities, differences in how work and personal life are blended, difficulties with emotion regulation, and the presence of mood and anxiety disorders are all hallmarks of this group. One of the main signs of social media addiction, according to a recent study, is FOMO [34].

The metaverse aspires to do what Internet gaming has successfully achieved for a considerable amount of time. Virtual reality gaming systems provide users with a three-dimensional immersive environment that closely resembles a real-life experience. Participants have the ability to engage in immediate and live interactions with each other within the virtual realm [35]. However, according to a study, most young individuals who show signs of gaming addiction have poor social skills and a strong tendency toward impulsive behavior [36]. Moreover, research has indicated that addictive conduct is more prone to causing heightened feelings of solitude, sadness, unease, social anxieties, and subpar academic achievement, rather than being triggered by these factors [36]. Furthermore, there have been numerous instances in Japan when persons, known as Hikikomori, have formed a strong emotional bond with virtual gaming and consequently resist the urge to leave their homes. Research has indicated that engaging in this behavior significantly raises the probability of acquiring mental health conditions such as despair and anxiety [37]. The addition of Internet gaming disorder to the DSM-5 and ICD-11 is due to the significant similarities found between the symptoms of gaming addiction and drug use disorder [38].

Cybercrime has been present for a substantial duration, with criminals utilizing sophisticated strategies. Despite global endeavors to avoid and mitigate the adverse impacts, cybercrime persists unabated without any decline [39]. Individualistic thought patterns and features have a substantial impact on the likelihood of engaging in fraudulent Internet activities [40]. Previous research has documented instances of sexual abuse in adolescents. Studies have demonstrated that teenagers who lacked both moral guidance and support from their families were more susceptible to this type of mistreatment. These vulnerable teenagers often sought validation from the Internet, which made it easier for sexual predators to exploit them [41, 42]. There was a recent incident reported on the VR social networking site, Horizon Worlds, involving a woman's 3D virtual avatar. The avatar experienced sexual harassment from nearby virtual avatars. The woman described the nature of the interaction as strange and emotionally unsettling. Prior studies have indicated that adverse, hostile, or maltreatment encounters in virtual settings can cause similar emotional and physical responses in a person's real life [43]. These occurrences can have a persistent adverse effect on the victim's mental well-being and heighten the likelihood of developing mental conditions such as depression, anxiety, posttraumatic stress disorder (PTSD), or insomnia [44].

Although the possibility of technology improving mental health support is fascinating, many individuals may face financial limitations and other restrictions that hinder their ability to obtain the required VR devices for accessing the metaverse. In addition, specific vulnerable population groups, such as elderly folks, may lack the inclination or ability to employ the innovative VR technology, despite its well-documented benefits [45].

9.6.6 *The Limitations of Using VR or the Metaverse Applications*

Although VR has great promise as a tool for mental health management, studies have shown that VR therapy, although better than nothing, falls short when compared to more conventional, evidence-based approaches. Currently, there is a lack of adequately trustworthy evidence, further investigation into the advantages of VR-based therapy is hindered by a scarcity of randomized controlled experiments, the absence of additional control or evaluation populations, variability, and publication bias.

9.7 Futuristics Technologies and Preventive Mentalcare Systems

The healthcare sector is experiencing a surge due to technological improvements. The emergence of digital health has facilitated the utilization of technologies such as blockchain, AR, and VR to enhance the visualization of transformations and significantly impact doctor–patient interaction. The rising prevalence of chronic illnesses and the expanding average lifespan pose significant challenges in terms of resource availability and cost. Healthcare services can use the rapid digital revolution in the metaverse environment. Both scholarly and business sources have confirmed that the architecture is appropriate for developing data-intensive digital health applications and transferring them to metaverse environments [46].

Continuous monitoring of individuals' health statuses is essential, and the collected data should be thoroughly evaluated. Continuous monitoring and analysis of individuals' health data would facilitate the maintenance of their physical and emotional well-being. In this hypothetical scenario, the data emitted by individuals' peripheral devices will be transmitted to their virtual counterparts in the metaverse. The level of physical activity one engages in has a significant impact on their health, along with their dietary habits and other contributing factors. By transferring daily activities and dietary habits to the virtual realm, it will be feasible to replicate real-world experiences within the metaverse. Through the retrieval and examination of data housed inside the metaverse, it is feasible to detect potential hazards to human well-being and implement precautionary steps to safeguard individuals against them. This technology enables individuals to access essential healthcare services and engage in discussions with advisors within the metaverse.

By utilizing algorithmic assessments on the state of the metaverse, we can ascertain the efficacy of therapy for real patients. The metaverse will enable individuals with the same ailment to overcome the barriers of physical distance and time, allowing them to communicate and exchange knowledge. The migration of individuals' daily routines and medical information to the digital domain forms the basis of the metaverse, a virtual reality. The utilization of Industry 4.0 technology is expected to considerably enhance the effectiveness of health applications in the metaverse. This advancement will be facilitated through the integration of several technologies, including those related to cyber defense, wearable sensors, wearable twins, high-speed data transmission systems, cloud computing, data storage, AR, and VR, facilitate the maintenance of mental and physical well-being. In this hypothetical scenario, data collected via wearable devices will be transmitted to virtual representations of themselves in the metaverse. Undoubtedly, a person's health is influenced by factors beyond their physical activity level, including their food. In the future, it will be feasible to transfer people's daily routines and dietary habits into the metaverse, enabling the replication of authentic real-life experiences.

9.8 Conclusion

The impact of Industry 4.0 on the health sector is already evident, and the recent outbreak has further accelerated this trend. Digital transformation is being utilized in the health sector to enhance efficiency and ensure long-term sustainability. The incorporation of the metaverse has brought about a revolutionary change in corporate operations, allowing transactions to take place without the constraints of time and space. Furthermore, the healthcare industry faces challenges in integrating with the metaverse due to the high costs and stringent testing protocols associated with obtaining licenses and developing technologies. Virtual systems are also inherently vulnerable to cybersecurity threats. Besides such constraints, there is still high requirement and strong necessity for rendering the healthcare services using the recent ICT-enabled initiatives. Also, in order to meet the acute shortage of highly skilled healthcare professionals, metaverse-related interventions are in high demand and acceptance. Web 3.0 is also expected to introduce a significant presence in the field of mental health in the near future, which might potentially revolutionize the entire mental health industry. Many socioeconomic sectors stand to benefit greatly from the metaverse, although it is unclear how it will grow in the future.

References

1. Calabrò, R. S., Cerasa, A., Ciancarelli, I., Pignolo, L., Tonin, P., Iosa, M., & Morone, G. (2022). The arrival of the metaverse in neurorehabilitation: Fact, fake or vision? Biomedicines, 10(10), 2602.
2. Abdelghafar, S., Ezzat, D., Darwish, A., & Hassanien, A. E. (2023). Metaverse for brain computer interface: Towards new and improved applications. In The Future of Metaverse in the Virtual Era and Physical World (pp. 43–58). Cham: Springer International Publishing.
3. Floridi, L. (2022). Metaverse: A matter of experience. Philosophy & Technology, 35(3), 73.

4. Chengoden, R., Victor, N., Huynh-The, T., Yenduri, G., H. Jhaveri, R., Alazab, M., Bhattacharya, S., Hegde, P., Maddikunta, P. K. R., & Gadekallu, T. R. (2023). Metaverse for healthcare: A survey on potential applications, challenges and future directions. IEEE Access, 11, 12764–12794.

5. Chengoden, R., Victor, N., Huynh-The, T., Yenduri, G., Jhaveri, R. H., Alazab, M., & Gadekallu, T. R. (2023). Metaverse for healthcare: A survey on potential applications, challenges and future directions. IEEE Access, 11, 12765–12795.

6. Park, S. M., & Kim, Y. G. (2022). A metaverse: Taxonomy, components, applications, and open challenges. IEEE Access, 10, 4209–4251.

7. Gadekallu, T. R., Huynh-The, T., Wang, W., Yenduri, G., Ranaweera, P., Pham, Q. V., & Liyanage, M. (2022). Blockchain for the metaverse: A review. arXiv preprint arXiv:2203.09738.

8. Colucci, A., Vermehren, M., Cavallo, A., Angerhöfer, C., Peekhaus, N., Zollo, L., & Soekadar, S. R. (2022). Brain–computer interface-controlled exoskeletons in clinical neurorehabilitation: Ready or not? Neurorehabilitation and Neural Repair, 36(12), 747–756.

9. Rahi, P., Sood, S. P., Dandotiya, M., Kalhotra, S. K., & Khan, I. R. (2023). Artificial intelligence of things (AIoT) and metaverse technology for brain health, mental health, and wellbeing. In Contemporary Applications of Data Fusion for Advanced Healthcare Informatics (pp. 429–445). IGI Global.

10. Nagel, S. (2019). Towards a home-use BCI: fast asynchronous control and robust non-control state detection (Doctoral dissertation, Universität Tübingen).

11. Stanica, I. C., Moldoveanu, F., Dascalu, M. I., Nemoianu, I. V., & Portelli, G. P. (2021). Advantages of telemedicine in neurorehabilitation and quality of life improvement. Revue Roumaine des Sciences Techniques, Série Électrotechnique et Énergétique, 66(3), 195–199.

12. Kao, C. C., Huang, C. J., Wang, M. Y., & Tsai, P. S. (2008). Insomnia: Prevalence and its impact on excessive daytime sleepiness and psychological well-being in the adult Taiwanese population. Quality of Life Research, 17, 1073–1080.

13. Chazelle, E., Chastang, J. F., & Niedhammer, I. (2016). Psychosocial work factors and sleep problems: Findings from the French national SIP survey. International Archives of Occupational and Environmental Health, 89, 485–495.

14. Stanica, I. C., Moldoveanu, F., Portelli, G. P., Dascalu, M. I., Moldoveanu, A., & Ristea, M. G. (2020). Flexible virtual reality system for neurorehabilitation and quality of life improvement. Sensors, 20(21), 6045.

15. Farina, D., Mohammadi, A., Adali, T., Thakor, N. V., & Plataniotis, K. N. (2021). Signal processing for neurorehabilitation and assistive technologies. IEEE Signal Processing Magazine, 38(4), 5–7.

16. Surya, N., Srivastava, A., Nagda, T., Palande, D., & Someshwar, H. (2021). Education, training, and practices of neurorehabilitation in India during the COVID-19 pandemic. Frontiers in Neurology, 12, 626399.

17. Chang, S. H., Tseng, S. C., Su, H., & Francisco, G. E. (2022). How can wearable robotic and sensor technology advance neurorehabilitation? Frontiers in Neurorobotics, 16, 1033516. doi: 10.3389/fnbot.2022.1033516

18. Ahlbom, A., Green, A., Kheifets, L., Savitz, D., Swerdlow, A., & ICNIRP (International Commission for Non-Ionizing Radiation Protection) Standing Committee on Epidemiology. (2004). Epidemiology of health effects of radiofrequency exposure. Environmental Health Perspectives, 112(17), 1741–1754.

19. Usmani, S. S., Sharath, M., & Mehendale, M. (2022). Future of mental health in the metaverse. General Psychiatry, 35(4), 1–5.
20. Wray, T. B., Kemp, J. J., & Larsen, M. A. (2023). Virtual reality (VR) treatments for anxiety disorders are unambiguously successful, so why are so few therapists using it? Barriers to adoption and potential solutions. Cognitive Behaviour Therapy, 52(6), 603–624.
21. Ifdil, I., Situmorang, D. D. B., Firman, F., Zola, N., Rangka, I. B., & Fadli, R. P. (2023). Virtual reality in metaverse for future mental health-helping profession: An alternative solution to the mental health challenges of the COVID-19 pandemic. Journal of Public Health, 45(1), e142–e143.
22. Hwang, T. J., Rabheru, K., Peisah, C., Reichman, W., & Ikeda, M. (2020). Loneliness and social isolation during the COVID-19 pandemic. International Psychogeriatrics, 32(10), 1217–1220.
23. Marroquín, B., Vine, V., & Morgan, R. (2020). Mental health during the COVID-19 pandemic: Effects of stay-at-home policies, social distancing behavior, and social resources. Psychiatry Research, 293, 113419.
24. Freeman, D., Lambe, S., Kabir, T., Petit, A., Rosebrock, L., Yu, L., & Waite, F. (2022). Automated virtual reality (VR) therapy (gameChange) treating agoraphobic avoidance and distress in patients with psychosis: A multicentre, parallel group, single-blind, randomised controlled trial in England with mediation and moderation analyses. Lancet Psychiatry, 9(5).
25. Falconer, C. J., Rovira, A., King, J. A., Gilbert, P., Antley, A., Fearon, P., & Brewin, C. R. (2016). Embodying self-compassion within virtual reality and its effects on patients with depression. BJPsych Open, 2(1), 74–80.
26. Bujnowska-Fedak, M. M., Mastalerz-Migas, A. (2014). Usage of medical internet and e-health services by the elderly. In Pokorski, M. (ed). Environment Exposure to Pollutants: Advances in Experimental Medicine and Biology, vol. 834. Cham: Springer.
27. Korte, M. (2020). The impact of the digital revolution on human brain and behavior: Where do we stand? Dialogues in Clinical Neuroscience, 22(2), 101–111.
28. Abbas, L., & Dodeen, H. (2022). Body dysmorphic features among snapchat users of "Beauty-retouching of selfies" and its relationship with quality of life. Media Asia, 49(3), 196–212.
29. Schulte, J., Schulz, C., Wilhelm, S., & Buhlmann, U. (2020). Treatment utilization and treatment barriers in individuals with body dysmorphic disorder. BMC Psychiatry, 20, 1–11.
30. Paul, I., Mohanty, S., & Sengupta, R. (2022). The role of social virtual world in increasing psychological resilience during the on-going COVID-19 pandemic. Computers in Human Behavior, 127, 107036.
31. Tayal, S., Rajagopal, K., & Mahajan, V. (2022, March). Virtual reality based metaverse of gamification. In 2022 6th International Conference on Computing Methodologies and Communication (ICCMC) (pp. 1597–1604). IEEE.
32. Franchina, V., Vanden Abeele, M., Van Rooij, A. J., Lo Coco, G., & De Marez, L. (2018). Fear of missing out as a predictor of problematic social media use and phubbing behavior among Flemish adolescents. International Journal of Environmental Research and Public Health, 15(10), 2319.
33. Gupta, M., & Sharma, A. (2021). Fear of missing out: A brief overview of origin, theoretical underpinnings and relationship with mental health. World Journal of Clinical Cases, 9(19), 4881.

34. Blackwell, D., Leaman, C., Tramposch, R., Osborne, C., & Liss, M. (2017). Extraversion, neuroticism, attachment style and fear of missing out as predictors of social media use and addiction. Personality and Individual Differences, 116, 69–72.
35. Kaimara, P., Oikonomou, A., & Deliyannis, I. (2022). Could virtual reality applications pose real risks to children and adolescents? A systematic review of ethical issues and concerns. Virtual Reality, 26(2), 697–735.
36. Gorman, T. E., Gentile, D. A., & Green, C. S. (2018). Problem gaming: A short primer. American Journal of Play, 10(3), 309.
37. Kim, M. (2015). The Good and the Bad of Escaping to Virtual Reality. The Atlantic.
38. Colder Carras, M., Shi, J., Hard, G., & Saldanha, I. J. (2020). Evaluating the quality of evidence for gaming disorder: A summary of systematic reviews of associations between gaming disorder and depression or anxiety. PLoS One, 15(10), e0240032.
39. Alghamdi, M. I. (2020). A descriptive study on the impact of cybercrime and possible measures to curtail its spread worldwide. International Journal of Engineering Research and Technology, 9, 731–5.
40. Monteith, S., Bauer, M., Alda, M., Geddes, J., Whybrow, P. C., & Glenn, T. (2021). Increasing cybercrime since the pandemic: Concerns for psychiatry. Current Psychiatry Reports, 23, 1–9.
41. Balasubramaniam, S, Kadry, S., & Kumar, K. S. (2024). Osprey gannet optimization enabled CNN based transfer learning for optic disc detection and cardiovascular risk prediction using retinal fundus images. Biomedical Signal Processing and Control, 93, 106177.
42. Kadry, S., Dhanaraj, R. K., & Manthiramoorthy, C. (2024). Res-UNet based blood vessel segmentation and cardio vascular disease prediction using chronological chef-based optimization algorithm based deep residual network from retinal fundus images. Multimedia Tools and Applications, 1–30.
43. Jonsson, L. S., Fredlund, C., Priebe, G., Wadsby, M., & Svedin, C. G. (2019). Online sexual abuse of adolescents by A perpetrator met online: A cross-sectional study. Child and Adolescent Psychiatry and Mental Health, 13, 1–10.
44. Basu, T. (2021). The Metaverse Has a Groping Problem Already. MIT Technology Review.
45. Balasubramaniam, S, Joe, C. V., Manthiramoorthy, C., & Kumar, K. S. (2024). ReliefF based feature selection and gradient squirrel search algorithm enabled deep Maxout network for detection of heart disease. Biomedical Signal Processing and Control, 87, 105446.
46. Lee, H. W., Kim, S., & Uhm, J. P. (2021). Social virtual reality (VR) involvement affects depression when social connectedness and self-esteem are low: A moderated mediation on well-being. Frontiers in Psychology, 12, 753019.

Chapter 10

Metaverse-Based Medical Disease Diagnosis: Cancer Detection Case Study

Sakthivel Sankaran, Suggala Lohitha, Shaik Reena, and Preethika Immaculate Britto

10.1 Introduction to Metaverse and Healthcare

10.1.1 Definition and Concept of the Metaverse

The metaverse is an interactive shared world where users may engage with virtual components and each other via collaboratively fusing digitally generated physical reality. Although the concept of the metaverse had been there for a while, Meta's rebranding has elevated it to the fore. The focus on this rebranding by Meta, the top big tech company in the metaverse industry, indicates a big move in the direction of creating mixed, virtual, and augmented reality [1].

The idea of the metaverse aims to bridge the gap between our fantasies and the real world, creating a transformed a location where people may uniquely experience through various available technologies. It facilitates enhanced virtual communication and offers a diverse range of experiences, including meetings, gaming, travel, adventures, and more [1].

DOI: 10.1201/9781003491668-10

10.1.1.1 Virtual Reality

Virtual reality (VR) technology enables users to fully submerge themselves in a virtual world, usually with the aid of motion-tracking sensors and headgear. Users can interact with virtual objects and witness events that appear to be happening in a different location or environment by donning VR headsets [1]. VR has many applications, including games, entertainment, education, training, rehabilitation, and even remote collaboration.

VR software includes all the apps and digital worlds that users may interact with. Virtual tours, educational experiences, productivity tools, and immersive simulations and games are few examples of what this might include. The capacity of VR to immerse users in environments that seem remarkably real is one of its primary characteristics [2]. VR may create the illusion of a user being physically present in the virtual world by utilizing stereoscopic 3D images, spatial sound, and responsive interactions.

10.1.1.2 Augmented Reality

The term "augmented reality" (AR) refers to the technology that superimposes digital data — like pictures, movies, or 3D models — on peak of the actual environment [1]. Through the inclusion of virtual features, AR improves the actual world as opposed to VR, which submerges users in a fully virtual environment. AR glasses, AR headsets, tablets, smartphones, and other gadgets may all enable users to experience this.

One type of AR experience is marker-based, in which certain patterns or markers in the real world — like QR codes or picture targets — trigger the display of digital material. Conversely, marker-less AR makes use of sensors such as cameras, accelerometers, and GPS to identify and enhance the physical environment without requiring pre-established markers [1]. As an outcome, AR experiences may be more dynamic and context-aware now.

AR is used in the consumer arena for social media filters that superimpose digital effects on users' faces or surroundings, gaming, and entertainment [1]. Digital try-on experiences for clothing and other items, as well as the capacity to see furniture and home décor in the user's living area, are made possible by AR in retail.

AR provides a count of obstacles in addition to its exciting potential [1]. These include the need to ensure that virtual material is accurately aligned with the actual environment, optimize performance across various devices, and manage privacy issues around the processing and capture of users' surroundings as shown in Figure 10.1 [1]. In order to enable intuitive interactions and prevent information overload, user interface design in AR also has to be carefully considered.

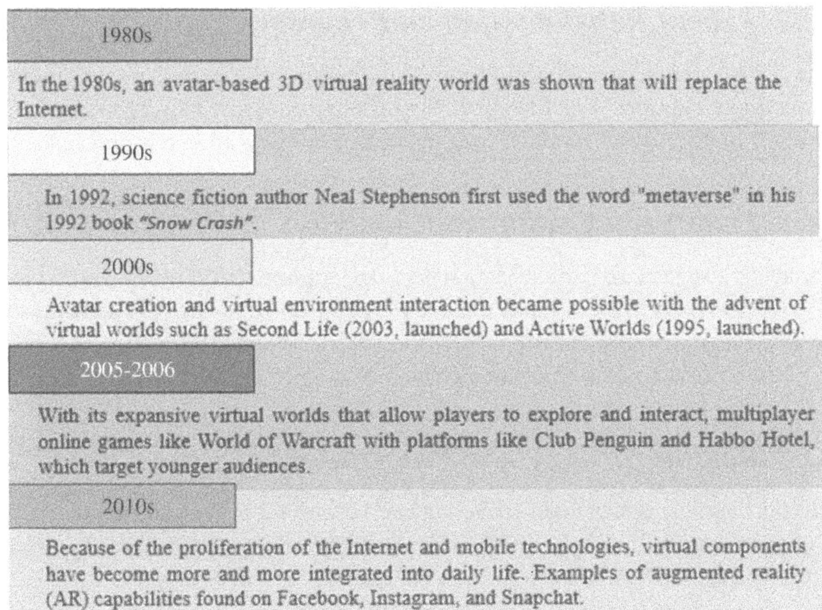

Figure 10.1   Evolution of the metaverse.

10.2 The Integration of Metaverse Technology in Healthcare

The rapid advancement of medical technology has undoubtedly resolved many medical issues, but challenges such as the scarcity of medical resources and the high cost of healthcare persist, leading to serious medical issues for patients. Access to quality medical services is crucial for sustaining the population's health, both physically and mentally, and is integral to societal development and stability. The quality of medical care directly influences the advancement and sustainability of society and the Earth's development [2].

The integration of metaverse technology in healthcare holds the promise of addressing some of the persistent challenges in the medical field. The following are some key areas where the metaverse could play a transformative role [2].

10.2.1 Virtual Health Consultations

With the assistance of the metaverse, patients can interact with the healthcare specialists virtually from their homes. This type of assistance can overcome the problem of receiving high-quality medical advice, mainly for those living in under-developed and rural locations [2].

10.2.2 Patient Rehabilitation and Therapy

In the aspect of patient rehabilitation and therapy, the experience of metaverse provides huge support. For instance, digital environments can be created in safe supervised surroundings to assist patients in overcoming anxieties and fears.

10.2.3 Data Visualization and Analysis

The analysis and visualization of data has a huge approach in the metaverse. Usually, this VR provides a three-dimensional representation by using VR settings. These three-dimensional representations provide better understanding for the medical practitioners and can help them make the best diagnosis [2].

10.2.4 Remote Surgery and Procedures

While performing operations, surgeons use lots of robotic equipment, thanks in part to metaverse technology. In situations and circumstances where access to specialized medical advice is limited, then the metaverse acts as a game-changer.

10.2.5 Patient Engagement and Compliance

The metaverse can enhance patient engagement by creating interactive and personalized healthcare experiences. Virtual platforms can be designed to educate patients about their conditions and treatment plans and encourage adherence to prescribed medications and lifestyle changes [2].

10.2.6 Global Collaboration and Research

The metaverse made global collaboration among researchers, health providers, and institutions possible. Innovative cures and medical research can be expedited through virtual conferences, cooperative research initiatives, and shared data spaces [1].

10.2.7 Health Data Security and Privacy

As the metaverse meets up with healthcare, then medical data security and privacy become critical. Implementing cryptography and blockchain technology in the digital settings might protect critical medical data.

10.2.8 Patient Support Communities

The metaverse helps establish patient support groups, where people with same health issues can interact, share their experiences, and offer emotional support to each other.

In healthcare, the metaverse provides many positive impacts. Even after having such positive impact, there are ethical, legal, and technological issues that are to be resolved to achieve safe, responsible, advanced application. Cooperation among tech developers, medical experts, and legislators is a necessary aspect to fully utilize the metaverse's potential [2].

10.3 Potential Benefits and Challenges

The metaverse includes immersive technologies like AI and VR that provide various applications in healthcare. VR technologies also access collaborative interactions among healthcare teams by providing real-time access to 3D representations of patient scans and improves decision-making and communication [3].

There are various issues related to virtual equity and access. These issues include ethical and legal considerations, security, privacy concerns, the accuracy of the application and quality of outputs, and technical hurdles. Overcoming these issues can be the open door for the grand launch of the metaverse into the healthcare. The integration of metaverse into healthcare allows its full potential to transform the treatment of patients and medical training [3].

10.3.1 Improved Patient Experience

Immersion VR and AR are becoming more and more popular in the medical industry, and their potential for education and therapeutic uses has been thoroughly studied. The term "augmented reality" describes how digital components are integrated and superimposed over the user's physical surroundings to allow for continuous attention to both [3].

10.3.2 Remote Consultations and Telemedicine

Patients may communicate electronically from home with healthcare professionals thanks to the metaverse. This kind of help can solve the issue of getting access to high-quality medical advice, especially for people who live in rural and impoverished areas. In such a way, metaverse makes ease of remote consultations possible [4].

10.3.3 Efficient Collaborative Decision-Making

The metaverse offers a wealth of ways for data analysis and visualization. Typically, this VR uses VR settings to generate three-dimensional representations. These three-dimensional depictions provide medical professionals a better understanding and enable the most accurate identification of disorders. This three-dimensional depiction results in an efficient decision-making process, even in typical difficult medical cases.

10.3.4 Legal and Ethical Considerations

There are various legal and ethical issues with the integration of metaverse technology in healthcare, such as consent for virtual treatments, liability in the case of virtual processes gone wrong, and the issue with accuracy of medical outputs, presented in virtual environments [4].

10.3.5 Technical Hurdles

Latency issues and high-quality Internet connections present some technological challenges. These hurdles impede the smooth operation of integration of metaverse technologies into healthcare systems [3].

10.4 Overview of Cancer Diagnosis

10.4.1 Types and Prevalence of Cancer

Cancer is the group of diseases characterized by the unusual growth and spread of tissues within the body. These aberrant cells have the ability to grow into tumors, infiltrate surrounding tissues, and spread to other areas of the body, affecting organ performance and general health. The development of cancer typically involves a combination of lifestyle, environmental, and genetic factors.

Cancers are categorized into various types based on certain parameters, including originating tissue or organ, kind of cell, the tumor's behavior, histological characteristics, clinical stage, genetics, and molecular characteristics. Based on the criteria presented in Table 10.1, cancer is categorized into various types.

10.4.2 Breast Cancer

The fast growth of cancerous cells within breast tissue is a major worldwide health hazard associated with breast cancer. Breast cancer is a complicated illness with many subtypes and side effects, making prevention, diagnosis, and therapy difficult.

Normal breast cells can become cancerous due to genetic abnormalities; this usually happens in the milk ducts or breast lobules, where the illness is most often found [4]. Tumors formed by these abnormal cells can be either benign (noncancerous) or malignant (cancerous). Breast cancer can present in a range of ways, from small, localized tumors to larger masses that have invaded nearby tissues or spread to distant organs. Early detection through screening and awareness of risk factors are essential for timely diagnosis and effective management of breast cancer.

Table 10.1   Classification of the Parameters of Cancer into Various Types

Parameters	*What it classifies*
Originating tissue or organ	This parameter categorizes the cancer by the organ or tissue from where it originated. For instance, lung cancer originated from lung tissue, breast cancer from breast tissue, and colon cancer from the cells lining the colon.
Kind of cell	This parameter categorized the cancer further within each tissue or organ, according to the sort of cells that give rise to them. Cancers that arise from epithelial cells are carcinomas. Cancers that arise from connective tissues cells are sarcomas. Cancers that arise from lymphomas are lymphocytes. Cancers that arise from blood forming cells are leukaemia. Cancers that arise from melanocytes are melanomas.
Tumor's behavior	This parameter classifies the cancer depending on the tumor behavior and its pattern of growth. For example, benign tumors are noncancerous growths that do not spread to other parts of the body, whereas malignant tumors are malignancies that have the capacity to do so and to penetrate nearby tissues.
Histological characteristics	Cancer categorization mostly relies on histology, the microscopic analysis of tissue samples. Pathologists can determine the kind and grade of a tumor by examining the unique morphological characteristics of several cancer cell types under a microscope.
Clinical stage	Cancer staging, which characterizes the disease's intensity based on factors such tumor size, involvement of lymph nodes, and metastasis, is an essential part of classification. Staging helps with provider communication, treatment planning, and prognosis prediction.
Genetic and molecular characteristics	Cancers are now categorized according to certain genetic alterations and molecular markers. Knowing the genetic changes causing cancer to spread can help tailor treatments and forecast patient outcomes.

Among women who report a breast lump to primary care, cancer is eventually diagnosed in about 8% of cases. The occurrence of breast cancer is notably higher among women aged 45 to 64 compared to those under 25, with approximately 15 times as many cases occurring in the former age group [5].

10.4.3 Lung Cancer

Lung cancer is one of the deadliest diseases and most well-known form of cancer. Lungs are the pair of spongy organs in the chest. These organs play a vital role in purifying the air. These smooth organs are surrounded by the rib cage for its protection. The left lung is smaller than right lung as it provides the place for the heart. Lung cancer is one of the types of cancer that begins with the unusual growth of lung cells. Each type of cancer has its own characteristics and differences in treatment and diagnosis [5].

Smoking is one of the main reasons for the occurrence of this dangerous disease. The heavy and worse cough that lasts for a long time, loss of appetite, unexplainable weight loss, shortness of breathing are most common symptoms seen in both male and female victim of this cancer. The early detection of any type of cancer gives the patient the greatest chance of success. Open communication with healthcare professionals is crucial for timely diagnosis of cancer [5].

10.4.4 Ovarian Cancer

The ovaries play a key role in female reproduction. Ovaries are the pair of glands that produce hormones like estrogen and eggs. The hormones have a huge role in breast development, menstrual cycle, growth of body hair, body shape, and pregnancy. Ovarian cancer is one of the most hazardous cancers among the various types of cancers. This cancer commences by unusual cell growth within these organs. This abnormal growth of ovarian cells leads a significant health risk. This cancer is considered as the most lethal, as the possibility of early detection of ovarian cancer is reduced and it is very aggressive.

This cancer is also known as "silent killer," as its symptoms are not known until it reaches its advanced stage. Ovarian cancer can affect women of all ages; it's often seen in postmenopausal women [6].

10.4.5 Other Cancers

There are various types of cancer aside from lung and ovarian. These various cancers include bladder cancer, pancreatic cancer, stomach cancer, kidney cancer, thyroid cancer, and esophageal cancer. There were 18,094,716 cancer cases reported in the year of 2020. Out all of them, 12.5% is the highest percentage of breast cancer reported, followed by lung cancer with 12.2%, prostate cancer with 7.8%, stomach cancer with 7.0%, liver cancer with 6.0%, esophageal cancer with 3.3%, pancreatic cancer with 2.7%, and thyroid cancer with 3.2% [6].

10.5 Traditional Methods of Cancer Detection

Specialists use various procedures to detect cancer. Traditional methods include treatment planning, utilizing a range of methodologies and techniques. These methodologies are often used to determine the cancer in early stages [7].

Traditional methods include imaging, such as CT scans, MRIs, and X-rays, providing detailed images of internal structures, which are essential for diagnosing and staging cancer [7].

PSA tests, which are similar to blood tests, are also commonly used in cancer detection. Regular screenings, endoscopy and ultrasound techniques are also valuable traditional methods for cancer detection. These methods are also considered the fundamental tests to be done while detecting the cancer.

10.5.1 Imaging Techniques

10.5.1.1 X-Ray

X-rays are the most commonly used imaging technique. The small dose of radiation is used to produce inside body images, including organs and tissues. These images capture every small detail of the organ and shows any irregularity that occurs. These irregularities are known as tumors. These tumors in X-rays often appear as lighter areas compared to the surroundings tissues.

The radiation is named as the X-ray beam. This X-ray beam is entered into the body, and by its specialized visualizing capacity it generates a digital image on a computer screen. These X-rays are mostly used for examining the bones and identifying abnormalities like breakage, tumors, cracks, and changes in bone density. In the aspect of cancer, they are used in identifying the bone cancer and lung cancer [7].

10.5.1.2 Computed Tomography (CT) Scans

Like X-rays, CT scans are a strong imaging tool used by medical professionals to visualize the body structure and internal organs in a detailed manner. The CT scans also display the size, shape, and location of tumors, which helps in accurate diagnosis and the best treatment [4].

10.5.1.3 Magnetic Resonance Imaging (MRI)

Although X-rays and CT scans have a well-known role in cancer detection, MRI imaging is most suitable for accurate diagnosis. This imaging technique uses radio waves and magnetic fields to produce the most detailed images of the organs inside the body. The X-ray detects the tumor and shows it in lighter shade as compared to the surroundings, but the MRI provides information about the tumor's size, location, and shape. From the information gained from the images generated, specialists may plan treatment and the forward procedures related to the diagnosis.

10.5.2 Biopsies

10.5.2.1 Needle Biopsy

A needle biopsy is used to extract a sample from the tumor for analysis. This is used to detect cancer in skin, lungs, thyroid gland, and breast. Once the needle is properly positioned, the sample is taken using vacuum. Biopsies can also be performed by patients.

10.5.2.2 Surgical Biopsy

Surgical biopsy is used to check cancerous cells. It detects the cells accurately. It is then sent to a pathology laboratory to exam the cancer cells under microscope. There are various types of surgical biopsies. They are as follows:

Incisional biopsy: It is a biopsy of collecting a sample from for analysis of large tumors.

Excisional biopsy: This biopsy removes in the entire tissue containing the tumor. This procedure is used for small tumors and involves the removal of a sizable sample of tissue during surgery to check for cancerous cells. This permits for a more accurate determination of the cancer's grade and aggressiveness. The biopsy sample is then sent to a pathological laboratory where it is processed, examined under a microscope by a pathologist, and checked for anomalies or cancer cells [7].

Open biopsy: An open biopsy involves making an incision to directly access the suspicious tissue for sampling. When more extensive tissue samples are needed for a diagnosis or when alternative biopsy techniques are impractical, an open biopsy could be essential [7].

10.5.3 Screening Test

10.5.3.1 Mammography

Mammograms are X-ray examinations of the breast tissue performed on women to check for breast cancer. Women should begin having screening mammograms at the age of 40, while specific risk factors and recommendations from various health organizations may influence this [7].

10.5.3.2 Pap Smear (Pap Tests)

These tests detect cervical abnormalities, which can sometimes lead to false or true positives and negatives. Women should be screened with this test at the age of 21 based on several considerations. The test also suggests the symptoms of cancer in the future. Early detection can help in curing cervical cancer.

10.5.3.3 Colonoscopy

Colonoscopies are performed to screen colorectal cancer. They also detect development of cancer in the intestine and rectum. This is a process which is done using a long flexible tube that has a camera that is moved into the colon. The test is taken on the regular basis for patients of ages above 45.

10.5.3.4 Fecal Occult Blood Test (FOBT) or Fecal Immunochemical Test (FIT)

These tests look for blood in the stool, which may indicate precancerous polyps or colorectal cancer. They may be completed at home and are noninvasive. Positive outcomes might lead to a colonoscopy for additional assessment [7].

10.5.3.5 Prostate-Specific Antigen (PSA) Test

The PSA test quantifies blood levels of PSA, which men with prostate tumors may have higher than normal. It is advised that men and their medical professionals collaborate to decide if screening is necessary in light of each person's unique risk factors.

10.5.3.6 Low-Dose Computed Tomography (LDCT) Scan

In high-risk patients, such as active smokers or those who have previously smoked, LDCT scans are utilized for checking for lung cancer. In high-risk groups, monitoring with LDCT scans has been demonstrated to lower lung cancer mortality.

10.5.3.7 Endoscopy

An endoscopy is a medical procedure where an endoscope — a flexible tube containing an imaging equipment and a light source — is used to see within the body. Endoscopy can be used for a number of diagnostic purposes, including the detection of cancer, as it offers a direct view of the internal organs and tissues [7].

10.5.3.8 Ultrasound

Using high-frequency sound waves, ultrasonic imaging, also known as ultrasonography, is a noninvasive diagnostic technique that produces images of the internal organs and tissues of the patient. Although ultrasound is not typically used as a standalone testing method, it is a valuable tool for cancer diagnosis, staging, and monitoring.

10.6 Limitations and Shortcomings

10.6.1 X-Ray

The main limitation of X-rays is that it does not show the difference between normal soft tissues and cancer tissues in early stages. Also, if a patient is exposed to X-rays too often, they may lead to development of cancer tissues and may also lead to produce radiations within the body. So, due to its disadvantages, some measures are to be taken.

10.6.2 Computed Tomography (CT) Scans

Like live X-rays, CT scans also expose the patients to ionizing radiation, which can increase the possibility of cancer. However, CT scans offer more advantages, such as it can easily and clearly resolve the soft tissues. They may sometimes cause allergic reactions.

10.6.3 MRI

MRI has more advantages than X-rays or CT scans, as it does not involve radiation. As MRI can be very helpful in imaging of soft tissues, it also has variable challenges. By improving the technology, these limitations can be resolved and increase its usage in the medical field.

10.6.4 Biopsies (Needle and Surgical)

Although biopsies are essential in verifying cancer diagnoses, they do have some drawbacks, as they can miss heterogeneous tumors.

According to the patient's resistance, biopsies should be taken appropriately. If the patient experiences discomfort, or if bleeding is a danger, imaging-based diagnostics on liquid biopsies can be used.

Tumor accessibility is difficult if it is situated in a deep-seated location. In this condition, supplementary diagnostic techniques, such as biomarker analysis, are used in cancer therapy.

10.6.5 Blood Tests (CBC, Tumor Markers)

Blood tests are an important part of tracking cancer. The complete blood count (CBC), which gives the number of blood cells, may not be very precise in identifying some cancers. The results frequently need to be validated by other diagnostic techniques such as biopsies. Multimodal strategy is crucial since blood tests may miss some tumors.

10.6.6 Screening Tests (Mammography, Pap Test, PSA)

Screening tests are invaluable, but they do have some drawbacks that are to be considered. Mammography, which is used to detect breast cancer, sometimes gives false positives. Mammograms do not detect cancer in dense breast tissue.

Pap tests detect cervical abnormalities but can yield false negatives and positives, which leads to tension in the patients. In prostate cancer screening, elevated PSA levels can occur in noncancerous conditions such as benign prostatic hyperplasia.

10.6.7 Endoscopy (Colonoscopy, Bronchoscopy)

Endoscopic procedures such as colonoscopy and bronchoscopy have limitations and challenges. Bronchoscopies, used for diagnosing lunch cancer, may have difficulty reaching peripheral lung lesions, which is challenging to access with bronchoscope. Therefore, careful patient selection and diagnostic approaches, such as CT endobronchial ultrasound (EBUS), are essential for diagnosis [8].

10.6.8 Ultrasound (Abdominal Ultrasound)

Ultrasound imaging is a good tool for abdominal examinations especially, due to its real-time visualization capability. Additionally, this tool has limitations in visualizing structures that can restrict its efficacy. Intestinal gas makes it difficult to see deeper abdominal structures. Compared to CT or MRI, ultrasound may have more difficulty identifying tiny lesions.

Avoiding the limitations, ultrasound remains valuable for its real-time imaging and avoiding ionizing radiation [8].

10.7 Metaverse Technology in Medicine

10.7.1 VR, AR, and Mixed Reality in Healthcare

In intensive care units (ICUs), VR is most widely used. It has proved its ability in various medical fields. It can make patients enjoy and feel the VR environment happily. It has been established and explained that the pain of patients can be reduced through captivating virtual landscapes. Especially for patients who are uncomfortable in the ICU, VR is very helpful.

AR can divert the patient's attention from suffering with the help of interactive activities. It can also be used to support the both physical and mental health of patients.

To improve patient care and clinical treatment, mixed reality (MR) is also used in healthcare. Whereas VR combines elements of AR and the components of MR to provide advanced facilities for patient care in the medical field. By delivering diversion and immersion in captivating virtual landscapes, VR has demonstrated its efficacy in mitigating pain and suffering. For patients in ICUs who may be in discomfort as a result of their treatments or illnesses, this can be very helpful [9, 10]. VR exposure treatment can be given via augmented reality (AR) to patients who suffer from post-traumatic stress disorder (PTSD) or anxiety associated with their ICU experience. In the medical field, mixed reality (MR) also used to the use of technology that combines the real and virtual worlds to improve patient care, medical education, and clinical processes. VR components are combined with augmented reality (AR) components that makeup the mixed reality (MR) to produce immersive experiences with a range of applications in the healthcare industry [11, 12]. By engrossing patients in soothing virtual worlds or interactive experiences, magnetic resonance imaging (MRI) technology can be utilized to divert patients' attention from their discomfort during surgeries or treatments.

10.7.2 Applications of Metaverse Technology in Medical Education, Training, and Diagnosis

10.7.2.1 Applications of Metaverse Technology in Medical Education

a. **Simulated Medical Procedures**

   VR simulations can replicate various medical procedures, offering students a realistic and risk-free environment to practice surgeries, injections, and other clinical tasks.

b. **Case-Based Learning in Virtual Environments**

   Case-based learning is an important aspect in virtual environments. It provides relevant opportunities to see the theory in practical applications, which also involve engaging in critical conditions, helping to improve problem-solving skills and decision-making abilities.

c. **Remote Collaborative Learning**

   Connecting people from different geographical locations in a single metaverse platform helps in learning new things. Collaborative learning helps people with communicational skills as well as interdisciplinary learning.

10.7.2.2 Applications of Metaverse Technology in Medical Training

a. **Surgical Simulations**

   Simulations provide great aid to surgeons, and simulations through VR are an excellent option to choose for surgeons to practice and improve their skills without any risks.

b. **Emergency Response Training**

   Emergency response training is most crucial for medical students as well as surgeons. Metaverse technology helps in simulating situations, which helps in improving the preparedness of a surgeon in different cases.

c. **Patient Interaction and Communication Training**

Communication between the patient and surgeon plays an important role. Thus, virtual scenarios are created that help in refining the communication of a surgeon in difficult situations, which includes breaking bad news.

d. **Pharmaceutical Training**

Pharmaceutical training through virtual metaverse technology is a great aid to pharma students. Which helps in exploring virtual labs and learning through technology helps in better understanding.

10.7.2.3 Applications of Metaverse Technology in Medical Diagnosis

a. **Virtual Diagnostic Imaging**

Virtual diagnostic imaging by metaverse technology helps in understanding the disease better in every dimension and also supports the intricate conditions.

b. **Telemedicine and Remote Diagnostics**

Metaverse platforms provide remote diagnostics and consultations, where healthcare professionals can remotely examine the patients' conditions using virtual tools.

c. **Data Vizualization for Decision Support**

Decision-making may be critical in medical field. But providing a better visualization technique of the patient helps in decision-making as it provides data in an integrated format. It improves accessibility of data and promotes experimental learning. The integration of metaverse technology in medical education, training, and diagnosis holds the potential to revolutionize the way healthcare professionals are educated, trained, and deliver patient care. It enhances accessibility, promotes experiential learning, and fosters collaboration across the healthcare ecosystem.

10.8 Metaverse-Based Cancer Detection

10.8.1 Conceptual Framework of Metaverse-Based Cancer Diagnosis

It is very crucial to develop the technology in the rapidly changing medical field to improve the positive outcome of the patient. The metaverse is one of the technologies that has great potential to revolutionize the present situation. It presents many prospects to transform cancer detection by implementing AI, AR, and digital reality. An outcome of the metaverse is the uncertain difference between the physical and virtual worlds.

The metaverse also provides a platform for the development of immersiveness in industries, including healthcare. The metaverse has the potential to completely change the method by which cancer is diagnosed and increase the effectiveness of the treatment.

10.8.1.1 Virtual Simulation Environments

On the basis of VR and AR, the metaverse was rooted in for the treatment of cancer. The framework is based on the lifelike systematic simulation environments that can behave like physiological structures and provide tumors environments. Virtual simulation can set up more treatment considerations by providing a 3D visual of complicated anatomical compartments through which spatial knowledge is improved.

10.8.1.2 Multidimensional Data Integration

For metaverse-based cancer detection, it is very important to record and study keenly the clinical records, genomics, and proteomics, and these are processed and given to AI to analyze. It provides data with specific information about patients. Through these data, medical professionals can provide suitable treatment for the patient [13].

10.8.1.3 Patient-Centered Engagement

The main feature of metaverse-based cancer diagnosis is the importance it places on sharing detailed treatment information with patients. This approach enables patients to make informed choices, enhancing their overall treatment experience. By fostering a sense of autonomy and empowerment, it can improve their quality of life and emotional well-being.

10.8.1.4 Predictive Modeling and Real-Time Data Analytics

This places emphasis on using predictive modeling and real-time data analysis to understand the condition of an individual patient. The ability of the doctors to make a neat and safe clinical decision is enhanced by using machine learning algorithms [13].

10.8.1.5 Surgical Diagnosis and Intervention through Immersion

With the use of the metaverse, this framework aims to provide immersive surgical preparation and intervention in the field of cancer. Surgeons may practice intricate operations, such as anatomical components, and practice surgical situations in an atmosphere without risks via VR simulators. The accuracy, surgical results, and precision are improved by the usage of AR in real time.

10.8.1.6 Advantages over Traditional Methods

The metaverse provides several traditional methods for detection of cancer, such as screening tests, biopsies, and imaging tools. They have benefits as well as risks that could be reflected in the metaverse. Traditional methods help in finding a minute sample or even single organisms. Thus, they are being used in many laboratories.

10.8.1.7 Improved Visibility

The metaverse provides many visualization capabilities, such as 2D imaging techniques. Position and location of a tumor can be detected by VR and AR by enabling 3D models. VR and AR technologies have helped significantly in modifying, altering, and creating virtual environments. Increased visibility helps make the information accurate. It also helps to depixelate blurred images.

10.8.1.8 Multiple Sensations

By utilizing VR and AR, the metaverse also offers other senses. As an example, audio cues let users interact with virtual tumors. AR and VR enable users to enter realistic stimulations of medical scenarios and interact with real scenarios. VR could enable five senses. So, these are used for public safety too [13].

10.8.1.9 Patient Empowerment and Education

Between patient and medical professionals in the metaverse, patient education plays a critical role. If the patient is knowledgeable enough about their condition, they too build trust and confidence. This deep link promotes cooperation and communication, which enhances the satisfaction of patient. Such empowerment helps patients to understand their situation and take self-care.

10.8.1.10 Individualized Risk Evaluation

Personalized risk assessment such as genetic predisposition and medical history is possible through the metaverse. This makes identification and treatment easier. It is very important to identify risks and hazards and eliminate them. This also prevents risk to patients.

Better results, such as increased survival rates and less morbidity from cancer diagnosis and treatment, can result from early intervention.

10.8.1.11 Case Studies and Research Findings

These techniques have been very beneficial in the detection of cancer, but they often have disadvantages, such as cost, accessibility, and invasiveness. With the emergence of the metaverse, researchers in academia and medicine are looking at a number of approaches that combine AI, VR, and data analytics to detect cancer early and enhance patient outcomes [14].

Researchers at Virtual Health Technologies created a virtual biopsy tool that enables medical professionals to replicate the procedure of removing tissue samples from tumors in a virtual setting, as reported in a groundbreaking study published in *The Journal of Medical Imaging*. Early clinical trial results for virtual biopsies have been positive, providing accuracy comparable with conventional procedures while reducing the risks involved for patients [15].

The group at Immersive Diagnostics, Inc., was the first to use immersive image processing methods in the diagnosis of cancer. This integrated strategy improves patient care and treatment planning by fostering collaboration among healthcare workers and improving diagnostic precision [16].

The innovative approach to emotional assistance not only reduces access barriers for patients living in remote or impoverished areas but also forges stronger connections among people facing similar challenges in their fight against cancer. Based on preliminary findings, participants in virtual support groups reported improvements in their overall quality of life, coping strategies, and mood [17].

Clinical studies have demonstrated the benefits of AR-guided operations for cancer patients, including decreased intraoperative complications, accelerated postoperative recovery, and improved postoperative results [18]. According to their research, deep learning models such as recurrent neural networks (RNNs) and convolutional neural networks (CNNs) performed better than other imaging modalities, such as mammography, colonoscopy, and dermatoscopy, in identifying early-stage cancer lesions.

Early tests carried out in association with preeminent medical facilities have shown encouraging findings, as the virtual screening tool has proven to have good sensitivity and specificity for a variety of cancer forms [19].

According to the study, trainees who got traditional didactic teaching alone were less accurate and efficient at identifying malignant lesions than those who received virtual reality simulation-based training [20].

The research also emphasized the significance of algorithm optimization, validation, and high-quality data in guaranteeing the clinical effectiveness and applicability of digital screening tools for population-wide cancer detection programs [21].

The study demonstrated how immersive visualization of data might be useful for cancer precision healthcare applications in identifying treatment targets, finding biomarkers, and formulating hypotheses [22].

The researchers had shortly concluded that it is very important to have a good collaboration among scientists, cancer specialists, and computer specialists for better impact of the metaverse on patients' health.

10.9 Development and Implementation

10.9.1 Design Considerations for Metaverse-Based Cancer Detection Platforms

Metaverse-based cancer diagnosis software requires a synthesis of cutting-edge technology, clinical knowledge, and user experience (UX) design. Here are some constraints.

10.9.1.1 Data Security and Privacy

Strict compliance with privacy laws such as the Health Insurance Portability and Accountability Act (HIPAA) is critical. To avoid unwanted access, every medical record must be securely kept and encrypted. HIPAA, a 1996 US federal law, is crucial for protecting sensitive medical data, also known as protected health information (PHI), related to a person's medical history, health status, future plans, healthcare provision, and payment for services.

10.9.1.2 Integration of Medical Knowledge

The platform's effectiveness depends on cooperation with radiologists, oncologists, and other medical specialists. With the additional data and insight, it offers to help with diagnosis. Radiologists and oncologists can use the platform as a decision support tool. For instance, the platform may give risk assessment based on the demographics of patients and clinical data, identify questionable areas in medical pictures, and make recommendations for differential diagnoses.

10.9.1.3 User-Friendly Design

This method is an easy way for patients and medical professionals to search and comprehend the findings. Detailed explanation and visualization are important. In the case of complicated medical data and finding patterns, visualization techniques using heatmaps, 3D versions, and graphs are used. Designing ideas with the idea in mind will ensure that people to use this technique.

10.9.1.4 Ethical Considerations

Maintaining trust and following ethical standards are crucial issues, like maintaining consent for data usage and availability of algorithmic decision-making. When it comes to complicated medical data, visualization is a crucial metric.

10.9.1.5 Regulatory Compliance

The healthcare platform must follow some regulations like Food and Drug Administration (FDA) clearances for medical equipment and software, as well as international standards and laws. Following these metrics ensures compliance with international and industry-based practices.

10.9.2 Technological Requirements and Infrastructure

The deployment of metaverse-based cancer detection systems requires careful consideration of various infrastructure and technology needs.

10.9.2.1 High-Performance Computing

High-performance computing (HPC) is crucial for processing large amounts of medical data, running complex algorithms, and creating lifelike virtual worlds in metaverse-based cancer detection systems. HPC systems use a strong computer infrastructure to resolve computational issues requiring substantial resources. They handle large and complicated medical data, such as genetic data and electronic health records, enabling faster and more precise cancer detection systems [23].

10.9.2.2 Infrastructure for Cloud Computing

Cloud computing platforms offer scalable and adaptable infrastructure for managing data storage, executing computational tasks, and implementing virtual healthcare solutions. Cloud computing platforms offer advanced analytics and machine learning technologies for cancer diagnosis and detection. They also ensure high availability and resilience in the event of system breakdowns or natural disasters.

10.9.2.3 Advanced Imaging and Sensing Technologies

Cancer diagnosis has been better recognized by advanced imaging sensing techniques, which are crucial. MRIs using the radio waves and magnets help identify tumors in the body, such as cerebral cortex, spine, abdomen, and pelvic tumors. There are multiple imaging sensing techniques like positron emission tomography (PET) imaging produce 3D views, and molecular imaging methods such as molecular MRI, bioluminescence, and fluorescence imaging.

10.9.2.4 Patient Engagement and Education Platforms

Patient engagement plays a crucial role in their healthcare journey, which may include cancer screening and treatment. Medline Plus, created by the National

Library of Medicine, offers clear information about illness, drugs, and wellness-related subjects. Several medical platforms such as cancer.net, which was created by the American Society of Clinical Oncology, offer patients educational materials such as articles, videos, and community forums and provide current and accurate information about cancer and also podcasts, films, and interactive tools. These sources help the patient understand their medical circumstances and help them make precise decisions during their medical journey.

10.9.3 Integration with Existing Medical Systems

The metaverse is a promising frontier in healthcare for cancer detection, treatment, and monitoring. It allows multidisciplinary teams to collaborate in real time, enabling more accurate diagnoses. The metaverse also offers opportunities for advanced treatment methods, such as simulation and tailored therapy planning. Oncologists can customize treatment plans based on individual patient needs, visualizing tumor features and physiological factors. Virtual simulations can optimize treatment regimens and reduce side effects by comparing different treatment modalities.

10.9.3.1 Data Analysis and Visualization in Virtual Environments

Medical experts used to analyze complex medical data, such as scanning reports; now pathology reports can be transformed into a 3D environment and interactive experience that enhances the real world with computer-generated perceptual information for better knowledge. They examine it by rotating images, zoom in on particular area of interest, and imitate surgical procedures.

10.9.3.2 Instruction and Modeling for Healthcare Workers

Simulations provide great aid to medical professionals and simulations through VR. It is a best option to choose for professionals to practice and improve their skills without any risks, which is a great opportunity through metaverse technology. This exposure helps to develop a strong knowledge base for clinical practices. Virtual simulations provide feedback systems, immediate direction, and evaluation. This shows continual progress and also helps in avoidance of minimal mistakes.

10.9.3.3 Integration of Machine Learning with Big Data Analysis

Cancer detection techniques and personalized treatment plans can improve by the metaverse's computing capacity. Data anonymization strategies and strong security protocols are necessary to protect patient privacy, as it is most important to protect and respect the ethical standards and to prioritize patients' privacy.

10.10 Data Gathering and Analysis

10.10.1 Utilization of Patient Data for Diagnosis

Patients data has a key role in detecting cancer using the metaverse. The following are the few issues related to patients' data utilization and the approaches.

10.10.1.1 Electronic Health Records

Electronic health records through metaverse technology function as digital archives of patient history. Electronic health records are much better than normal paper records as they help to maintain a vast range of data essential for efficient healthcare provision. Such health records help to maintain information about prior diagnosis, treatments, prescription, drugs, test results, imaging accounts, surgical operations, and much more. These records are maintained through the patient's contact with the healthcare system.

10.10.1.2 Imaging Scans

As a recent breakthrough in medical imaging technology, imaging sensing techniques like PET imaging produce 3D views, and molecular imaging methods such as molecular MRI, bioluminescence, and fluorescence imaging have emerged. Cancer diagnosis has been better recognized by advanced imaging sensing techniques, which is crucial. MRI using radio waves and magnets helps to identify the tumors in the body like cerebral cortex, spine, abdomen, and pelvic tumors [24].

10.10.1.3 Image Segmentation

Within medical imaging, tumor zones may be properly defined by machine learning algorithms, which can also quantify factors like size, volume, and form. Tumor volumetry, rate of growth evaluation, and therapy response evaluation are made easier by this computerized segmentation, which also streamlines clinical operations and lowers interobserver variability [25].

10.10.1.4 Computer-Aided Diagnosis

Computer-aided diagnosis (CAD) systems help radiologists evaluate images in real time by integrating predictive algorithms into their workstations for radiology. These systems provide decision assistance according to qualitative analysis of images and clinical data integration, flag worrisome results, and rank cases for evaluation [25]. CAD improves the efficiency and accuracy of radiologists' diagnoses, especially in screening programs and high-volume imaging environments.

10.10.1.5 Genetic Profiles

The discovery of certain mutations in genes, biomarkers, and molecular signatures linked to different forms of cancer has been made possible by genetic testing, which has completely changed the field of oncology. These genetic insights give important details regarding the molecular features of a patient's tumors as well as their propensity to develop cancer [26].

10.10.1.6 Identification of Hereditary Cancer Symptoms

Genetic testing can reveal inherited abnormalities in genes linked to genetic cancer disorders, such as Lynch's syndrome in cancer of the colon or BRCA1/2 mutations in cancers of the breast and ovary. Early detection and preventive efforts are facilitated by the recognition of these genetic predispositions, which allows for focused screening techniques for those at risk and their families.

10.10.1.7 Predictive Biomarkers for Treatment Response

Certain genetic alterations or biomarkers can be used as predictors of how a patient would react to particular cancer treatments. For instance, BRAF mutations influence the usage of targeted therapy in melanoma and cancer of the colon, whereas alterations in the estimated glomerular filtration rate (EGFR) chromosome indicate susceptibility to inhibitors of EGFR for non-small cell lung cancer (NSCLC) [26].

10.10.2 Privacy and Security Concerns

10.10.2.1 Data Privacy

Ensuring the security of patient data in the metaverse is crucial for maintaining patient privacy and adhering to legal requirements that include HIPAA. It is ethically required of healthcare professionals and information technology (IT) developers to protect patients' autonomy, privacy, and dignity. By ensuring that patient interests are given priority during the development and implementation of digital health technologies, safeguarding patient data inside the metaverse demonstrates a dedication to ethical values [27], [28].

10.10.2.2 Data Security

In the metaverse ecosystem, strong cybersecurity measures are necessary to protect patient data from cyberattacks, unauthorized access, and data breaches. Healthcare companies may reduce the risk of breaches of information inside the metaverse ecosystem by putting strong cybersecurity measures in place, such as encrypting and access limits [29]. Frequent audits and monitoring assist in identifying and resolving possible security flaws before malevolent actors may take advantage of them.

10.10.2.3 Strategies for Data Privacy and Data Security

Data privacy and data security play important roles. To protect the patient data, we put a strong encryption measure in place. It puts a strict access control to avoid unauthorized entry, protect sensitive information, and restrict data access to authorized people only. Open communication and proper use of patients' data promotes ethical and professional standards. This technique also helps in ensuring equitable treatment for all patients, regardless of their background.

10.10.3 Machine Learning Techniques and AI in Data Analysis

AI and machine learning (AIML) play an essential role in sorting the huge volumes of data produced in the metaverse to find cancer. This technology provides integrated tools for pattern detection, generating data, and giving useful ideas.

10.10.3.1 Types of Machine Learning Algorithms

10.10.3.1.1 Supervised Learning

Supervised learning [30] algorithms are the crucial methods for the diagnosis of cancer because these algorithms use labeled data in the training of an algorithm. This method will accurately identify tumors, provide related predictions, and give us treatment strategies. The following will help in understanding of the role of supervised learning in the field of cancer detection.

10.10.3.1.2 Labeled Data

Supervised learning always uses labeled data. In the field of cancer detection, such as genetic mutations and medical images, this will be linked to details such as kind, stage, and presence or absence of cancer among patients.

10.10.3.1.3 Feature Extraction

Features need to be removed before training the model. These features include size, form, and state of tumors in the images. Features in the data may correspondence to certain mutations.

10.10.3.1.4 Model Training

Model training is done using labeled datasets. We use supervised learning techniques like decision tree, support vector machine, and deep neural network, which are trained using labeled data. By changing some of the internal parameters, the pattern will gain the ability to change the input data similar to output labels during the training process.

10.10.3.1.5 Classification and Prediction

This model can recognize and divide datasets into separate data such as labeled and unlabeled datasets after it gets trained. In the process of cancer detection, it divides patients into categories such those having cancer and not having cancer, using the help of medical image analysis or genetic data analysis.

10.10.3.1.6 Unsupervised Learning

Unsupervised learning algorithms play a vital role in the area of cancer. It involves revealing the hidden structure and patterns and unlabeled datasets of the patients suffering from cancer.

10.10.3.1.7 Identifying the Hidden Patterns

To identify unlabeled patient data, we can use the method named unsupervised learning. This algorithm includes clustering, principal components analysis, and dimensionality reduction methods. These patterns indicate disease subtypes, underlying biological processes, and other variables linked to the reason for spread of cancer.

10.10.3.1.8 Finding Anomalies

To find anomalies or patterns in patients that may include the presence of malignant tumors or other conditions, we can also use anomaly detection techniques. Outliers found in images of the patients show the presence of cancer growth.

10.10.3.1.9 Analyzing Exploratory Data

There are many helpful methods for examining data analysis, like unsupervised learning, which helps in understanding the connections and patterns of cancers by medical experts [31]. By visualizing important elements or clusters of data, this can also help in decision-making in clinical areas.

10.10.3.1.10 Deep Learning

A CNN is a type of deep neural network that is suitable for processing grid-like input, such as images, etc. There are various layers in CNN, such as convolutional, pooling and fully linked layers. This is a very good option to use in learning the spatial hierarchies of the characters.

10.10.3.1.11 Segmenting Tumors

Preprocessing techniques like reduction, normalization, and scaling are used in medical imaging before feeding the image into the neural network. The UNet architecture is the most used adaptation for tumor segmentation. It is made as the path for precise localization and path detection for capturing contextual information. Various medical image segmentation, such as lung nodule identification and brain tumor detection, can be effectively completed [32].

10.10.3.1.12 Clinical Applications

The foundation of a computer-aided diagnostic system, CNN helps radiologists diagnose patients accurately by tutoring them in understanding medical pictures. Radiologists' productiveness and diagnosis are increased by a computer-aided detection system. It can be identified as a problematic area and provides frequent measuring. By recognizing these unique characters to each patient and forecasting the course, and by mixing genetic and clinical data with imaging data, CNN enables precise medical strategies for each patient [32, 33].

10.11 Challenges and Future Directions

10.11.1 Addressing Technical Challenges and Limitations

It is really a difficult task to maintain the data information of patients securely. Also, developing new techniques in the treatment of cancer in the metaverse is a more difficult task.

Data Privacy and Security: The fusing of metaverse usually involves the usage and sharing of sensitive data.

Accuracy and Reliability: It is not an easy task to develop accurate and reliable methods for cancer detection [34, 35].

10.11.2 Scaling Up and Widespread Adoption

Infrastructure: The infrastructure of the metaverse requires abundant funding, and it requires a great collaboration between technical companies and medical institutions for a successful outcome.

User Training: It is mandatory to check that the professionals are educated in how to use this metaverse technology for better outcomes.

Regulatory Approval: For regulatory approvals, in the metaverse a navigation system has been used.

10.11.3 Future Directions and Innovations

The accuracy of cancer treatment can be improved by advanced techniques like AR and VR. But in the metaverse, real-time collaboration between professionals all over the world can increase the results of a patient in a more effective way with less cost. It also increases the knowledge of doctors [36–38].

10.12 Conclusion

Metaverse technology has both advantages and disadvantages. It can be more effective in diagnosis of cancer. It also provides a better platform for medical students to learn medicine without any risk [39, 40].

10.12.1 Recap of Key Points

The metaverse uses both AR and VR, which provides a great environment to the patients to recover soon and healthily. It helps professionals to study the cases that are very risky to handle in virtual world without any risk, therefore increasing their confidence and knowledge about the case [41–43].

10.12.2 Summary of Benefits and Challenges

10.12.2.1 Benefits

- The metaverse creates a virtual environment that helps the patient to recover soon.
- It also helps the doctors to study complex cases without any risk.
- It also allows the professionals to work together for any particular case.
- It also helps people to get medical service who are living in remote areas.
- Due to its 3D virtual representation, it helps professionals to perform surgery more easily [44, 45].

10.12.2.2 Challenges

Metaverse technology in healthcare faces many challenges.

Legal and Social Considerations: Due to the development of the metaverse in the medical field, many legal and social problems may arise.

Security and Privacy: Ensuring the safety of patients' data is also a great challenge.

Protecting patient data is a difficult task in the digital environment to guarantee privacy and security in healthcare.

Accuracy and Reliability: It is also very essential to balance the quality and accuracy of treatment in the metaverse for better results.

Technical Conflicts: To avoid technical hurdles such as latency issues and for the correct process and great outcomes, high-quality Internet service is required.

Accessibility and Equity: Some people can't access the metaverse due to various reasons like Internet service and financial ability.

10.12.3 Future Outlook for Metaverse-Based Medical Disease Diagnosis

There is a great possibility for advanced treatment of patients due to the metaverse in the medical field.

Due to this, the patient will be offered personalized treatment by individual professionals who can analyze the data of individual patient with the help of virtual simulations. The involvement of AI in the metaverse really helps the doctors to understand the individual patterns and healthcare data of patients, which helps in providing a better diagnosis. If the metaverse is developed more, it can provide a platform for research all over the world to study complex cases together. Also, it provides medical education and advanced treatment for professionals. It offers great data about patients to doctors and also provides a virtual environment to the patients. In the future, for the usage of metaverse by the individual it requires a robust moral and framework to get access. Though it has many advantages like better diagnosis of diseases and cost-effectiveness, it also has disadvantages. These disadvantages will need to be managed or resolved as well.

References

1. Bale, A. S., Ghorpade, N., Hashim, M. F., Vaishnav, J., & Almaspoor, Z. (2022). A comprehensive study on metaverse and its impacts on humans. Advances in Human–Computer Interaction, 2022, Article ID 3247060. https://doi.org/10.1155/2022/3247060
2. Shao, L., Tang, W., Zhang, Z., & Chen, X. (2023). Medical metaverse: Technologies, applications, challenges and future. World Scientific, 23(02), 2350028. https://doi.org/10.1142/S0219519423500288
3. Yazdipour, A. B., Saeedi, S., Bostan, H., Masoorian, H., Sajjadi, H., Ghazisaeedi, M., et al. (2023). Opportunities and challenges of virtual reality-based interventions for patients with breast cancer: A systematic review. BMC Medical Informatics and Decision Making, 23, Article number: 17. https://doi.org/10.1186/s12911-023-02108-4
4. Allam, Z., Sharifi, A., Bibri, S. E., Jones, D. S., & Krogstie, J. (2022). The metaverse as a virtual form of smart cities: Opportunities and challenges for environmental, economic, and social sustainability in urban futures. Smart Cities, 5(40). https://doi.org/10.3390/smartcities5030040
5. Hamilton, W. (2009). Cancer diagnosis in primary care. British Journal of General Practice, 60(571), 121–128. https://doi.org/10.3399/bjgp10X483175
6. National Institute for Health and Excellence. (2015). Suspected cancer: Recognition and referral (ISBN: 978-1-4731-5438-4).
7. Iqbal, S., Siddiqui, G. F., Rehman, A., Hussain, L., Saba, T., Tariq, U., & Abbasi, A. A. (2021). Prostate cancer detection using deep learning and traditional techniques. IEEE Xplore, 9, ISSN: 2169-3536. https://doi.org/10.1109/ACCESS.2021.3057654

8. Lone, S. N., Nisar, S., Masoodi, T., Singh, M., Rizwan, A., Hashem, S., et al. (2022). Liquid biopsy: A step closer to transform diagnosis, prognosis, and future of cancer treatments. BioMed Central, 21, Article number: 79. https://doi.org/10.1186/s12943-022-01543-7

9. Bruno, R. R., Wolf, G., Wernly, B., Masyuk, M., Piayda, K., Leaver, S., et al. (2022). Virtual and augmented reality in critical care medicine: The patient's, clinician's, and researcher's perspective. BioMed Central, 26, Article number: 326. https://doi.org/10.1186/s13054-022-04202-x

10. Halbig, A., Babu, S. K., Gatter, S., Latoschik, M. E., Brukamp, K., & Mammen, S. (2022). Opportunities and challenges of virtual reality in healthcare – A domain experts inquiry. Frontiers, 3, Article 837616. https://doi.org/10.3389/frvir.2022.837616

11. Ara, J., Bhuiyan, H., Bhuiyan, Y. A., Bhyan, S. B., & Bhuiyan, M. I. (2021). AR-Based Modern Healthcare: A Review. ResearchGate.

12. Kamińska, D., Zwolińsksi, G., Laska-Leśniewicz, A., & Coelho, L. P. (2022). Virtual Reality in Healthcare. ResearchGate. https://doi.org/10.4018/978-1-7998-8371-5.ch001

13. Shinde, D., & Shrivas, P. (2021). Augmented reality in healthcare. International Research Journal of Engineering and Technology, 08(08), 4204–4208.

14. Kolecki, R., Pręgowska, A., Dąbrowa, J., Skucinski, J., Pulanecki, T., Walecki, P., et al. (2022). Assessment of the utility of mixed reality in medical education. Translational Research in Anatomy. Elsevier, 28, 100214. https://doi.org/10.1016/j.tria.2022.100214

15. Steyaert, S., Pizurica, M., Nagaraj, D., Khandelwal, P., Hernandez-Boussard, T., Gentles, A. J., & Gevaert, O. (2023). Multimodal data fusion for cancer biomarker discovery with deep learning. PubMedCentral, 5. https://doi.org/10.1038/s42256-023-00633-5

16. Aliwi, I., Schot, V., Carrabba, M., Duong, P., Shievano, S., Caputo, M., et al. (2023). The role of immersive virtual reality and augmented reality in medical communication: A scoping review. SAGE Journals, 10, 1–10. https://doi.org/10.1177/23743735231171562

17. Butpheng, C., Yeh, K.-H., & Xiong, H. (2020). Security and privacy in IoT-cloud-based e-health systems – A comprehensive review. Symmetric, 12, 1191. https://doi.org/10.3390/sym12071191

18. Tretter, M., Samhammer, D., Ott, T., & Dabrock, P. (2023). Towards an ethics for the healthcare metaverse. Journal of Metaverse, 3(2), 181–189. https://doi.org/10.57019/jmv.1318774

19. Bouslama, A., & Laaziz, Y. (2018). AWS For Healthcare System. ResearchGate.

20. Mbonihankuye, S., Nkunzimana, A., & Ndagijimana, A. (2019). Healthcare data security technology: HIPAA compliance. Wireless Communications and Mobile Computing, 2019, Article ID 1927495. https://doi.org/10.1155/2019/1927495

21. Harrington, R. L., Hanna, M. L., Oehrlein, E. M., Camp, R., Wheeler, R., Cooblall, C., & Perfetto, E. M. (2020). Defining patient engagement in research: Results of a systematic review and analysis: Report of the ISPOR patient-centered special interest group. Elsevier, 23(6), 677–688. https://doi.org/10.1016/j.jval.2020.01.019

22. Almeida, S. (2013). An introduction to high-performance computing. World Scientific, 28(22n23), 1–9. https://doi.org/10.1142/S0217751X13400216

23. Hansberry, D. R., Agarwal, N., Gonzales, S. F., & Baker, S. R. (2014). A critical review of the readability of online patient education resources from RadiologyInfo. Org. American Journal of Roentgenology, 202(3), 566–575. https://doi.org/10.2214/AJR.13.11223

24. Kanas, G., Morimoto, L., Mowat, F., O'Malley, C., Fryzek, J., & Nordyke, R. (2010). Use of electronic medical records in oncology outcomes research. ClinicoEconomics and Outcomes Research: CEOR, 2, 1–14. https://doi.org/10.2147/CEOR.S8411

25. Sebastian, A. M., & Peter, D. (2022). Artificial intelligence in cancer research: Trends, challenges and future directions. Life, 12, 1991. https://doi.org/10.3390/life12121991

26. Singh, D. N., Daripelli, S., & Bushara, M. O. E. (2023). Genetic testing for successful cancer treatment. PubMed Central, 15. https://doi.org/10.7759/cureus.49889

27. Zhang, B., Shi, H., & Wang, H. (2023). Machine learning and AI in cancer prognosis, prediction, and treatment selection: A critical approach. Journal of Multidisciplinary Healthcare, 16. https://doi.org/10.2147/JMDH.S410301

28. Rasool, A., Bunterngchit, C., Tiejian, L., Islam, M. R., Qu, Q., & Jiang, Q. (2022). Improved machine learning-based predictive models for breast cancer diagnosis. International Journal of Environmental Research and Public Health, 19, 3211. https://doi.org/10.3390/ijerph19063211

29. Gupta, U. C. (2013). Informed consent in clinical research: Revisiting few concepts and areas. PubMed Central, 4. https://doi.org/10.4103/2229-3485.106373

30. Nasr, M. M., Nasr, M. M., & Shehata, L. H. (2022). Cybersecurity in health systems: Challenges, and proposals. International Journal of Progressive Sciences and Technologies (IJPSAT), 35, 195–208.

31. Choudhury, A., Balasubramaniam, S, Kumar, A. P., & Kumar, S. N. P. (2023). PSSO: Political squirrel search optimizer-driven deep learning for severity level detection and classification of lung cancer. International Journal of Information Technology & Decision Making, 1–34.

32. Ha, J., Parekh, P., Gamble, D., Masters, J., Jun, P., Daniels, T., & Halai, M. (2021). Opportunities and challenges of using augmented reality and heads-up display in orthopedic surgery: A narrative review. Journal of Clinical Orthopaedics and Trauma, 18, 209–215. https://doi.org/10.1016/j.jcot.2021.04.031

33. Balasubramaniam, S, Syed, M. H., More, N. S., & Polepally, V. (2023). Deep learning-based power prediction aware charge scheduling approach in cloud based electric vehicular network. Engineering Applications of Artificial Intelligence, 121, 105869.

34. Whalley, L. J. (1995). Ethical issues in the application of virtual reality to medicine. Computers in Biology and Medicine, 25(2), 107–114. https://doi.org/10.1016/0010-4825(95)00008-r

35. Halbig, A., Babu, S. K., Gatter, S., Latoschik, M. E., Brukamp, K., & Mammen, S. (2022). Opportunities and challenges of virtual reality in healthcare – A domain expert inquiry. Frontiers, 3, Article 837616. https://doi.org/10.3389/frvir.2022.837616

36. Kadry, S., Dhanaraj, R. K., & Manthiramoorthy, C. (2024). Res-UNet based blood vessel segmentation and cardiovascular disease prediction using chronological chef-based optimization algorithm based deep residual network from retinal fundus images. Multimedia Tools and Applications, 83, 1–30.

37. Mistry, D., Brock, C. A., & Lindsey, T. (2023). The present and future of virtual reality in medical education: A narrative review. Cureus, 15(12), 1–6. https://doi.org/10.7759/cureus.51124

38. Gupte, N. (2019). Augmented reality and health informatics: A study based on bibliometric and content analysis of scholarly communication and social media. Digital Commons LIU, 1–255.

39. Mazurek, J., Kipper, P., Kipper, A., Cieslik, B., Rutkowski, S., Rutkowski, E., mehlich, K., Rutkowski, B., Turolla, A., & Szcepanska-Gieracha, J. (2019). Virtual reality in medicine: A brief overview and future research directions. Human Movement, 20(3), 16–22. https://doi.org/10.5114/hm.2019.83529

40. Hasegawa, T., Chatani, S., Sato, Y., Murata, S., Yamaura, H., Tsukii, R., Yoshihara, T., Machida, M., Nagasawa, K., & Inaba, Y. (2021). Percutaneous image-guided needle biopsy of musculoskeletal tumours: Technical tips. Interventional Radiology, 6(3), 75–82. https://doi.org/10.22575%2Finterventionalradiology.2020-0030

41. Sharib, A. (2022). Where do we stand in AI for endoscopic image analysis? Deciphering gaps and future directions. npj Digital Medicine, 5, Article number: 184. https://doi.org/10.1038/s41746-022-00733-3

42. MurthyT, S. D., & Sadashivappa, G. (2019). An analytical research study of MRI brain tumour modalities and classification techniques. Semantic Scholar, 8, 357–376. https://api.semanticscholar.org/CorpusID:212456330

43. Ramalingam, V., Revathidevi, S., Shanmuganayagam, T., Muthulakshmi, L., & Rajaram, R. (2016). Biogenic gold nanoparticles induce cell cycle arrest through oxidative stress and sensitize mitochondrial membranes in A549 lung cancer cells. RSC Advances, 6(25), 1–16. https://doi.org/10.1039/C5RA26781A

44. Balasubramaniam, S, Joe, C. V., Manthiramoorthy, C., & Kumar, K. S. (2024). ReliefF based feature selection and gradient squirrel search algorithm enabled deep Maxout network for detection of heart disease. Biomedical Signal Processing and Control, 87, 105446.

45. Faheem, B., Kumar, B. K., Sekhar, K. V. G. C., Kunjiappan, S., Jamalis, J., Balaña-Fouce, R., Tekwani, B. L., & Sankaranarayanan, M. (2020). Druggable targets of SARS-CoV-2 and treatment opportunities for COVID-19. Bioorganic Chemistry, 104, 1–25. https://doi.org/10.1016/j.bioorg.2020.104269

Chapter 11

Metaverse-Based Autism Spectrum Disorder Social Skills Training: Case Study

K. Suresh, V. Kavitha, S. Poonkodi,
and Jayaraj Ramasamy

11.1 Introduction

11.1.1 Autism and the Metaverse

In the autism metaverse, people with autism can access digital worlds that help them grow. Often, folks with autism find it hard to talk and connect with others. They may act, socialize, and feel in different ways. The metaverse lets them meet their needs and wants through online spaces and ways to chat. Here, people with autism might find new and easy ways to talk with others. This can help them with troubles they face in normal social spots. The virtual world can give a steady and expected space, good for those who are extra sensitive to senses. This way, autistic people can talk in ways that match what they like and are good at. Also, the metaverse can make a kinder community where people with different brain setups are liked for their unique views and help. In the metaverse, autistic folks can chat with others in more free and new ways, skipping the hard parts they might hit in regular social places. To make a convivial metaverse for all, especially for those with autism, it's key that experts in autism, creators, and everyone work together. Many things linked to autism spectrum disorder (ASD)

DOI: 10.1201/9781003491668-11

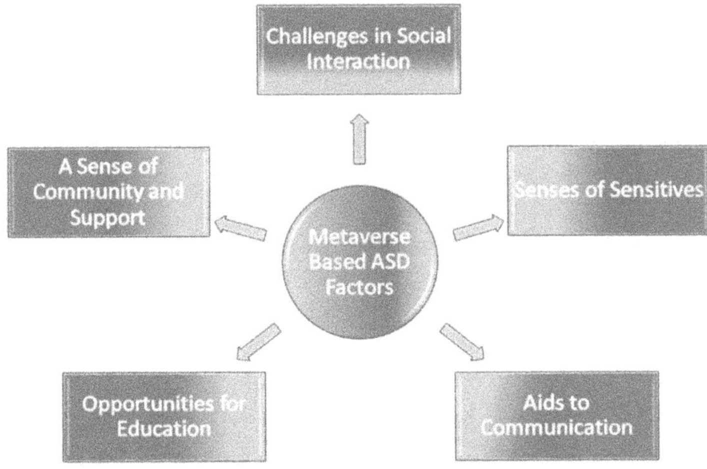

Figure 11.1   Factors associated with ASD.

need to be thought about when thinking of the metaverse. Figure 11.1 shows different aspects tied to ASD.

Challenges in Social Interaction:
In real life, meeting and talking to others can be hard for many people with autism. With the metaverse, users can join in on social activities in a way that's easy for them, in a place that's easy to manage.

Senses of Sensitivity:
Autism often means feeling things very deeply, and many people with autism experience this. When making the metaverse, these feelings can be thought of. This lets users change their online world to fit what they want to feel.

Aids to Communication:
The digital space can be made with special tools and hands-on features just for people with autism. These tools are picked to match what each person needs.

Opportunities for Education:
People with autism can learn in the metaverse in ways that fit how they like to learn best. Interactive places and virtual reality setups let us make learning more fun and tailored for each person.

A Sense of Community and Support:
In this view, the metaverse ought to have special groups for building friendships, sharing thoughts, and helping each other.

11.1.2 Challenges in Social Interaction in the Metaverse with Autism

The difficulties that people with autism have in social interaction are depicted in Figure 11.2. When it comes to interacting socially in the metaverse, autistic people face a number of challenges, including the following:

Communication Based on Nonverbal Cues:
The majority of interactions that take place online are conducted through nonverbal cues such as body language and facial expressions. These nonverbal cues create social behaviors that are always challenging for people who have autism to comprehend.

Overload with Sensory Information:
In case of sensory hypersensitivity people, such a feeling of the intensive sensory stimuli created in a virtual reality (VR) environment may be too much stimulation for them. When colors are vivid, sounds are loud, or tasks require urgent responses in due time, it often ends up that such people disable their ability to actively interact with the metaverse.

Interpretation in the Literal Sense:
Individuals who have autism have a tendency to view the linguistic component as "crude," which results in them having difficulty comprehending figurative and metaphorical language, which is an essential component of successful social interaction.

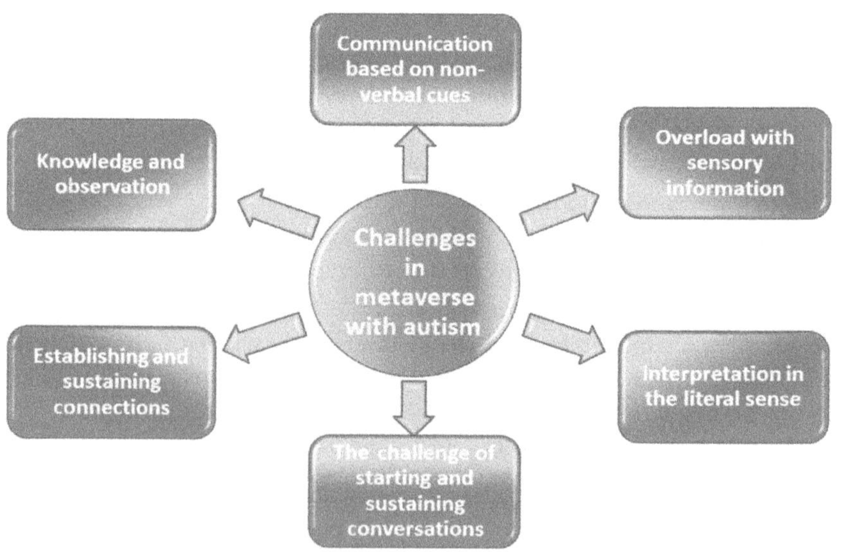

Figure 11.2 Challenges in social interaction in the metaverse with autism.

The Challenge of Starting and Sustaining Conversations:
If you have the feeling of autism, you will realize that it will be hard for you since the beginning to start a conversation. Digital abuses of various kinds could, however, be heightened by the involved lack of synchrony and the anonymous character of online discourses, since the differences might hinder communications.

Establishing and Sustaining Connections:
The way we build relationships in the virtual world may be unique, just as it is when people interact in real life, reflecting the essence of how we connect with others. Due to the uniqueness of meeting in the metaverse, for people with autism, the more socializing it gets, the more challenging and complex it can be for them than just thinking about socializing in the real world.

Knowledge and Observation:
The education of people who spend their time in a metaverse for the purpose of developing empathy and understanding of neurodiversity and autism can result in positive outcomes. The implementation of crucial campaigns and job training programs within online communities has the potential to be very effective in reducing the impact on the environment.

11.1.3 Metaverse: Educational Prospects for Children with Autism

The metaverse uses immersive technology, including augmented reality (AR) and VR, to provide children with autism with a wide range of educational opportunities While catering to their individual learning preferences and challenges, these programs must provide a more personalized and enjoyable educational experience for children with autism. Social interaction situations, such as group activities or discussions, can be created so that children can practice and learn in a safe environment. VR scenarios can be developed to teach and practice real-world skills such as cooking, shopping, and navigating public spaces in a safe and repeatable environment. Children with autism can benefit from using simulations to improve their skills and apply them to real-world contexts. Speech therapy and communication exercises can be combined with a mixture of engaging and stimulating elements. The use of AR can provide visual and interactive support for the acquisition of communication skills.

Virtual environments can be suited to satisfy specific needs and sensitivities of each child. VR can be used as a therapeutic tool for interventions such as exposure therapy, desensitization, and relaxation techniques. VR is one tool that therapists, psychologists, educators, parents, and their kids are embracing to help individuals with autism connect and communicate with others, and the outside world is better than before. It's also being used to educate nonautistic people about what it means to live with the condition. Children with autism have also benefited from

VR preparation for public speaking. Through the use of avatars as the audience, who vanish if the speaker fails to make eye contact, kids were encouraged to look around the room instead of just forward. Participants responded well to the game in which they had to keep their avatars on screen.

With the ongoing advancement of technology, there are more opportunities to apply AR and VR in the field of mental health. The treatment of neurodevelopmental disorders is one area in which these technologies show great promise. When discussing the impact of the metaverse on mental health, we also need to consider how it can be used to treat neurodevelopmental disorders. The mainstay of treatment for neurodevelopmental disorders has historically been in-person interactions between patients and therapists.

11.1.4 Motivations for the Development of the Metaverse

There are many factors that contributed to development at the beginning of metaverse development. These factors include technological advancements, business goals, and a desire to create new, fully immersive online experiences. The data presented in Figure 11.3 suggest that the creation of the metaverse offers many potential benefits in the treatment of neurodevelopmental disorders.

Involvement
VR and AR are two forms of entertainment that can be interesting for people with arthritis. By creating a space of safe and permanent exit, this project has the potential to encourage sharing, healing, and learning.

Individualization
When it comes to mental health, the metaverse makes it possible to cater to each individual's needs and wishes, which in turn enables personalized treatment and therapy.

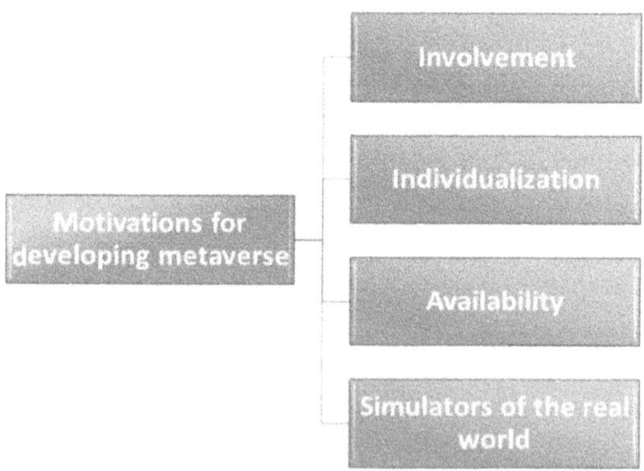

Figure 11.3   Motivations for the development of the metaverse.

Availability

The costs associated with accessing treatment can be reduced with the help of metaverse platforms that also enable live or remote treatment, and individuals who may not have easy access to conventional treatment can benefit from it based on the metaverse. These treatments can be very beneficial.

Simulators of the Real World

There is a wide range of advantages connected with this simulation, two of which are an enhanced simulation of data from the real world and an increased level of reliability. The metaverse is a healthcare platform that offers people with neurodevelopmental disabilities the safest and most organized environment possible, giving them with the opportunity to develop skills in areas such as problem-solving activities of daily living and life skills.

11.1.5 Important Things to Think about When Creating a Metaverse for Mental Health

Regarding the treatment of neurodevelopmental disorders, the goal in order to design functional psychotherapy, it is necessary to take into consideration a number of important factors. Figure 11.4 shows how key ideas have grown regarding making a virtual world for therapy use.

Privacy and Ethics:

Integrating measures to protect the privacy and well-being of client data are a fundamental part of metaverse applications.

Techniques Based on Evidence:

To find lasting success in the metaverse, mediations should be supported by examination and data.

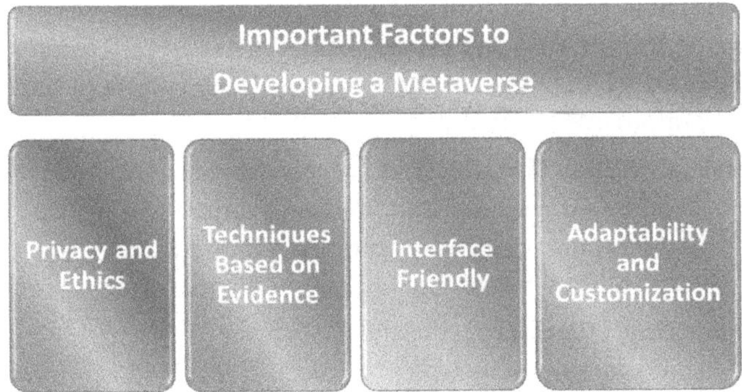

Figure 11.4   Important factors to developing a metaverse.

Interface-Friendly:
Applications intended for the metaverse should have a point of interaction that is easy to understand and straightforward to work. It is feasible to further develop client commitment and experience by giving clear guidelines and elements that are easy to understand.

Adaptability and Customization:
It is important that individuals who have neurodevelopmental disabilities have the ability to use the metaverse in a manner that is adaptable to their specific capabilities and requirements.

11.1.6 Common Characteristics of Neurodevelopmental Disorder

A collection of illnesses known as neurodevelopmental disorders impact how the brain develops and functions in an individual. These conditions usually start in early childhood and last the entirety of a person's life. ASD is one of the many conditions that fall under the umbrella of neurodevelopmental disorders. Depending on the particular condition, neurodevelopmental disorders can present with a variety of symptoms. Nonetheless, a few typical signs and symptoms are social interaction challenges, communication deficits, recurrent actions, hyperactivity, impulsivity, and issues with learning and academic achievement. These symptoms may range from mild to severe in extent, and some people will need ongoing help and support. Common characteristics or forms of neurodevelopmental disorders (as shown in Figure 11.5) include the following:

Autism Spectrum Disorder (ASD)
Social interaction problems, communication issues, repetitive behaviors, and narrow interests are characteristics of ASD. Since it is a spectrum disorder, people with it may exhibit a broad range of symptoms at different intensities.

Attention-Deficit/Hyperactivity Disorder (ADHD)
Hyperactivity, impulsivity, and persistent patterns of inattention are characteristics of ADHD. ADHD sufferers may have trouble focusing, setting priorities, and limiting impulsive behavior.

Intellectual Disability (Intellectual Developmental Disorder)
Limitations in adaptive behavior and intellectual functioning are characteristics of this disorder. It is characterized by problems in practical skills, reasoning, and problem-solving abilities, which make daily living difficult.

Specific Learning Disorder
Academic achievement is impacted by specific learning disorders, which are typified by difficulties with learning and applying academic skills. Dyslexia in reading, dyscalculia in math, and dysgraphia in writing are a few examples.

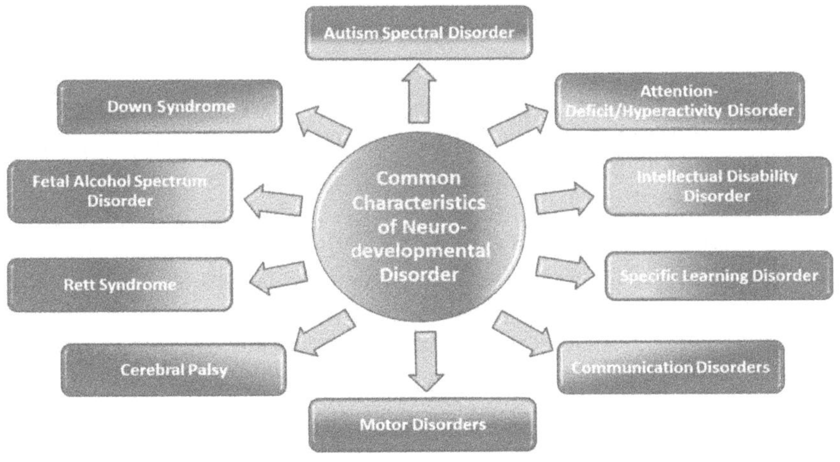

Figure 11.5   Common characteristics forms of neurodevelopmental disorders.

Communication Disorders

Impairments in spoken or written language comprehension and usage. Difficulty producing speech sounds, which causes articulation problems.

Motor Disorders

Impairment in the motor coordination development and challenges in the motor development and execution.

Cerebral Palsy

A collection of conditions that impact posture and movement and are typically brought on by harm to the establishing brain. It may lead to problems with control and coordination of the muscles.

Rett Syndrome

A rare genetic disorder that primarily impacts girls and is characterized by repetitive hand movements, loss of targeted hand skills, and developmental regression.

Fetal Alcohol Spectrum Disorders (FASD)

Disorders caused by alcohol exposure during pregnancy, which can cause a variety of behavioral and cognitive deficits.

Down Syndrome

There are genetic disorders that are carried by new copies of chromosome 21, and these disorders can result in mental retardation, a unique appearance, and other health problems.

It's vital to remember that each neurodevelopmental disorder can have wildly varying symptom severity, and that support and early detection are essential for those who suffer from these conditions. Furthermore, continued research could result in revisions to the categorization and comprehension of neurodevelopmental disorders.

11.2 Literature Survey

For children with high-functioning autism spectrum disorder (HFASD), this is the first pilot randomized controlled trial (RCT) intended to show off a metaverse-based social skills training program. The use of the metaverse in the classroom, which aims to teach real-life social skills such as soccer, has the potential to increase social skills and reduce cognitive behavioral issues in children who have problems, according to the findings of the study carried out by the researchers. Autism is an extremely uncommon condition. The findings of this study suggest that interventions aimed at improving home life appear to have the potential to be extended to include a larger population, targeting those suffering from chronic diseases [1]. ASD is a progressive developmental disorder characterized by difficulties with language, nonverbal communication and socialization, and restricted or repetitive behaviors [2]. The purpose of this research is to determine the business procedures that can be utilized in order to implement the metaverse in the field of healthcare services. Published and Internet sources were searched for relevant statistical data [3].

Planning strategically to create business opportunities of metaverse services is among the most essential activities in the healthcare industry. The presence of multiple critical factors complicates the planning and implementation of developing a plan for the creation of business opportunities, as numerous qualitative and quantitative factors need to be taken into account. Numerous studies pertaining to the metaverse in the healthcare sector have been investigated [4].

A universe of VR called the metaverse is being developed to enable user interaction, virtually in a highly immersive manner that resembles real-life situations. The metaverse has the potential to have an impact on a number of industries, including digital anti-aging in healthcare, even though its main goals are social interaction and entertainment [5]. Using avatars to engage and converse with professors and fellow students, students can virtually attend lectures using Edu-Metaverse's application [6]. Studies on Edu-Metaverse were mostly focused on higher education. We do not, however, know if the metaverse is more useful than undergraduate students for assisting secondary students in particular or general learning contexts because no further information is supplied [7]. Throughout the categories of cognitive research and surgical interventions, VR and AR can optimize patient results and quickly create effective patient management. There needs to be more immersive digital technology clinical trials [8]. We have examined how these newly developed technologies can help students with learning difficulties receive an inclusive education, as well as the requirements for instruction and assistance that arise from a student's educational challenges. We have located papers from conferences and articles in journals that are pertinent to our investigation by searching a variety of online digital libraries. Our review of the pertinent literature revealed that assistive technologies pertaining to extended reality (XR), the Internet of Things (IoT), and the metaverse have not received much attention. Compared to other technologies, AI and human–computer interaction (HCI) are used as assistive technologies more frequently [9]. This study is an innovative attempt to use the current metaverse trend as a platform for delivering training courses on job readiness, adaptability, and employment maintenance [10]. Autism provided an example of machine learning models for recognizing the initial phase of ASD. Performance was evaluated on the converted ASD dataset using various classification algorithms and the feature development (FT) method. The key ASD characteristics were examined using the ASD dataset. A good performance rate is determined by a number of metrics, including sensitivity, log loss, area under the ROC curves (AUROC), sensitivity, specificity, and accuracy. Using a classifier model, this ASD dataset was predicted with 97.10% accuracy. Early detection of ASD is possible with the help of machine learning techniques [11].

11.3 Methodology

Since social skills are a part of most people's developmental stages, most of us haven't received any kind of specialized training in them. Body language, tone, and eye contact are examples of social cues that we are naturally good at reading. Additional complex elements like metaphors, idioms, and sarcasm aid in our understanding of the discourse. However, people with ASD are not able to pick up on these, which can cause communication gaps. Autism-related social skills training is necessary for a person's development. Early-intervention behavioral treatments intended to promote "correct" behavioral development make up social skills development training. The basic concept is to create a system of rewards and incentives to teach kids on the autism spectrum about socializing with other people. Since every child is different and has different issues, they will also need different treatments, which is what kind of training is taught.

11.3.1 Social Skills Training

The program for social skills training is based on the metaverse. Socialization along with peers is crucial for kids who have HFASD to form relationships with friends and participate in constructive transfers. On interactive game platforms that are based in the metaverse, kids can take part in a variety of group activities. PEERS, a metaverse-based social skills training program, has been released for kids with ASD on the metaverse platform. There were four sessions in the curriculum for the program. The introduction and awareness of the necessity of guidelines and outcomes took place in the first session. In the second session, team-building exercises and an understanding of the scenarios based on behavior were involved. In the third session, we talked about how to react to unpleasant feelings and behavioral experiences. The topic of the fourth session was recognizing and valuing personal differences. Each session included homework, feedback, and metaverse practice in addition to theoretical classes. The following are some essential elements of social skills instruction for autistic people.

11.3.2 Evaluation and Customized Planning

Start by evaluating the person's existing social skills and pinpointing the precise areas in which they require development. Create a personalized plan based on the person's age-appropriate social expectations, strengths, and challenges. Efficient support and intervention for individuals with autism require the implementation of assessment and individualized planning. Understanding a person's strengths, weaknesses, and particular needs is crucial to creating interventions that are tailored to meet those needs, as presented in Figure 11.6. In the context of autism, evaluation and customized planning are broken down as follows:

Diagnosis
An official diagnosis of ASD by licensed medical professionals, such as child development specialists, psychologists, or psychiatrists, is usually at the beginning of the screening process.

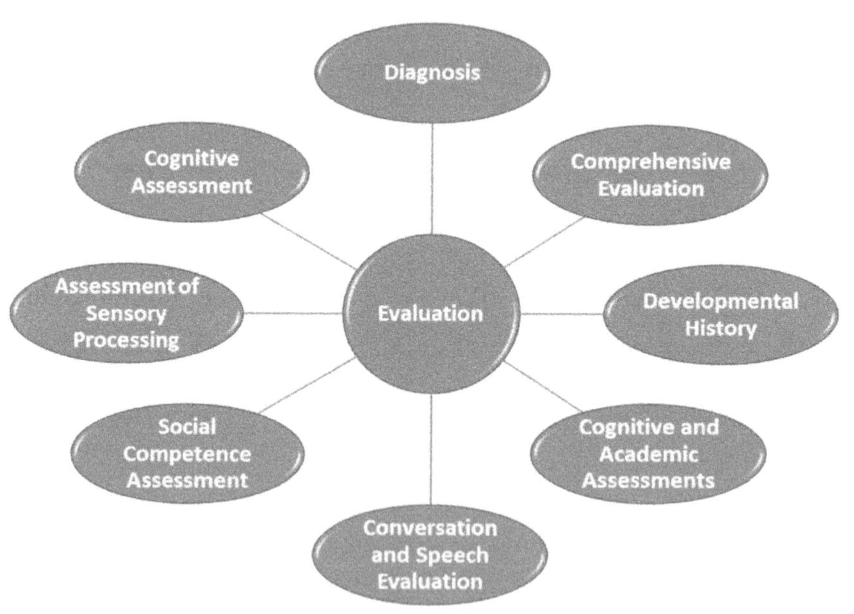

Figure 11.6 Evaluation and customized planning.

Comprehensive Evaluation

Data are collected from various sources for comprehensive analysis. These sources include the person's parents, guardians, teachers, and in many cases the direct caregiver.

Developmental History

Collecting a complete developmental history before surgery begins help to understand the individual's initial performance, complications, and any signs of developmental delay.

Cognitive and Academic Assessments

Academic skills and intellectual functioning tests (IQ tests) can be used to determine a person's intelligence (IQ) as well as weaknesses. This includes identifying any potential learning difficulties.

Conversation and Speech Evaluation

As part of this position, the individual's communication and speaking skills are tested. The aim of this study is to provide support for interventions that will best support successful communication. This assessment also takes into account the individual's expression of receptive language.

Social Competence Assessment

By evaluating social skills and gaining an understanding of social indicators, it is possible to identify particular areas of strength and suggest strategies for the development of projects that are specifically targeted.

Assessment of Sensory Processing

Some people with autism may experience difficulties or sensitivities with their senses. In order to better understand sensory processing difficulties and develop strategies for regulating sensory input, assessments in this field are helpful.

Cognitive Assessment

Cognitive assessments facilitate the creation of behavior intervention plans by assisting in the identification of problematic behaviors, their triggers, and possible purposes.

11.3.3 Clear Guidance

Give social skills instruction that is clear. Divide up difficult social behaviors into smaller, more doable steps. To demonstrate proper social behaviors and expectations, use visual aids, social stories, or video modeling. In the framework of autism, explicit instruction refers to a methodical, direct teaching strategy that is organized, clear, and concentrated on giving students explicit information. People with ASD, who frequently benefit from explicit and concrete information, will find this method especially helpful. By confirming that the student has understood the intended concept or skill, explicit instruction seeks to increase transparency in the

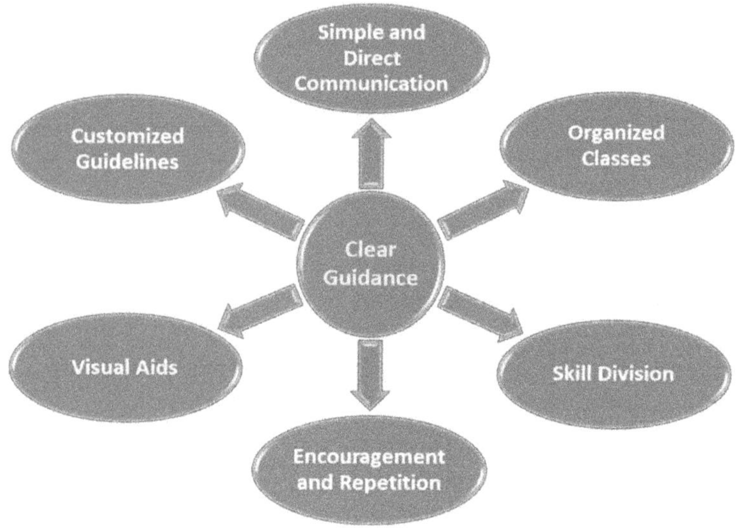

Figure 11.7 Clear guidance.

learning process. Figure 11.7 gives the essential elements of autism clear guidance, which are:

Simple and Direct Communication
- To prevent ambiguity, instructions are written in an easy-to-understand, succinct style.
- Information is stated clearly by teachers or instructors, minimizing opportunity for misunderstanding.

Organized Classes
- Lessons have a defined structure and are well organized, usually consisting of an introduction, explicit instruction, guided practice, and independent practice.
- Schedules and charts are examples of visual aids that can be used to improve the organization and predictability of the learning environment.

Skill Division
- Difficult skills are divided into easier-to-manage smaller parts. To ensure a step-by-step understanding, each component is explicitly taught before going on to the next.
- Before combining skills into a whole, the breakdown of skills enables autistic learners to understand the constituent parts of a task or concept.

Encouragement and Repetition
- An essential part of explicit instruction is repetition. To improve learning, ideas and abilities are reviewed and strengthened.

- Praise and rewards are examples of positive reinforcement that can be used to inspire students and increase their involvement in the learning process.

Visual Aids
- In order to strengthen comprehension and improve clarity, it is common practice to incorporate visual aids such as charts and diagrams.
- Individuals with autism can benefit from the use of visual aids when it comes to information processing and navigating the classroom.

Customized Guidelines
- Explicit instruction is frequently customized to meet the unique requirements and abilities of students with autism.
- Educators can utilize evaluation results to pinpoint particular areas of weakness and modify their lessons accordingly.

To meet the learning needs of people with autism, specific guidance is frequently used in educational settings, including special education programs. For students on the autism spectrum, this method can help with skill acquisition, independence, and generalization. It also conforms to evidence-based practices.

11.3.4 Playing Responsibilities

In the context of autism, role-playing is a therapeutic or educational approach in which people, frequently those with ASD, participate in fictitious social situations or exchanges. This method is intended to assist people in practicing and growing a range of social skills in a safe and encouraging setting. Therapists, educators, and caregivers can effectively address the social challenges that individuals with autism often face by utilizing role-playing as a valuable tool. Figure 11.8 visualizes the key elements of role-playing in the context of autism, including the following:

Implementing Real-life Social Scenarios
In role-playing activities, people with autism are assisted in engaging in situations that replicate authentic social contexts. These scenarios could involve commonplace exchanges like greetings, group activities, and conversations with peers.

Established and Encouraged Environment
Often run by a therapist or educator, role-playing sessions take place in a structured and encouraging environment. Without the constraints or worries that come with social situations in the real world, this environment promotes the development of specific skills.

Social Skills Practice
People with autism frequently struggle to comprehend and react to social cues, communicate nonverbally, and exhibit acceptable social behaviors. A safe and regulated environment for honing these abilities is offered by role-playing.

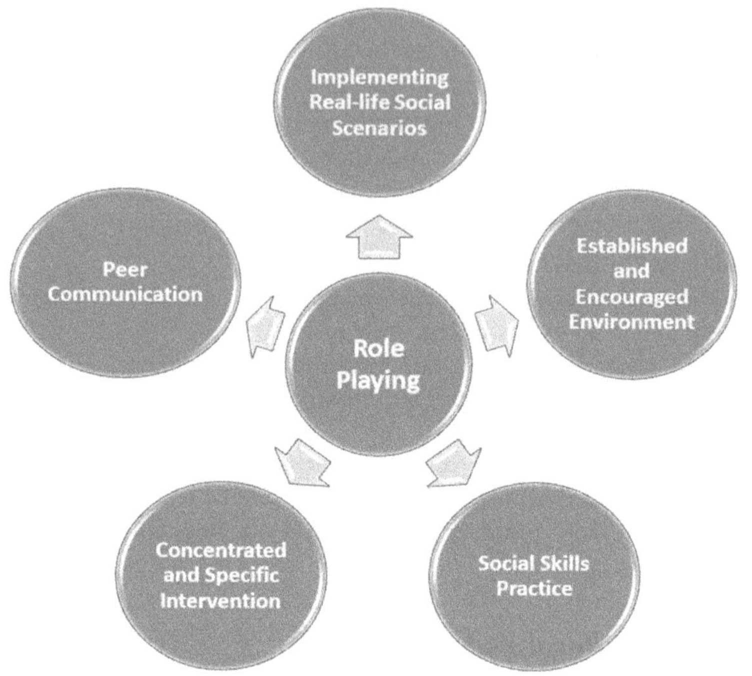

Figure 11.8 Playing responsibilities.

Concentrated and Specific Intervention
Role-playing interventions can be tailored to a person's unique social challenges. Therapists can modify scenarios to concentrate on skills like striking up a conversation, maintaining eye contact, sharing, or comprehending feelings.

Peer Communication
Playing roles with peers can foster communication and social interaction in a group environment. People are encouraged to use and modify their social skills in a social setting by this collaborative feature.

11.3.5 *Working Together with Parents and Guardians*

In order to reinforce learning at home and in the community, involve parents and other caregivers in the social skills training process. One of the most important aspects of supporting people with ASD is working in tandem along with parents and caregivers. The consistency, comprehension, and general well-being of people with autism are greatly enhanced by the involvement of parents and other caregivers

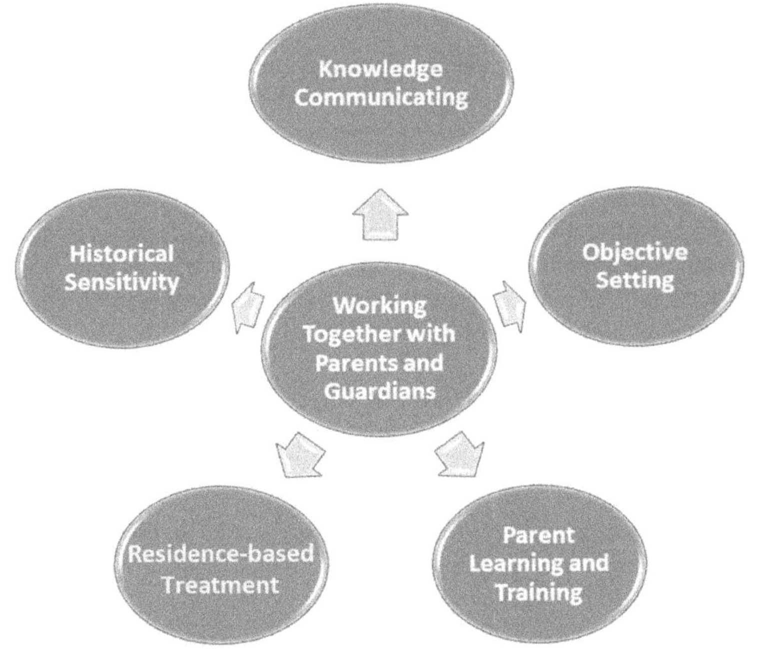

Figure 11.9 Working together with parents and guardians.

in the intervention and care process, which are presented in Figure 11.9. In the context of autism, the following are some essential elements of working in tandem with parents and caregivers:

Knowledge Communicating
A more thorough understanding of the child or individual with autism is produced by sharing information about the person's strengths, challenges, preferences, and unique needs.

Objective Setting
An intervention plan can be developed in a more comprehensive and customized manner by working together with parents and caregivers during the goal-setting process.

Parent Learning and Training
Providing parents and other caregivers with knowledge about autism makes it possible for them to provide better support for their child at home.

Residence-Based Treatments
Advancement and implementation in the home by providing opportunities for parents and other caregivers to be actively involved in the treatment process also provide these opportunities.

11.3.6 Historical Sensitivity

Historical sensitivity is designed to meet the individual's needs. Furthermore, ongoing reinforcement and support are essential to maintaining the acquisition and application of life skills. Working together with specialists in the field, like occupational therapists, behavioral therapists, and speech therapists, can improve how well social skills training works for people with autism. Groups for social skills programs for teaching social skills are typically run through recovery-oriented support groups. These are settings where people (of all ages) with autism can regularly practice social skills. Consider these settings their support system. Activities for social groups with autism include certain features.

1. Working in groups or pairs to encourage collaboration and partnership.
2. Simplifying language and classifying people according to their language comprehension level.
3. Offering structure.
4. Minimizing the complexity of abstract ideas to make them more approachable.
5. Offer a variety of learning opportunities.
6. Encourage self-awareness and self-esteem.

11.4 VR and AR

AR and VR are two examples of how modern social skills training tools have shown promise in assisting individuals who have ASD. In this particular setting, VR and AR can be useful in a few different ways. People with autism are able to experience anxiety that is similar to that which they would experience in real-life situations and use it in social interactions through the use of VR, which provides a safe and regulated virtual space. By using the overlaying of digital data on the real world, AR provides context and guidance for social interactions that occur in the moment. It is possible for VR to provide real-life scenarios, such as job interviews, casual conversations, or public speaking, which enable individuals with autism to develop and impart their complex social skills that they have developed under a variety of circumstances.

Through the utilization of real-time compression, social scripts, or visual tools, AR has the potential to facilitate communication, thereby making it convenient and more productive for individuals. With the help of VR, users can practice verbal and nonverbal communication in interactive scenarios, enhancing their expressive and receptive communication abilities. There is a lot of promise for developing individualized, successful, and entertaining interventions that can enhance the social interactions and general standard of daily life for those who have autism through the integration of VR and AR into social skill training. But in order to guarantee the creation of applications that are both ethically sound and grounded in evidence, cooperation with other experts in the field — such as psychologists, therapists, and educators — is crucial. A managed supportive atmosphere is crucial when interviewing children with autism who are focused on social skills and training. The objective is to evaluate their present social skills, pinpoint areas in which they can grow, and comprehend their particular requirements.

11.5 Interview Instructions for Children with Autism: Social Ability and Guidelines

Interviewing children with autism requires a careful, customized strategy to meet their special communication and sensory requirements. Figure 11.10 shows interview instructions for children with autism. The following are recommendations and directions for interviewing autistic children.

11.5.1 Knowledge in Communication

Verbal Communication
- Assess the coherence and clarity of the speech.
- Take note of any scripting or echolalia used.
- Assess expressive language proficiency.

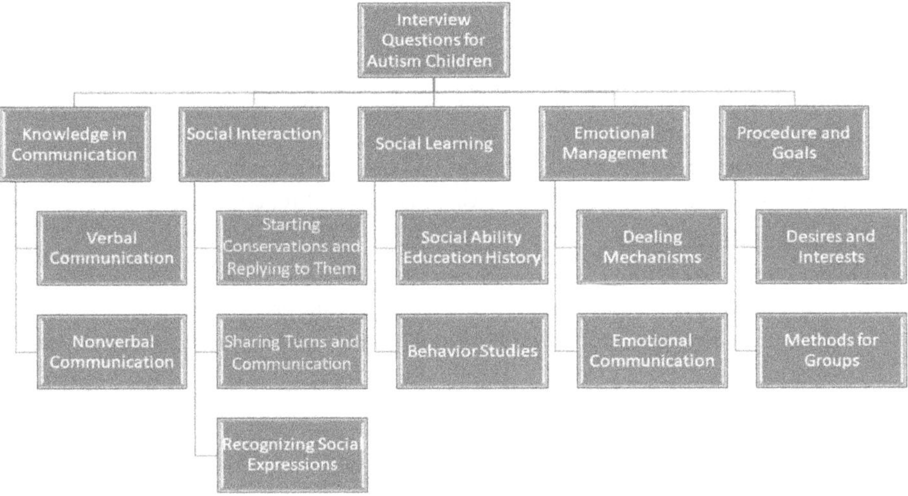

Figure 11.10 **Interview instructions for children with autism.**

Nonverbal Communication
- Give attention to facial expressions and eye contact.
- Examine your body language and gestures.
- Take note of any usage of augmentative and alternative (AAC) devices or other alternative communication methods.

Social Interaction
Starting Conversations and Replying to Them
- Pay attention to the child's conversation-starting skills.
- Evaluate how receptive they are to the advances made by others.

Sharing Turns and Communication
- Assess the child's capacity for sharing and taking turns during a conversation.
- Evaluate sharing behaviors in situations involving both words and nonwords.

Recognizing Social Expressions
- Pay attention to how people react to various social cues, like how one speaks and facial expressions.
- Evaluate a capacity for appropriate interpretation and response.

Social Learning
Social Ability Education History
- Find out if there has been any prior social skills instruction or therapy.
- Determine whether the child is aware of their social strengths and weaknesses.

Behavior Studies
- Pay attention to how people behave in planned social situations.
- Assess the child's flexibility and adaptability in various social situations.

Emotional Management
Dealing Mechanisms
- Determine the child's coping strategies for handling stress or anxiety.
- Evaluate how self-regulation techniques are being applied.

Emotional Communication
- Pay attention to the child's emotional communication.
- Assess the suitability and strength of emotional reactions.

Procedures and Goals
Desires and Interests
- Talk about the child's passions and areas of interest.
- Examine the potential contributions these interests may make to social interactions.

Methods for Groups
- Evaluate group activity participation.
- Assess the child's capacity for peer cooperation.

Through the integration of these elements, the social skills training program based in the metaverse seeks to provide people with ASD a thorough and immersive educational experience that promotes enhanced social interactions and communication skills and abilities.

11.6 Dataset

There are numerous datasets available to diagnose ASD. The UCI Machine Learning Repository, Kaggle, and Figshare data repositories are the regular sources of the autism dataset. The UCI repository, which is accessible to the public, provided these datasets [12–15]. The description of the datasets is shown in Figure 11.11. There are three sets of data: AQ10 for kids (ages four to 11), AQ-10 for AQ-10 has been developed for adults (18 years of age and older) and adolescents (12–17 years old). The Kaggle data repository stored the dataset for toddler autism screening, which was made available in July 2018. It has six different authors as of this moment, and it was first released in November 2018. The basic structure of the dataset is the toddler ASD screening QCHAT-10 tool [16]. The file contains a total of 1,054 instances in it. The datasets, in particular the Adult ASD Screening Data, Child, and Adolescence developed from the UCI Machine Learning Respiratory, are presented in Tables 11.1–11.3. The dataset for adults contains 21 attributes and 704 cases; for children, it contains 292 instances and 21 attributes; and for adolescents, it contains 104 instances and 21 attributes. In all datasets (AT1 to AT30), the screening questions are expressed by ten binary attributes [13–15].

This dataset collects data on children who have been identified as having ASD. A broad variety of variables, including characteristics of behavior, developmental history, clinical assessments, and demographic data, have been included in the

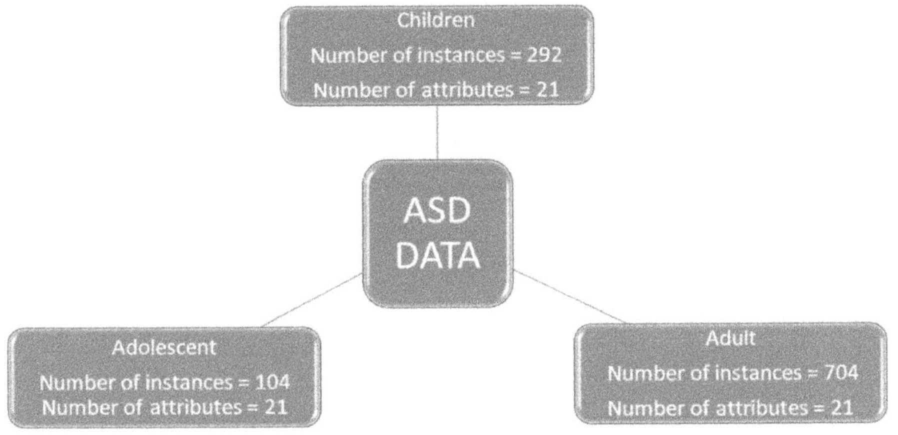

Figure 11.11   **The details of the ASD dataset.**

Table 11.1   Description of the ASD Child Dataset

Attribute No.	Corresponding AQ-10-Child Features
AT1	He or she frequently hears little noises that others miss.
AT2	Typically, she or he pays more attention to the larger context than to the little things.
AT3	He or she is capable of following multiple conversations between individuals in a social environment.
AT4	It is effortless for the child to move between various tasks,
AT5	He or she does not have the ability to maintain a conversation with peers.
AT6	He or she is skilled at making conversation.
AT7	When reading a story, she or he finds it difficult to determine the motivations or sensations of the characters.
AT8	He or she enjoyed playing pretend games with other kids when they were children in preschool.
AT9	He or she finds it easy to determine someone's opinions or feelings purely by observing their gestures.
AT10	Making new friends can be challenging for them.

data. Clinical evaluations, parent interviews, teacher reports, and in-person observations are all used to gather data. To guarantee consistency in the gathering of data, standardized assessments are employed. Tables 11.1–11.3 list the attributes of the dataset.

We gathered information using databases from ACM, IEEE Xplore, Scopus, and WoS ProQuest, EBSCO, ERIC, Science Direct [17].

11.7 Discussion

We believe that running children with ASD will benefit from the peer program in the metaverse by developing their social skills. Research findings indicate that PEERS programs have a notable impact on enhancing social competencies knowledge, a routine of social interaction and overall social abilities, all while preventing symptoms of ASD. The integration of healthcare services within a metaverse setting presents many kinds of advantages. This study's major objective was to demonstrate how social skills instruction in the medical field can

Table 11.2   Description of the ASD Adolescent Dataset

Attribute No.	Corresponding AQ-10-Adolescent Features
AT11	He or she continually searches for patterns in things.
AT12	Usually, he or she pays more attention to the big picture than to the particulars.
AT13	In a community, he or she can easily follow the conversations of various individuals.
AT14	If there is a disruption, they can quickly return to their previous task.
AT15	When someone starts talking to me, I am able to read between the lines.
AT16	He or she is skilled at making conversations.
AT17	When the individual in question was younger, they used to take satisfaction in engaging in pretend games with other kids.
AT18	He or she discovers it difficult to visualize stepping into another person's footwear.
AT19	Social situations appear easily to him or her.
AT20	It can be challenging for them to find friends who are new to them.

be beneficial while incorporating the metaverse environment. The ASD prediction model uses three different dataset types, including adult, child, and adolescent ASD screening data. An item pool of ten questions was created in order to assess the participants' interviewing abilities. From this pool, one-on-one mock interviews, also known as simulated interviews, were conducted, and the results were compared using a screening procedure. The interview rubric utilized by [18], which has been revised and expanded upon to examine the impact of interview preparation for individuals with intellectual disabilities, served as the basis for the analysis of the simulated interview screening procedure. Ten questions (AT1 through AT10, AT11 through AT20, and AT21 through AT30) are represented as attributes in all datasets that survey respondents answered during the screening test. Tables 11.1–11.3 list the attributes of the dataset. Performance can be assessed using the following metrics: sensitivity, specificity, accuracy, and precision, which are presented in Table 11.4.

Table 11.3   Description of the ASD Adult Dataset

Attribute No.	Corresponding AQ-10-Adult Features
AT21	I frequently hear small disturbances while other people do not.
AT22	Typically, I focus less on the minute details and more on the larger picture.
AT23	It appears undoubtedly to me to do multiple things.
AT24	In the case of an interruption, I can quickly return to my previous task.
AT25	I can read the thoughts of others easily when they're speaking to me.
AT26	I am able recognize when someone becomes more uninterested in what I am saying.
AT27	When studying a story, I have issues determining what the intentions of a character are.
AT28	I enjoy what I do gather data about various groups of objects, such as various kinds of motor vehicles, animals, transport, trees, and so on.
AT29	Simply by observing someone's face, I can usually tell what they are considering or feeling.
AT30	I have trouble seeking out what people are trying to say.

Table 11.4   Evaluation Metrics

Accuracy	$Accuracy = \dfrac{TRP + TRN}{TRP + TRN + FAP + FAN}$
Specificity	$Specificity = \dfrac{TRN}{TRP + TRN}$
Sensitivity	$Sensitivity = \dfrac{TRN}{TRN + FAN}$
Precision	$Precision = \dfrac{TRP}{TRP + FAP}$

11.8 Conclusion

According to this case study, social skills training based on the metaverse can be a successful and well-liked intervention for people with ASD. Targeted skill development is made possible by the virtual environment, which offers a safe and encouraging setting for practicing social interactions [19, 20]. To generalize these results and investigate the long-term effects of metaverse-based procedures on people with ASD, more studies with higher sample sizes and extended follow-ups are required. This study utilizes an exploratory meta-analysis approach to examine the uses to provide the metaverse services within the medical field sector. When utilizing an online metaverse gaming platform, research apparatus and Internet connectivity can lead to issues. Although research on the metaverse's effects on autism is still in its infancy, preliminary findings point to a great deal of promise for improving the lives of people with autism in a variety of ways. To improve and optimize these applications for the autism community, more research, ongoing user feedback, and collaboration between technology developers and medical professionals will be essential.

References

1. J. H. Lee et al., "Metaverse-Based Social Skills Training Programme for Children with Autism Spectrum Disorder to Improve Social Interaction Ability: An Open-Label, Single-Centre, Randomised Controlled Pilot Trial," eClinicalMedicine, vol. 61, p. 102072, 2023, doi: 10.1016/j.eclinm.2023.102072.
2. F. Svenaeus, "Diagnosing Mental Disorders and Saving the Normal," Med. Health Care and Philos., vol. 17, pp. 241–244, 2014, doi: 10.1007/s11019-013-9529-6.
3. C. W. Lee, "Application of Metaverse Service to Healthcare Industry: A Strategic Perspective," Int. J. Environ. Res. Public Health, vol. 19, no. 20, 2022, doi: 10.3390/ijerph192013038.
4. A. Albujeer and M. Khoshnevisan, "Metaverse and Oral Health Promotion," Br. Dent. J., vol. 232, p. 587, 2022, doi: 10.1038/s41415-022-4255-1.
5. M. Damar, "What the Literature on Medicine, Nursing, Public Health, Midwifery, and Dentistry Reveals: An Overview of the Rapidly Approaching Metaverse," J. Metaverse, vol. 2, no. 2, pp. 62–70, 2022, doi: 10.57019/jmv.1132962.
6. H. Guo and W. Gao, "Metaverse-Powered Experiential Situational English-Teaching Design: An Emotion-Based Analysis Method," Front. Psychol., vol. 13, pp. 1–9, 2022, doi: 10.3389/fpsyg.2022.859159.
7. M. T. Sarıtaş and K. Topraklıkoğlu, "Systematic Literature Review on the Use of Metaverse in Education," Int. J. Technol. Educ., vol. 5, no. 4, pp. 586–607, 2022, doi: 10.46328/ijte.319.
8. S. Ray, S. Tawar, N. Singh, and G. Singh, "Transition toward Technological Transformation: Challenges of Implementing Virtual Reality and Augmented Reality in the Health Sector," J. Mar. Med. Soc., vol. 26, no. 2, pp. 161–164, May–Aug 2024, doi: 10.4103/jmms.jmms_89_23.

9. G. Yenduri et al., "From Assistive Technologies to Metaverse – Technologies in Inclusive Higher Education for Students with Specific Learning Difficulties: A Review," IEEE Access, vol. 11, pp. 64907–64927, 2023, doi: 10.1109/ACCESS.2023.3289496.

10. S. Lee, Y. Lee, and E. Park, "Sustainable Vocational Preparation for Adults with Disabilities: A Metaverse-Based Approach," Sustain., vol. 15, no. 15, pp. 1–12, 2023, doi: 10.3390/su151512000.

11. T. Akter et al., "Machine Learning-Based Models for Early Stage Detection of Autism Spectrum Disorders," IEEE Access, vol. 7, pp. 166509–166527, 2019, doi: 10.1109/ACCESS.2019.2952609.

12. "Autism Screening Data for Toddlers," [Online]. Available: https://www.kaggle.com/fabdelja/autism-screening-fortoddlers, (2018). Accessed on January 2024.

13. F. Thabtah, Autistic Spectrum Disorder Screening Data for Children [Dataset]. UCI Machine Learning Repository. 2017, doi: 10.24432/C5659W.

14. F. Tabtah, Autistic Spectrum Disorder Screening Data for Adolescent [Dataset]. UCI Machine Learning Repository. 2017, doi: 10.24432/C5V89T.

15. F. Thabtah, Autism Screening Adult [Dataset]. UCI Machine Learning Repository. 2017, doi: 10.24432/C5F019.

16. S. Raj and S. Masood, "Analysis and Detection of Autism Spectrum Disorder Using Machine Learning Techniques," Procedia Comput. Sci., vol. 167, no. 2019, pp. 994–1004, 2020, doi: 10.1016/j.procs.2020.03.399.

17. X. Chen, D. Zou, H. Xie, and F. L. Wang, "Metaverse in Education: Contributors, Cooperations, and Research Themes," IEEE Trans. Learn. Technol., vol. 16, no. 6, pp. 1111–1129, 2023, doi: 10.1109/TLT.2023.3277952.

18. F. Thabtah, F. Kamalov, and K. Rajab, "A New Computational Intelligence Approach to Detect Autistic Features for Autism Screening," Int. J. Med. Inform., vol. 117, pp. 112–124, 2018.

19. S. Balasubramaniam, C. V. Joe, C. Manthiramoorthy, and K. S. Kumar, "Relief Based Feature Selection and Gradient Squirrel Search Algorithm Enabled Deep Maxout Network for Detection of Heart Disease," Biomed. Signal Process. Control., vol. 87, p. 105446, 2024.

20. S. B. Kadry et al., "Res-Unet Based Blood Vessel Segmentation and Cardio Vascular Disease Prediction Using Chronological Chef-Based Optimization Algorithm Based Deep Residual Network from Retinal Fundus Images," Multimed. Tools Appl., 2024, doi: 10.1007/s11042-024-18810-y.

Chapter 12

MultiSense Diagnosis: Navigating Disease Diagnosis with Metaverse Multimodal Interaction

Ashwini A, Shamini G. I, Banu Priya Prathaban, and Balasubramaniam S

12.1 Introduction to MultiSensor Diagnosis

The emergence of novel innovations is redefining developed methods to identifying illnesses in the rapidly shifting clinical landscape. At the point of intersection of multidimensional communication and the wider universe, MultiSense Diagnosis is an innovative breakthrough that offers a revolutionary method for conquering the obstacles that accompany diagnosing medical disorders [1]. Fundamentally, MultiSense Diagnosis uses a wide range of sensory inputs and highly immersive virtual environments in order to offer an enjoyable and dynamic diagnosis procedure. This novel approach goes beyond the bounds of traditional diagnostic techniques by using modalities like speech, gesture, and haptic input, allowing healthcare workers to interact with individuals in ways that were previously unthinkable. Customized diagnostic and treatment regimens are made achievable by the integration of multiple modes of interaction and personalized medical care. However, difficulties regarding security of data, moral issues, and technical advancements remain crucial areas of concentration for enhancing the confidence and wide adoption of MultiSense Diagnosis. It has created entirely novel, fully interactive experiences that take place in real time and promote relationships.

MultiSense Diagnosis introduces a new paradigm in healthcare by fusing multimodal interaction with the abilities of the metaverse, developing the way of recognizing illness. This chapter explores the groundbreaking advantages of MultiSense Diagnosis and how technology might help healthcare move toward an additional precise and patient-oriented diagnostic system. The growth of the metaverse will enable novel ways for offering healthcare and will lead to significant improvements in the administration of long-lasting problems. The main intention for MultiSense Diagnosis is concentrated on providing the diagnosis experience on a comprehensive scale to their own clients taking only the list of the passive consumers on the prominent medical evaluation. These clients are enabled to develop the active participation of the passive consumers having an online meeting with the medical specialist on such medical evaluations.

Figure 12.1 shows the overall MultiSense Diagnosis framework. Moreover, MultiSense Diagnosis improves the evaluation method through using modern innovations like intelligent technology (AI) and machine learning to improve results [2]. This helps in determination of high degree of realistic participation to the virtual world. More significant connections between customers and healthcare practitioners are made possible by these realistic and interactive surroundings, which encourage participation and working together. Artificial intelligence (AI)

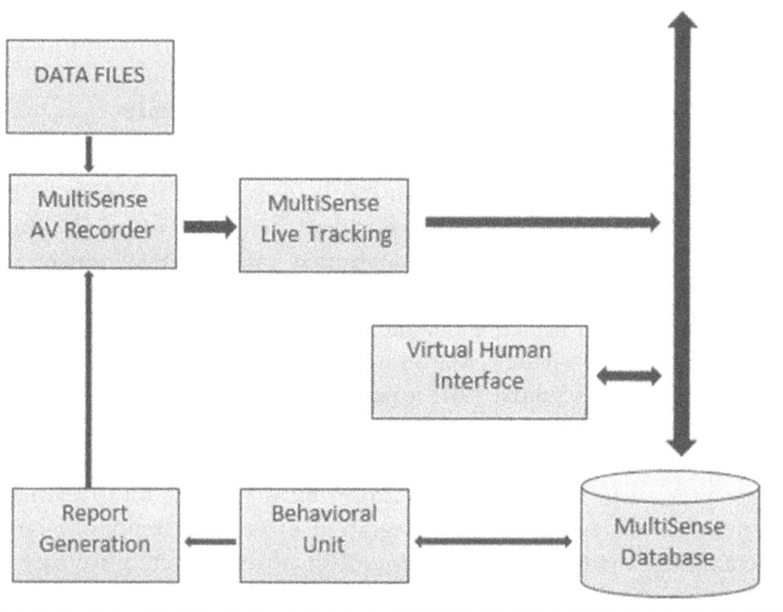

Figure 12.1   Framework for MultiSense Diagnosis.

can help healthcare professionals rate patient information, identify trends, and make precise diagnoses employing real-time multiple forms of analysis. The merging of technical development and human ability not only enhances testing efficiency and accuracy yet additionally creates new opportunities for personalized and unique healthcare services. AI is capable to provide these sorts of advice. This revolutionary system allows for an evolving and interactive dialogue among healthcare providers and patients, minimizing geographic obstacles and expanding access for qualified evaluation. This chapter examines the elements of the virtual world for multidisciplinary collaboration and demonstrates the use of health technologies in the field of medicine. Additionally, it facilitates an increased awareness of patient conditions, hence enhancing the level of precision in medical examinations.

This chapter will examine the technology foundations, medicinal uses, legal problems, and possible future advances of MultiSense assessment in greater depth throughout this implementation. This research work helps in developing the potential of changing diagnostic patterns on distributed health-based services over a period of years to achieve the proper and deeper investigation of various strengths.

12.2 Role of Multimodal Interaction in Healthcare

Multimodal sets of collaboration are meant to provide minimized operations with enhanced communication transforming the means of providing proper healthcare advice. This can help in meeting the specific unique demands of both the workers and the patients with the prominent means of gesture, sound, reach, and graphical interfacing tasks [3]. Additionally, it offers a new range of options for engaging patients with the medical educational contents and home-based medical providers, thus enabling multimodal interfaces to bring about an active participation in the medical journey.

Furthermore, irrespective of physical distance, multimodal contact in telemedicine promotes confidence and connection among patients and clinicians by enabling online meetings that resemble in-person conversations. Healthcare institutions may improve patient engagement, optimize treatment delivery, and ultimately improve individual and community health effects by employing a variety of technological advances. Multimodal involvement performs a substantial part in healthcare, delivering a range of strengths and uses that increase patient care, streamline clinical procedures, and encourage interaction between providers and patients. Figure 12.2 shows the significant elements explaining how multidisciplinary communication works within the field of medicine.

Enhanced User Experience:
In order to offer natural and interesting user interactions for healthcare applications, the use of multimodal interaction includes several different input and output modalities that include speaking commands, actions, displays, and tactile input [4].

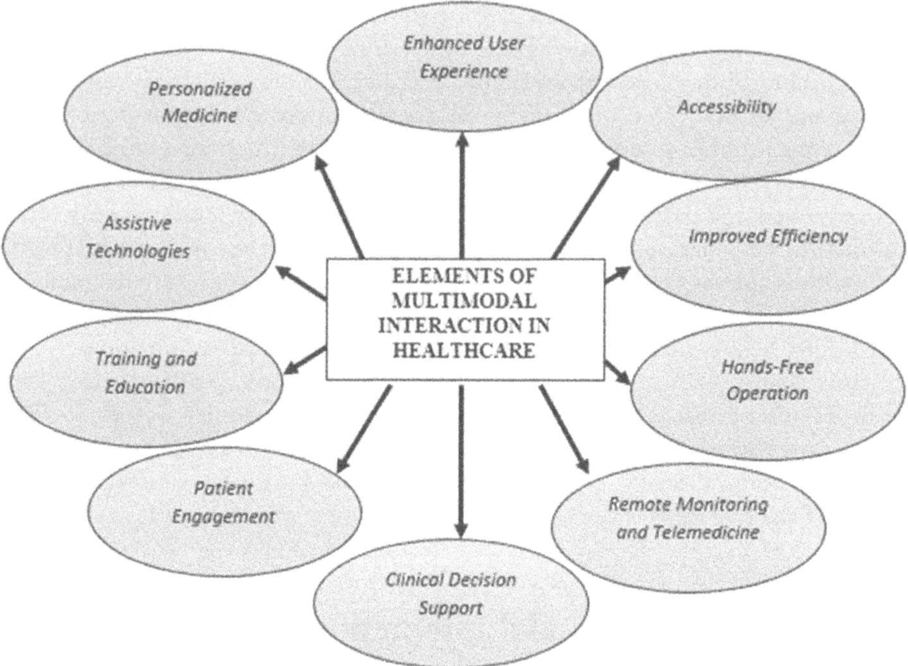

Figure 12.2   Elements of multimodal interaction in healthcare platform.

Accessibility:
By allowing additional input techniques beyond typical keyboard and mouse connections, multimodal user interfaces serve a number of customer individuals, including those having difficulties or poor skills.

Improved Efficiency:
By facilitating quicker and more intuitive conversations with healthcare organizations, multimodal communications speed up clinical activities by cutting down on the time needed for input of data, travel, as well as data extraction.

Hands-Free Operation:
Voice-based communications provide free use during clinical tasks and patient meetings by permitting healthcare professionals to communicate with electronic patient records, medical supplies, and other hospitals devoid requiring input from the user.

Remote Monitoring and Telemedicine:
Multimodal interaction improves visual connection between consumers and doctors and nurses, facilitating immediate assessment, evaluations, and calls. This enables for online surveillance and telemedicine visits.

Clinical Decision Support:
In order to advance informed choices and improve patient security, multiple modes of interaction link with clinical decision-support platforms (CDSS) to give health professionals useful data, alarms, as well as suggestions at the time of care [5].

Patient Engagement:
By presenting consumers with simple user interfaces that enable communication with medical providers, giving them access to information on health and the handling of their medication, a variety of methods can foster patient ownership and involvement.

Training and Education:
Healthcare workers' access to interactive training simulations, instructional parts, and experiences in virtual reality is made practical by multidimensional user interfaces, which improve health education, skill training, and continuous professional development.

Assistive Technologies:
Screen customers, gesture-based devices for input, programs that recognize voices, and other assistive devices that help people with limitations or disabilities are built on the base of multisensory communication.

Personalized Medicine:
By giving customized relationships, suggestions, and treatment based on unique individual features, tastes, and requirements, interfaces that are multimodal advertise personalized health objectives [6]. Ultimately, multichannel communication is critical for contemporary medical care because it makes an assortment of clinical and managerial tasks easier to perform, productive, and easy to use, and thus improves the results for patients and delivery of care.

12.3 Technological Framework of Disease Diagnosis

An innovative approach can be envisioned that uses technology such as virtual reality (VR), augmented realities (AR), intelligent technology (AI), and data analytics to reinvent how medical professionals evaluate and manage illnesses by imagining a technological structure for identifying diseases within the realm of metaphysics [7]. A complex powered by an AI diagnostic tool that continuously examines a huge amount of information about patients, comprising genetic information, wireless sensor information in immediate time, medical records, and fingerprint data, is at the focal point of this designing. This AI system functions in the metaverse, a virtual world where people engage through VR and AR devices with environments that computers create and interact with one another. Figure 12.3 shows the features of MultiSense disease diagnosis.

Healthcare professionals may explore cells, tissues, and biological functions in extraordinary depth by immersing themselves in highly detailed models of human

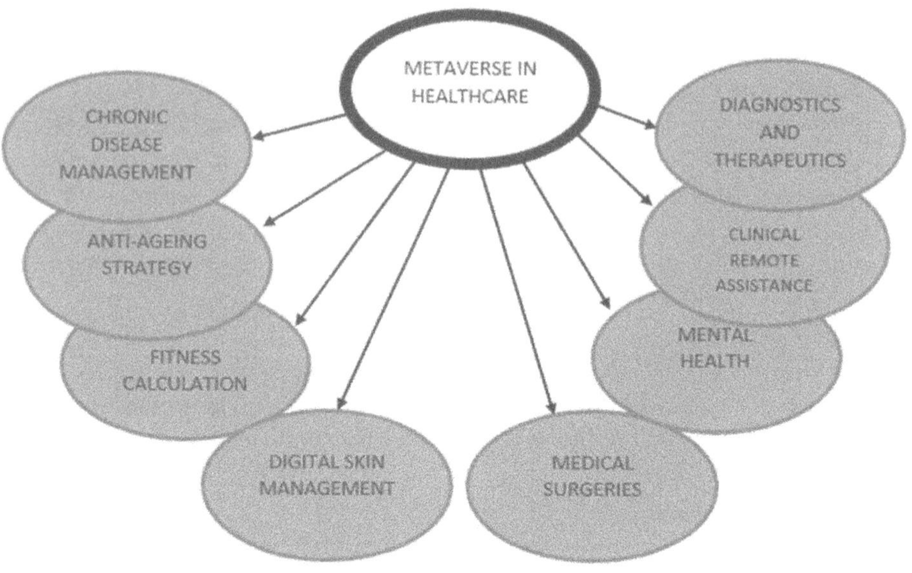

Figure 12.3   Features for metaverse disease diagnosis.

tissue in this virtual space. They may see data about patients immediately in these simulated images with AR overlays, which enable more understanding of intricate healthcare issues. These modern AI algorithms help common physicians to evaluate the accuracy in biological irregularities and imagery forecasting the key ailments. Practitioners in the medical field may receive immediate feedback and make more timely interventions with the help of these AI-driven tools for diagnosis that can quickly assess imaging scans, pathological slides, and other types of diagnostic procedures [8]. This metaverse-based diagnostic paradigm not only aids physicians but also enables people to take greater in regard to their wellness treatment.

People can research alternatives to treatment, learn more concerning their health concerns, and establish peer support communities with people going through similar difficulties by using interactive virtual reality interactions. Moreover, the technology framework has made it easier for scholars, developers, and healthcare experts from throughout the world to work with one another. Experts may work cooperatively on difficult issues, share expertise, and co-design creative approaches to important health-related issues via shared virtual environments [9]. All things thought out, the metaverse's technical foundation for illness identification has enormous potential to transform healthcare delivery, raise the benchmark for clinical precision, and possibly enhance the results for patients in ways that were previously unimaginable.

12.4 Learning Models for Diagnosis Improvement

Improved intelligence methods, interactive environments, and full immersion can all increase the models of learning for evaluation advancement across the metaverse. These are a few key components of models of learning developed for the metaverse's greater assessment:

Immersive Training Simulations:
VR environments enable doctors and nurses to participate in extremely lifelike simulations of patient visits. These risk-free simulations emulate a wide range of medical scenarios, giving medical professionals a chance to hone their diagnostic competencies, improve their decision-making methods, and get acquainted with uncommon or complicated ailments. Clinicians can become more proficient and confident in their ability to diagnose a variety of medical problems through holographic encounters.

Interactive Case Studies:
Active investigations may be built within the realm of metaphysics to pose difficult diagnostic conundrums to medical professionals. Healthcare workers can examine diagnostic test the results, go over histories with patients, and work with colleagues virtually to make correct evaluations by using AR interfaces [10]. Professionals learn from these engaging investigations by developing their analytical thinking, resolving issues, and honing collaborative abilities, which eventually increases the precision of diagnoses.

AI-Powered Diagnostic Support:
Smart neural networks can be built into the virtual world to give medical practitioners on-the-spot medical assistance. Through extensive analysis of client information, encompassing imaging scans, testing outcomes, and patient records, systems based on AI can provide recommendations, highlight pertinent discoveries, and spot possible errors in diagnosis.

Collaborative Learning Environments:
Doctors and nurses at different geographical regions and various locations can gather in work by providing an alternate universe, thus helping to exchange information, even in complex situations, and insights with their counterparts [11]. Thus, clinicians can voluntarily participate in various types of conversations, sharing their insights and retaining their speed in all such diagnostic forms of procedures on various conferences, training courses, and discussions.

Continuous Feedback and Evaluation:
The models pertaining to the virtual world can learn the various assessment models with the peculiar feedback conditions, creating a monitory level of monitoring using feedback and assessment and enabling a mode of development over time [12].

12.5 Design Interface and User Centered Design Principles

A design interface in the metaverse is a visual user interface or the total user experience that enables users to interact with elements or other users inside the metaverse, navigate virtual surroundings, and access digital material. The metaverse's design interface consists of a number of components, including chat interfaces, options, switches virtual characters, 3D environments, and navigation tools. These components are all intended to improve user immersion, usability, and interest [13].

The requirements, choices, and activities of individuals are given priority through the creative process by user-centered design concepts, which are frequently used in the creation of metaverse design interfaces. These guidelines are meant to make the virtual environments that users engage with easy to understand, fun, and accessible. The following shows the application of virtual world:

- The layouts are designed based on user preferences and thus satisfying the keen motives, objectives, and viewpoints.
- These interfaces are precisely designed by people who are very knowledgeable about online environments in such a way that users can easily comprehend the interfaces' correct use [14].
- The systems are perfectly accessible to persons with vision impairments, cognitive limits, and disabilities with movement.
- Developing captivating and dynamic experiences promotes involvement, cooperation, and metaverse discovery for all the users.
- User evaluations and usability assessments provides design-based decisions and layouts that are periodically improved.
- Users are granted the ability to alter settings, choose selections based on personal tastes, and customize images in order to make their online journey more unique.
- Enhancing the performance, adaptive design, and productivity of design interfaces guarantees fluid and easy user interactions even in virtual settings with limited resources.

Developers as well as artists may produce intuitive, captivating, and inclusive design interactions in the metaverse by following these user-friendly design principles, which will ultimately increase users' enjoyment of virtual settings [15].

Accessibility:
Everyone must be able to effortlessly navigate and engage with the multiverse through the provision of a system that is suitable to users of various skill sets. This includes functions like modifiable oversight, compatibility with assistive devices, and textual, auditory, and visual clues that clearly convey ideas. Figure 12.4 shows how to put these ideas into practice.

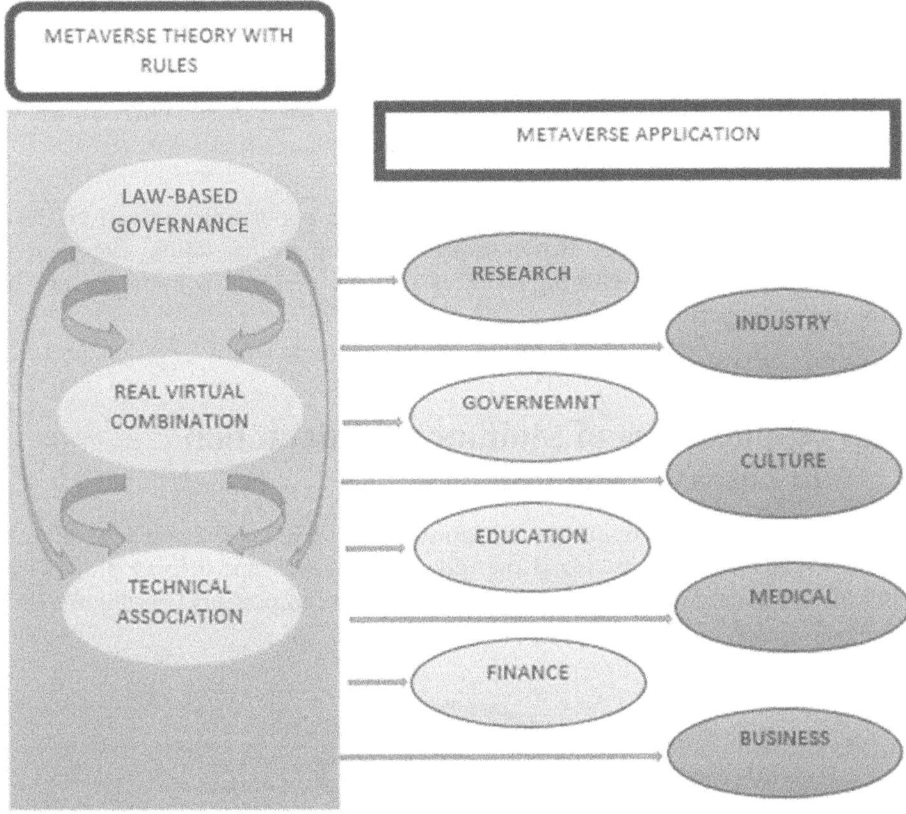

Figure 12.4   Theory rules of the metaverse with applications.

Intuitiveness:
Without having to look for in-depth guides or lessons, users should to be able to navigate and engage relatively the realm of possibility with ease. It should be straightforward for consumers to find elements and take action through using well-known style guidelines and features in the experience [16].

Customization:
It must be accessible to users to alter their preferred design according with their own requirements and tastes. For the sake of enhancing user expertise, this contains choices to change visual solution, login strategies, translation habits, and screen layout.

Feedback and Responsiveness:
When clients interact with the user interface, they ought to get prompt, unambiguous input that validates the information they provide and indicates system replies. This consists of sense, aural, and optical signals to recognize behaviors and smoothly navigate users around the metaverse.

Consistency:
It is imperative for the interface's designers to uphold uniformity in terms of design features, user behavior, and language throughout various sections of the virtual world. Stability reduces strain and assists users in creating representations of the device functions [17].

Engagement:
Clients interact with the interface, providing an opportunity to actively take part in the virtual world. This entails recognizing results, adding engagement components, and establishing chances for interpersonal communication in online settings [18].

12.6 Applications of Multimodal Interaction in Disease Diagnosis

With its state-of-the-art resources and immersive experience, the potential of multimodal stages has revolutionized the way of diagnosis, thus helping professionals with accurate identification and precise treatment to patients [19]. Figure 12.5

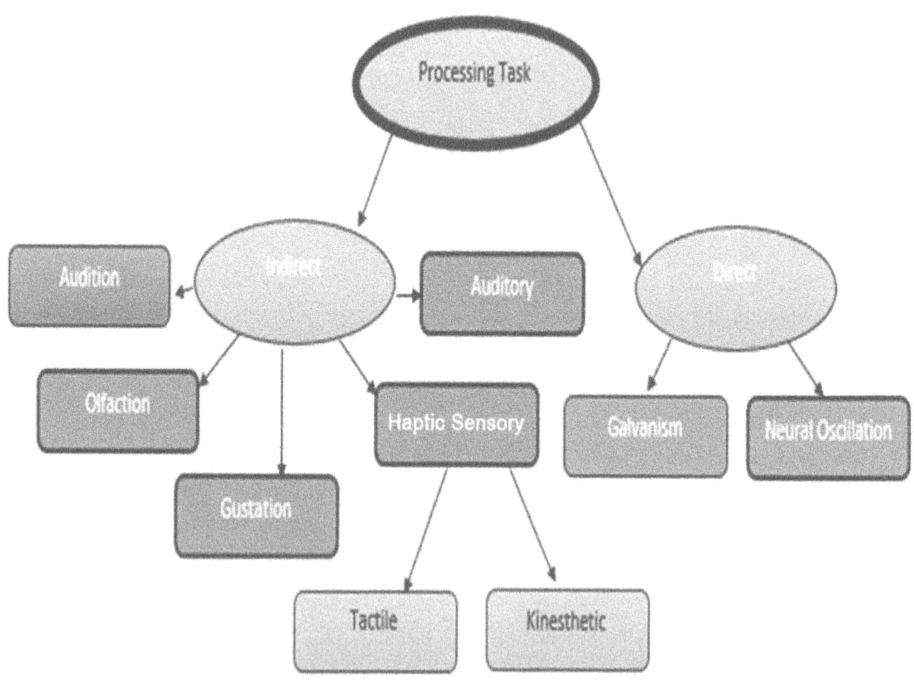

Figure 12.5   Multimodal communication in disease detection.

shows the way in which the metaverse and multimodal communication help in detection of illnesses.

Immersive Diagnostic Imaging:
Imaging specialists and other experts can modify and understand medical photos, such as MRI, CT, and X-ray scans, in three dimensions by using augmented and virtual reality interfaces. Professionals may study anatomical features, collaborate more effectively with colleagues, and identify issues throughout the diagnostic process by using speech, gesture recognition, and touch-based instructions [20, 21]. By employing VR simulations that replicate the environment of a surgical procedure, for example, surgeons may practice challenging procedures and view the anatomy for patients before they even arrive at the surgery center.

Immersion imaging technology additionally boosts the accuracy of diagnoses and therapy planning. Immersion-based diagnostic imaging has enormous potential to transform medicine, enhance the results for patients, and progress the science of diagnostic imaging as immersive technology continues to advance and become more widely available.

Interactive Medical Data Visualization:
Complex clinical information may be actively seen in the metaverse with the help of multifunctional systems. Healthcare professionals may see data related to patients in realistic three-dimensional locations using VR and AR tools, encompassing genetic data, laboratory findings, and digital health records. Therapists can search through databases, collect important information, and obtain deeper insights into their patients' health state to aid in diagnostic selections by combining spoken words, gestures of the hands, and eyes tracking.

Figure 12.6 shows the machine learning based diagnosis system. In order encourage deeper comprehension and analysis, dynamic visualization enables users examine data from different perspectives, explore into specific factors, and modify graphics elements in real-time. Managers of healthcare may use visualizations for tracking important measures of performance, consumption of resources, and public health trends, while healthcare providers can use these to follow illness development over time or discover irregularities in medical imaging data [22]. Graphical medical information visualization also improves interprofessional teams' interactions and collaboration, facilitating more effective transfer of information, analysis, and decisions.

Collaborative Diagnostic Workspaces:
Medical staff can work together in real time, in addition to borders of distance, in cooperative diagnosis places of work rendered viable by multimodal communication [23]. Together, therapists may create action plans for difficult situations, share clinical findings, and conduct integrative discussions in virtual reality settings.

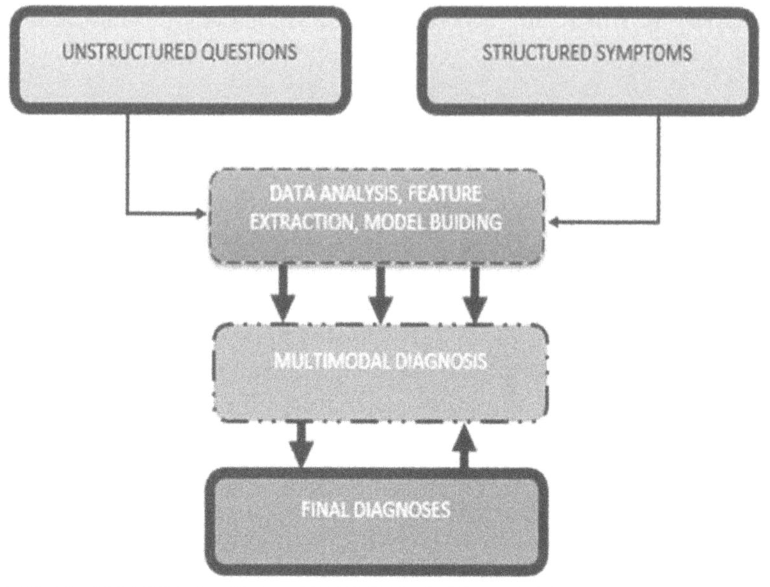

Figure 12.6   Machine learning–based diagnosis system.

By breaking down obstacles and promoting cooperation, joint healthcare organizations reduce diagnostic errors, enhance the well-being of patients, and boost diagnosis correctness. Furthermore, these networks allow medical professionals to share information globally, overcome regional barriers, and apply collective expertise to difficult clinical problems [24].

Training and Education:
Through multidimensional involvement, healthcare workers can gain from comprehensive education and alternate dimension learning experiences. These solutions reduce geographic obstacles to continuing education by allowing healthcare practitioners to participate in online sessions, access educational materials, and role-play real-world clinical scenarios from any location at any time [25].

12.7 Comparison with Traditional Diagnostic Methods

Numerous major differences as well as advantages emerge when combining multimodal interactions in the realm of possibility [23, 26–28] with standard approaches for illness assessment:

■ Remote cooperation, learning, and education are made possible for healthcare workers by the ability to utilize virtual diagnosing settings in any location with a link to the web. Figure 12.7 shows the metaverse with the technology and challenges.

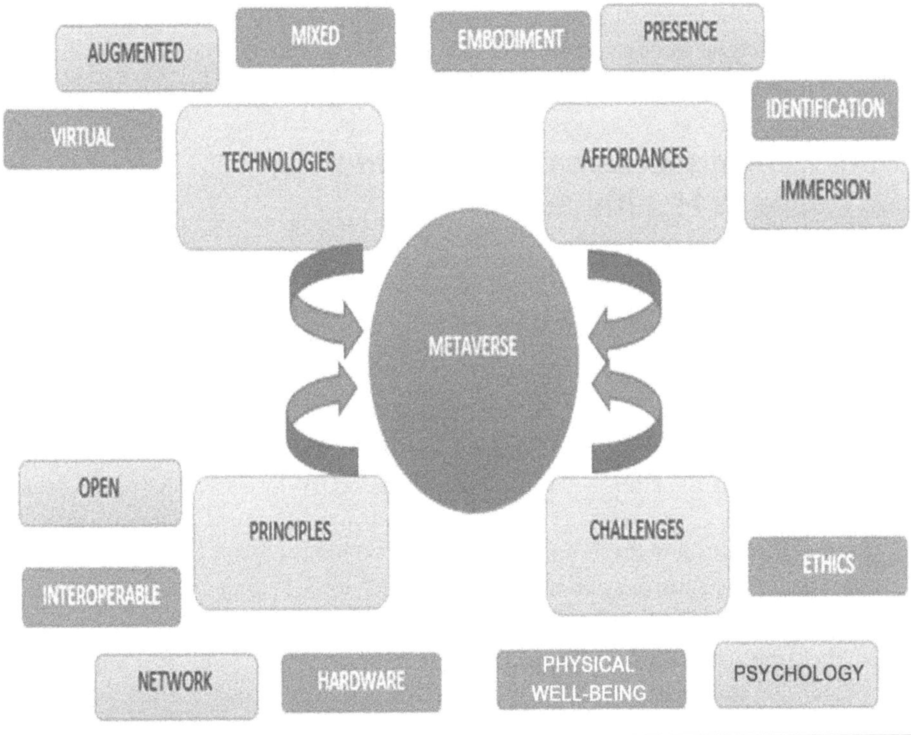

Figure 12.7   Metaverse with technological development and challenges.

- Improved healthcare data and imaging diagnostic study visualization is made possible by multidisciplinary collaboration in the metaverse.
- This is particularly helpful in underprivileged communities or in circumstances where there may be restricted direct interaction with healthcare providers.
- Data may be examined and evaluated in ways that are not feasible with conventional two-dimensional photographs or physical models by physicians using VR and AR screens. These interfaces offer multidimensional visualizations of organs and pathologies.
- Shared virtual environments and immediate interaction technologies enable physicians to collaborate on decisions in the metaverse.
- These solutions reduce geographic obstacles to continuing education by allowing healthcare practitioners to participate in online sessions, access educational materials, and role-play real-world clinical scenarios from any location at any time [25].
- The procedure of diagnosis can have AI techniques and information analysis applications seamlessly integrated into the metaverse.

■ Using AI-powered diagnostic systems, large volumes of health information can be analyzed, trends can be spotted, and immediate guidance on choices to improve the effectiveness and precision of diagnoses can be provided to doctors.

12.8 Ethical Guidelines for Technology Use in Healthcare

To ensure that beneficial effects can be fully utilized, the establishment of rules for technology within the medical field is considered essential. Important moral precepts and directives are as follows:

Privacy and Confidentiality:
Protecting identities of individuals and private information is crucial. Healthcare organizations must implement robust security procedures to safeguard confidential patient data in the metaverse. These safety measures have to include encryption, entrance restrictions, and data anonymization. Customers must be informed about how their personal data will be handled and given the choice to consent to its collection and sharing.

Informed Consent:
Medical personnel must obtain patients' consent before using inventions from the parallel universe to treat them. It is critical that patients receive comprehensive education on the kind of devices being used, potential benefits and hazards, and any workable alternatives [29]. They must also have the freedom to refuse or withdraw permission at any time.

Equity and Accessibility:
Fairness and affordability for all people should be given first priority in the creation and implementation of innovations inside the metaverse, regardless of their physical ability, socioeconomic status, or place of birth. This entails allowing some individuals with disabilities and those living in impoverished areas to obtain electronic medical care [30].

Transparency and Accountability:
Healthcare organizations view openness on the use of technology in treating patients virtually as essential. Customers should be informed about any computer algorithms or artificially intelligent systems employed in the diagnostic and treatment process, as well as their personal medical records and the ability to review and correct inaccuracies.

Clinical Validity and Safety:
When using metaverse technology for medical reasons, it must adhere to safety regulations and undergo empirical evaluation. Before integrating virtual diagnostic tools, therapeutic approaches, and decision-making systems into clinical practice, physicians should appropriately assess the reliability, accuracy, and efficacy of these technologies [31].

Professional Integrity:
Healthcare professionals must uphold moral principles and reliable behavior when utilizing breakthroughs in the parallel universe. This means safeguarding the privacy of individual patients, preventing conflicts of interest, and ensuring that digital patient interactions are managed with the same level of decency and thoughtfulness as those that occur in traditional healthcare settings.

Patient Autonomy and Informed Consent:
Respect the patient's independence and freedom while providing them with care. Ensure that individuals comprehend the benefits, risks, and reasoning for using innovations in their care [32]. Obtain their express consent before using technology to assist customers or collecting their medical information.

Beneficence and Nonmaleficence:
Patients' health and safety should be the first priority in the development and use of medical technology. Ensure that any technology solutions are safe for patients, supported by documentation, and professionally proved. Monitoring the impact of innovation on patient outcomes, evaluating it often, and adjusting course of action as needed to optimize benefits and minimize risks.

Collaboration and Stakeholder Engagement:
Promote communication and cooperation among many groups, including the general public, lawmakers, information technology (IT) companies, and medical professionals. Include customers in the development, implementation, and evaluation of technology-enabled medical solutions to ensure that they meet their needs and preferences.

Continuing Education and Training:
Healthcare professionals should get ongoing education and training about the ethical use of technology for healthcare inside the metaverse [33]. This means staying informed about new technological advancements and the best methods to integrate them into healthcare settings while maintaining patient safety and confidentiality. It also means being aware of the ethical risks associated with giving therapy online.

12.9 Limitations in Practical Implementation

Although the concept of using the parallel world for medical has a lot of potential, there are a few problems that may prevent it from being implemented in practice, as described in Table 12.1.

Technological Infrastructure:
Substantial technological infrastructure, such as rapid Internet access, advanced processing abilities, and ubiquitous platforms, is required for the widespread application of the virtual world in medicine. However, the vast majority of

Table 12.1 Limitations in Practical Implementation

Limitations	Explanations
Technological infrastructure	Rapid Internet access, advanced processing abilities, and ubiquitous platforms
Digital divide	Digital literacy and access to technology expression
Data security and privacy concerns	Collection, storage, and sharing of health data
Regulatory challenges	Data privacy, telemedicine reimbursement, and certification laws
Cost and resource constraints	Technology with the developed software

localities remain without the necessary equipment to ensure smooth digital medical encounters, especially places that are suffering from being underserved.

Digital Divide:

The knowledge gap acts as the differences in digital literacy and access to technology expression [34] and is the major barrier to the use of the Internet in therapy. In the case of patients missing the access to Internet-connected devices or the sufficient level of technological literacy, the opportunity to benefit from VR healthcare services will not be available, which will only increase the existing health disparities.

Data Security and Privacy Concerns:

The adoption is also limited by concerns about security and privacy regarding the collection, storage, and sharing of health data in the parallel world. For instance, to protect access to the personal and sensitive medical information, healthcare organizations are expected to employ strong data encryption, control access, and comply with the privacy policies, such as the Health Insurance Portability and Accountability Act (HIPAA) [35].

Regulatory Challenges:

Due to the relatively young age of the regulatory framework for the implementation of virtual treatments in the real world, there are probable deployment difficulties and uncertainties. In particular, health professionals are constrained by intricate rules and laws that apply differently across countries, including data privacy, telemedicine reimbursement, and certification laws [36].

Cost and Resource Constraints:
The cost and resources in the Metaverse environment is highly dependent on the software developed for a particular application. These technologies can be too high for practices with fewer resources [37, 38].

12.10 Conclusion

The virtual world helps in transforming and providing intense solutions that keenly focus on longstanding issues, which prominently improves patient outcomes. Healthcare companies provide advanced technologies that greatly leverage VR, along with AI, creating personalized, real-time experiences on the effective diagnosis, treatment, and various forms of engagement. The metaverse on real-time healthcare, however, has various limitations. Addressing these obstacles, with the use of technological infrastructure and regulatory impediments, helps in patient security, maintaining equality in access. The metaverse platform empowers addressing health concerns using easily accessible, patient-centered healthcare systems. This way, the metaverse has the potential to create an impact on the future healthcare, enhancing global well-being.

References

1. Chengoden, R., Victor, N., Huynh-The, T., Yenduri, G., Jhaveri, R. H., Alazab, M., & Gadekallu, T. R. (2023). Metaverse for healthcare: A survey on potential applications, challenges and future directions. *IEEE Access, 11*, 12765–12795.
2. Moztarzadeh, O., Jamshidi, M., Sargolzaei, S., Jamshidi, A., Baghalipour, N., Malekzadeh Moghani, M., & Hauer, L. (2023). Metaverse and healthcare: Machine learning-enabled digital twins of cancer. *Bioengineering, 10*(4), 455.
3. Elhenawy, I., AL-Baker, S. F., & Mohamed, M. (2023). Intelligent healthcare: Evaluation potential implications of metaverse in healthcare based on mathematical decision-making framework. *Neutrosophic Systems with Applications, 12*, 9–21.
4. Yang, Y., Zhou, Z., Li, X., Xue, X., Hung, P. C., & Yangui, S. (2023). Metaverse for healthcare: Technologies, challenges, and vision. *International Journal of Crowd Science, 7*(4), 190–199.
5. Gupta, O. J., Yadav, S., Srivastava, M. K., Darda, P., & Mishra, V. (2023). Understanding the intention to use metaverse in healthcare utilizing a mix method approach. *International Journal of Healthcare Management, 12*(2), 318–329.
6. Ullah, H., Manickam, S., Obaidat, M., Laghari, S. U. A., & Uddin, M. (2023). Exploring the potential of metaverse technology in healthcare: Applications, challenges, and future directions. *IEEE Access, 11*, 69686–69707.
7. Bashir, A. K., Victor, N., Bhattacharya, S., Huynh-The, T., Chengoden, R., Yenduri, G., & Liyanage, M. (2023). Federated learning for the healthcare metaverse: Concepts, applications, challenges, and future directions. *IEEE Internet of Things Journal, 15*, 21873–21891.

8. Athar, A., Ali, S. M., Mozumder, M. A. I., Ali, S., & Kim, H. C. (2023, February). Applications and Possible Challenges of Healthcare Metaverse. In *2023 25th International Conference on Advanced Communication Technology (ICACT)* (pp. 328–332). IEEE.

9. Kumar, V., Joshi, K., Kumar, R., Anandaram, H., Bhagat, V. K., & Baloni, D. (2023). Multi modalities medical image fusion using deep learning and metaverse technology: Healthcare 4.0 a futuristic approach. *Biomedical and Pharmacology Journal, 16*(4), 1949–1959.

10. Ashwini, A., & Sriram, S. R. (2023). Quadruple spherical tank systems with automatic level control applications using fuzzy deep neural sliding mode FOPID controller. *Journal of Engineering Research*.

11. Bang, J., & Kim, J. Y. (2023). Metaverse Ethics for Healthcare Using AI Technology: Challenges and Risks. In *International Conference on Human-Computer Interaction* (pp. 367–378). Cham: Springer Nature Switzerland.

12. Ashwini, A., Purushothaman, K. E., Rosi, A., & Vaishnavi, T. (2023). Artificial intelligence based real-time automatic detection and classification of skin lesion in dermoscopic samples using DenseNet-169 architecture. *Journal of Intelligent & Fuzzy Systems*, (Preprint), *45*(4), 6943–6958.

13. Zhang, T., Shen, J., Lai, C. F., Ji, S., & Ren, Y. (2023). Multi-server assisted data sharing supporting secure deduplication for metaverse healthcare systems. *Future Generation Computer Systems, 140*, 299–310.

14. Ashwini, A., & Sangeetha, S. (2024). IoT-Based Smart Sensors: The Key to Early Warning Systems and Rapid Response in Natural Disasters. In *Predicting Natural Disasters with AI and Machine Learning* (pp. 202–223). IGI Global.

15. Kim, E. J., & Kim, J. Y. (2023). The metaverse for healthcare: Trends, applications, and future directions of digital therapeutics for urology. *International Neurourology Journal, 27*(Suppl 1), S3.

16. Ashwini, A., Sriram, S. R., Manisha, A., & Prabhakar, J. M. (2024). Artificial Intelligence's Impact on Thrust Manufacturing with Innovations and Advancements in Aerospace. In *Industry Applications of Thrust Manufacturing: Convergence with Real-Time Data and AI* (pp. 197–220). IGI Global.

17. Letafati, M., & Otoum, S. (2024). Digital healthcare in the metaverse: Insights into privacy and security. *IEEE Consumer Electronics Magazine. 13*(3), 80–89.

18. Ashwini, A., & Kavitha, V. (2023). Automatic skin tumor detection using online tiger claw region based segmentation – A novel comparative technique. *IETE Journal of Research, 69*(6), 3095–3103.

19. Ashwini, A., Vaishnavi, T., Rosi, A., Shahila, D. F. D., & Nalini, N. (2023, December). Deep Learning Based Drowsiness Detection with Alert System Using Raspberry Pi Pico. In *2023 International Conference on Data Science, Agents & Artificial Intelligence (ICDSAAI)* (pp. 1–8). IEEE.

20. Zhang, G., Dai, Y., Wu, J., Zhu, X., & Lu, Y. (2023). Swarm learning-based secure and fair model sharing for metaverse healthcare. *Mobile Networks and Applications, 28*(4), 1498–1509.

21. Akbari, A. A., & Teymouri, M. (2023). The role and position of metaverse in health care. *Medical Law Journal, 17*(58), 839–850.

22. Çeçen, Z., & Yüksel, O. Metaverse and healthcare sector. *International Journal of Engineering and Innovative Research, 5*(3), 280–290.

23. Al Kuwaiti, A., Nazer, K., Al-Reedy, A., Al-Shehri, S., Al-Muhanna, A., Subbarayalu, A. V., & Al-Muhanna, F. A. (2023). A review of the role of artificial intelligence in healthcare. *Journal of Personalized Medicine, 13*(6), 951.

24. Ashwini, A., & Murugan, S. (2023). Automatic skin tumour segmentation using prioritized patch based region – A novel comparative technique. *IETE Journal of Research, 69*(1), 137–148.
25. Stephanie, V., Khalil, I., & Atiquzzaman, M. (2024). DSFL: A decentralized SplitFed learning approach for healthcare consumers in the metaverse. *IEEE Transactions on Consumer Electronics, 70*(1), 2107–2115.
26. Shahila, D. F. D., Ashwini, A., Vaishnavi, T., Rosi, A., & Evangelin, D. L. (2023, August). IOT Based Object Perception Algorithm for Urban Scrutiny System in Digital City. In *2023 International Conference on Circuit Power and Computing Technologies (ICCPCT)* (pp. 1788–1792). IEEE.
27. Ashwini, A., Purushothaman, K. E., Prathaban, B. P., Jenath, M., & Prasanna, R. (2023, April). Automatic Traffic Sign Board Detection from Camera Images Using Deep Learning and Binarization Search Algorithm. In *2023 International Conference on Recent Advances in Electrical, Electronics, Ubiquitous Communication, and Computational Intelligence (RAEEUCCI)* (pp. 1–5). IEEE.
28. Li, Y., Gunasekeran, D. V., RaviChandran, N., Tan, T. F., Ong, J. C. L., Thirunavukarasu, A. J., & Ting, D. S. (2023). The next generation of healthcare ecosystem in the metaverse. *Biomedical Journal, 47*(3), 100679.
29. Balasubramaniam, S, Kadry, S., & Kumar, K. S. (2024). Osprey Gannet optimization enabled CNN based transfer learning for optic disc detection and cardiovascular risk prediction using retinal fundus images. *Biomedical Signal Processing and Control, 93*, 106177.
30. Wu, T. C., & Ho, C. T. B. (2023). A scoping review of metaverse in emergency medicine. *Australasian Emergency Care, 26*(1), 75–83.
31. Yang, E. (2023). Implications of immersive technologies in healthcare sector and its built environment. *Frontiers in Medical Technology, 5.*
32. Balasubramaniam, S, Arishma, M., & Dhanaraj, R. K. (2024). A comprehensive exploration of artificial intelligence methods for COVID-19 diagnosis. *EAI Endorsed Transactions on Pervasive Health and Technology, 10.*
33. Huang, H., Zhang, C., Zhao, L., Ding, S., Wang, H., & Wu, H. (2023). Self-supervised medical image denoising based on WISTA-net for human healthcare in metaverse. *IEEE Journal of Biomedical and Health Informatics, 28*(11), 6329–6337.
34. Balasubramaniam, S, Nelson, S. G., Arishma, M., & Rajan, A. S. (2024). Machine learning based disease and pest detection in agricultural crops. *EAI Endorsed Transactions on Internet of Things, 10.*
35. Ramamurthy, S., Yammahi, A. S., & Rahim, A. A. (2023). The role of the metaverse in transforming healthcare. *Research Journal of Pharmacy and Technology, 16*(11), 5506–5513.
36. Balasubramaniam, S, Prasanth, A., Kumar, K. S., & Kavitha, V. (2024). Medical Image Analysis Based on Deep Learning Approach for Early Diagnosis of Diseases. In *Deep Learning for Smart Healthcare* (pp. 54–75). Auerbach Publications.
37. An, P. H. (2023). Exploring the digital healthcare product's logistics and mental healthcare in the metaverse: Role of technology anxiety and metaverse bandwidth fluctuations. *iRASD Journal of Management, 5*(4), 223–241.
38. Tripathi, A., Chauhan, N., Choudhary, A., & Singh, R. (2023). Augmented Reality and Its Significance in Healthcare Systems. In *Meta-Learning Frameworks for Imaging Applications* (pp. 103–118). IGI Global.

Chapter 13

Virtual Realities: The Influence of the Metaverse on Healthcare E-Governance

N. Bindu, R. Ajith Kumar, T. Radhakrishnan, T. K. Manoj Kumar, and K. Satheesh Kumar

13.1 Introduction

The metaverse is a transitional tool capable of reshaping the future of public services and civic life. The advanced techniques and the virtual tools used in the metaverse are marking a radical shift from traditional bureaucratic governance processes, ushering in a new era of streamlined bureaucracy radically different from conventional bureaucratic processes. The corresponding e-governance revolution in the metaverse will change how the government delivers its services by creating virtual civic spaces for citizens. Its impact ranges from public administration to education. Singapore leads in incorporating virtual spaces in e-governance. For example, 'Virtual Singapore' integrates metaverse technologies that simulate urban scenarios, optimize traffic flow and plan infrastructure improvements. Metaverse-based e-governance helps citizens better engage with public services in a lively and inclusive environment. Through metaverse-assisted virtual governance, administrative procedures like permitting or licensing have become more intuitive and efficient today. Virtual government offices allow citizens to navigate through digital representations, interact with AI-powered virtual assistants, and participate in real-time

DOI: 10.1201/9781003491668-13

Table 13.1 Main Areas of Metaverse Application in Healthcare Sector

Sl No.	Applications Areas
1.	Medical education and training
2.	Remote patient monitoring
3.	Telemedicine and telehealth
4.	Therapeutic interventions
5.	Collaborative research and development
6.	Health and wellness programs
7.	Data visualization and analysis
8.	Population health management

consultations. The integrating of the metaverse into healthcare can enable the establishment of virtual health clinics, providing access to virtual appointments, consultations as well as wellness programs for enhanced accessibility and preventive care.

This section enumerates various applications of the metaverse in the healthcare field as well as several aspects of the metaverse-based e-government on the healthcare sector. The concept of the metaverse could speed up medical treatment as well as inform international health organizations through research sharing and data processing mechanisms. The decentralized nature, enhanced user experience and user engagement removes barriers within a bureaucratic process, which has potential for revolutionizing healthcare. Multidisciplinary teams across borders have much potential for achieving positive outcomes toward global health equity when enabled by technology. What implications does this have for healthcare in various ways? When adopted, this technology will significantly affect patient monitoring, telemedicine, education, training and many other aspects. Metaverse-enabled digitalizing medical education may offer students from all around the world an inclusive learning platform taking place without geographical boundaries.

It can make healthcare domain more democratic through its engaging capabilities that make it accessible, interactive and efficient. A few of the trust areas for healthcare in the metaverse are given in Table 13.1.

13.2 Medical Education and Training

The metaverse, which combines virtual and augmented reality (VR and AR), can give medical education and training to students and healthcare practitioners in a real-world setting, enhancing their learning experience. The hands-on training provided in the metaverse is free from risks and offers better surgical simulations and continuous learning.

13.2.1 Simulations and Training

Integration of metaverse into healthcare governance introduces a new approach to medical education through realistic experience of surgeries or procedures without pain or suffering [1]. The advantage is that it can generate complex medical scenarios for training which will help trainees acquiring decision-making skills when encountering medical emergencies. It is a revolutionary medical training method which enhances the involvement of participants and provides a safe environment to conduct surgical procedures, avoiding the risk involved in traditional training methods [1]. These modern training conditions enhance the confidence of the trainees by providing experience conducting complex procedures which would ultimately help provide better patient care. One advantage mentioned in particular is that the trainees can carry out detailed surgeries or other complicated medical procedures without risking a patient's life. It will also reduce the number of years spent by physicians acquiring knowledge. Another important aspect is that these procedures will not inflict pain to the patients, which is more significant than physicians gaining skills. This scenario is more patient-centric, rooted in empathy rather than compassion. Further advancements in this field are expected to completely alter the way medical knowledge is acquired and bring competence, empathy and precision into medical practice. The virtual training ground offered by the metaverse has several benefits. It definitely enhances the modes of medical training and physician's proficiency levels [1]. As a result, technical skills and thinking capabilities within a controlled environment of learners can be enhanced. The provision of collective learning provided by metaverse can encourage teamwork through full-blown tutorials and simulation of complex procedures such as surgeries. Thus physicians can virtually encounter and experience various situations of healthcare problems at various clinical levels.

However, there are challenges in integrating these healthcare metaverse simulation techniques and training. These challenges include the inferiority of nonliving computerized simulations to deal with sick people. In addition, even though these simulations provide real-life-like environments, they might lack emotional elements as well as the unpredictability of real medical situations. Additionally, creating highly complex healthcare models for the metaverse based on sophisticated technologies can be very expensive for many medical institutions [1]. In virtual environments of training, safeguarding the privacy and confidentiality of patients' sensitive data requires strong measures. Thus, one needs to consider both pros and cons before introducing simulation and training in the healthcare sector in metaverse environments.

As mentioned earlier, the learning facilitated by remote management using simulation in the metaverse makes it possible for healthcare providers to practice real-world scenarios with more preparedness and competence [2]. That is, medical teams can learn how to cooperate, communicate and coordinate their actions in a collaborative virtual environment. This advantage of the metaverse has a remarkable impact on medical education since it can build individual competencies as well as prepare experts for efficacious functioning under real-life clinical situations as a team [3].

13.2.2 Continuous Education

Current VR platforms enable ongoing training and education for healthcare providers updating more with medical innovations. These facilities provide an unconventional way of keeping the students of medicine informed about their training progress [4, 5]. In addition, they also facilitate experiential learning, which is useful to healthcare professionals to develop diagnostic expertise as well as decisiveness under safe conditions, ensuring that they become conversant with the most up-to-date medical practices. This approach also encourages effective teamwork, collaboration and communication in interdisciplinary training sessions [6]. This facility enhances the efficiency of general health service delivery and caters for the escalating importance of interdisciplinary collaboration in modern medicine.

13.2.3 VR-Based Learning

The notable advantage of VR is that it can create high-fidelity yet risk-free training scenarios, particularly in risk-laden industries like healthcare, aviation and emergency services. It will help individuals to improve their decision-making skills and practice overcoming obstacles they might face in their lives. In the healthcare sector, VR can provide deep learning experiences, which is not at all possible with traditional methods. It helps the learner understand complex concepts much more easily by allowing simulations that mirror real-life situations. Further, these platforms can offer on-demand training to professionals. They can access them anytime and learn at their own pace, which is significant as healthcare providers can adapt to changes caused by advancements in medical treatments.

13.3 Remote Patient Monitoring

Remote monitoring patients has several advantages, including proactive healthcare management, timely detection of diseases and individualized, real-time intervention for preventative measures. The VR/AR devices are valuable in this, as they can help to share real-time health data with healthcare providers for consistent monitoring of patients' vital signs, medication adherence and other health indices. The use of the metaverse in healthcare could reshape patient care through virtual clinics creation and virtual consultations, giving room for distant interaction between patients and their carers, thus reducing physical visits and addressing accessibility and convenience [7]. The platform including the metaverse helps to set up virtual clinics where patients may ask questions on medical problems, take part in simulated procedures or receive guidance from physicians who communicate from a distance, leading to enhanced personalized care [8].

One advantage is that the environment can be designed to provide more exciting and interactive experiences for patients while participating in virtual consultations. For medical professionals, the advantage is that it allows them to go beyond their imaginable boundaries. They can reach out to those who live in remote areas like inaccessible rural areas, simplifying treatment access and optimizing healthcare resources [9, 10]. The move from in-person to online consultations highlights how telemedicine is changing and becoming important, efficient and accessible. It is expected to improve overall efficiency across various levels of healthcare. From smart watches to health-tracking sensors, wearable gadgets can effortlessly link up with the metaverse, resulting in significant improvements in healthcare and new ways of continuous patient monitoring. These gadgets offer a comprehensive platform for people to share real-time updates on their daily routines and health patterns. Healthcare professionals can tackle concerns early by pairing the wearable devices with the metaverse. These wearable gadgets can help in measuring various health parameters such as heart rate more reliably [11, 12]. Apart from that, the accurate measurements of health parameters of a person using wearable gadgets are invaluable for preventive care and swift responses [13]. Because metaverse technology lowers the frequency of hospital visits, it will be a game changer in the healthcare industry for patients with chronic conditions [14]. VR in the metaverse eliminates the need for cadavers [15] and helps surgeons improve their skills in carrying out complex surgeries for better service [16]. As a result, the overall efficiency of the healthcare system is expected to witness large-scale improvement. The combination of wearable devices and the metaverse is expected to have profound influence in the future of healthcare systems.

13.4 Telemedicine and Telehealth

The metaverse provides virtual clinics and telemedicine systems, allowing patients to consult with doctors in interactive virtual settings. Telemedicine and telehealth increase access to medical treatment, particularly for remote residents, by providing a simple and secure means of contact for fast response consultations. This is highly important in the case of patients with disabilities and at times of emergency. Thus, telemedicine and telehealth break the barriers of distance, transport costs and time in the case of healthcare service delivery.

The fact that people can get medical advice without having to physically go to a doctor is a remarkable benefit of telemedicine. They can consult with medical personnel virtually from the comfort of their own homes. The main biorefineries of telemedicine are the people from remote areas with limited healthcare facilities. With mild symptoms, people may hesitate to consult a doctor by visiting physically, but with easy virtual consultation, people will be encouraged to discuss their medical problems at an early stage. This practice could help medical professionals intervene at an early stage, which in turn increases early recovery. Another advantage of remote access devices is that they enable patients to become active participants in their own disease care. However, it has a detrimental influence. For example, technological failures during consultations might result in patient disconnection or poor service quality, jeopardizing patient safety. This is also important when transmitting sensitive medical information online. Another concern is data privacy and security. Regulatory and license concerns may also develop in multinational healthcare delivery systems with disparate legal frameworks. Telemedical consultations do not include a physical examination. There is a risk of misdiagnosis and missing critical indications and symptoms. As a result, in some circumstances, telemedicine must be combined with traditional face-to-face treatment to provide full health service delivery.

13.4.1 Virtual Clinics

Within the metaverse, virtual clinics are expected to transform healthcare delivery by creating a digital space where patients can quickly locate doctors. Patients appreciate the ease of accessing health services without being limited by physical boundaries. Implementation of this alternative is influenced by new telemedicine trends that allow medical providers to meet patients using online portals even in remote areas and emergency conditions [17, 18]. It allows patients to share safely their medical history, test results and other important details with healthcare providers so that a care plan can be developed based on his or her requirements and provide the most accurate information about their patients' health to the doctors. Usage of VR technologies can equip healthcare professionals to perform physical examinations via simulation, thereby giving rise to more engaging and comprehensive healthcare interactions [8]. They would also be able to give personalized advice, follow-up care plans and even run virtual wellness programs where people could join online meetings from their own homes, as they might do with any video-chat service on demand. In virtual clinics like these, the metaverse becomes a flexible platform for providing patient-centered care that may be accessed remotely or onsite depending on the individual needs of each case. Remote health monitoring is an innovative way of approaching healthcare through integration of VR and AR devices within the metaverse. With VR/AR devices, users are able to provide real-time health data such as vitals, activities among other relevant health metrics, which help in continuous monitoring hence proactive interventions. As it relates to telehealth's dynamic landscape, this novel approach presents as a dynamic platform for remote patient care within immersive settings [19–21]). These techniques thus enable early detection of problems and timely intervention in chronic disease management through remote patient care. This approach will improve patient adherence to monitoring protocols by increasing their involvement in the process [22]. AR-based solutions allow health professionals to see a complete picture of their patient's conditions because they improve data visualization. For example, the emerging platform of computer–human environment interaction (HCI), which refers to any combination of humans, computers or the physical environment, is a highly recommended system in healthcare.

Computer input methods and the ability to perceive the environment in HCI have been revolutionized by the Internet of Things (IoT) and other advances in processing capacity sensing and GSM network speed (e.g., 5 G GPRS). The sensors that function over a high-speed GSM network have the potential to enhance the mobile interactions of users with both physical and virtual objects [23]. With the progression of remote health surveillance, it becomes increasingly evident that the metaverse functions as a dynamic framework that enhances the efficiency and availability of healthcare provision.

13.5 Therapeutic Interventions

The metaverse broadens the scope of therapeutic interventions by deploying immersive and interactive technologies, which create personalized and engaging mental health experiences. In the metaverse, virtual environments are used as platforms for interventions like exposure therapy, mindfulness exercises and immersive relaxation techniques enabling individuals to access novel mental healthcare affordably.

VR revolutionizes addressing mental health with specific regards to exposure therapy that is even more potent and flexible when applied within the boundaries of the metaverse. For instance, [24] found out that VR-based exposure therapy can be effective for various psychological conditions like anxiety disorders and post-traumatic stress disorder (PTSD). This technology means that in a virtual environment, patients are exposed to levels determined by therapists so they can learn to manage their symptoms without getting overwhelmed but still get better over time. The benefits of VR therapy do not end at exposure therapy alone; it is capable of extensively dealing with a range of mental health problems. VR can create an environment that gives an individual calmness, thereby allowing them to relax and become more mindful. According to [25], VR facilitates emotional regulation, enhances therapies and improves mental well-being. As technology advances, VR therapy could replace conducting some psychotherapies such cognitive behavioral therapies (CBTs) or drug treatments like ibogaine for psychiatric disorders.

VR-based rehabilitation systems for physical therapy create an immersive environment that puts patients in control of their treatment and improves adherence to prescribed exercises, leading to better rehabilitation outcomes. It has also been shown to improve patient enjoyment and motivation during exercise sessions. Customizing exercises is achievable through VR-based rehabilitation, thus making them suitable for patient-specific needs as they progress toward full recovery. It may contain VR interventions involving task-specific training enhancing motor skill development and ultimately contributing to better physical recovery outcomes among people undergoing physical therapy. For instance, this means specific impairments of patients will be addressed through customized sets, hence leading to an improved recovery process that is not only better but also more effective [26]. Hence, VR-based rehabilitation systems may make it easier for patients to exercise at home.

13.6 Collaborative Research and Development

A metaverse is where researchers and professionals worldwide come together, making collaborative research and development grow beyond their usual boundaries. The net of digital interconnectivity enables seamless sharing of insights, data and simulations among scientists in real time, thus speeding up breakthroughs in various fields and transforming the research and development space.

13.6.1 *Global Collaboration*

The metaverse enables scientists or medical professionals to work from anywhere in the world. This could be helpful for fast, efficient medical treatments as well as technological developments. The metaverse marks a turning point for scientific community members, putting them at an advantage to push for global collaboration. Despite distances that separate them on the map, the metaverse offers a common virtual space for research within the healthcare delivery sector. Scientists may collaborate in real time with one another across boundaries when they are researching medicine or related areas. Working together in real time is possible through this platform. It would enable doctors to share their ideas faster and more efficiently, providing an enabling environment for healthcare advancements. It improves how fast healthcare studies can be carried out. Healthcare research conducted within simulated environments could also be made more efficient by the use of VR technology [2, 27, 28]. Researchers have access to virtual experimental labs via the metaverse without any limitations, thus improving their efficiency. This technology was used to conduct realistic simulations of medical procedures to test hypotheses better [29]. Therefore, medical researchers might find benefits through having a 'virtual' environment where physical barriers do not exist anymore, resulting in improved efficacy and innovation in conducting studies. We cannot ignore how much the metaverse has done in shaping collaborative research as we proceed.

13.6.2 Drug Discovery

The use of virtual laboratories integrated into a metaverse represents a new approach toward collaborative drug discovery and testing toward creating dynamic simulation spaces that will reshape the pharmaceutical industry forever. Usually traditional processes of drug discovery are time-consuming and expensive, involving a lot of lab work. On the other hand, the metaverse creates a new way, for example through blockchain and cloud computing, that enables researchers to collectively design, simulate and test virtual drug compounds. Researchers will have access to new possibilities not available elsewhere, and this will reduce knowledge gaps in their research work. Virtual labs can be established where biologists or chemists from multiple disciplines can collaborate. A number of diverse interactions have been shown when studying drugs alone with even more variables introduced. Utilizing the metaverse for collaborative drug discovery taps into distributed scientific communities, yielding better solutions that are robust and innovation inclined.

13.7 Telemedicine and Telehealth

Telemedicine and telehealth in the metaverse provide virtual access to doctors and patients. Healthcare delivery can now be done from one's home through envisioning digital representation of the vital information of the patient. This technology has enhanced telehealth into real-time interactions, virtual examination as well as collaborative decision-making among patients and healthcare providers. It alters how patients engage with doctors. The goal of universal healthcare is based on these services being available to everyone, and this is what the metaverse does for us.

If successfully implemented, virtual clinics could provide a novel platform for patients to communicate with medical professionals online while sharing medical records within the metaverse. This concept represents a significant advancement in healthcare delivery by providing a dynamic and accessible communication platform. Virtual clinics may disrupt our traditional method by providing remote services, allowing patients to receive the required care without physically visiting a health center or hospital [30]. These new working models will enable us to communicate with healthcare professionals instantly when we need them the most. The convenience alone is groundbreaking.

This platform could also improve coordination among healthcare professionals, ensuring comprehensive care. Building this space would allow doctors and nurses of various specialities to collaborate on individual cases without being in close proximity [31]. When patients can digitally transform information across servers, having multiple doctors in the same room is no longer necessary.

13.7.1 Remote Health Monitoring

VR/AR devices enable patients and providers to share live health data outside of traditional hospitals through continuous monitoring technology in the metaverse. Continued monitoring has shown great promise because early detection leads to early intervention, promoting personalized care and patient outcomes while lowering long-term costs [32]. This new technology can significantly reduce the overall costs of the healthcare system and streamline the system. In addition, the utilization of VR/AR devices to enable patients to transmit critical health data in real time, including pulse rate, blood pressure, and activity levels, to healthcare providers facilitates the transition of the medical sector from reactive to preventative care. By adopting a proactive approach, doctors can identify ways to assist individuals well before the start of any illness − known as preventive healthcare [33]. With VR/AR devices in the metaverse, doctors can provide personalized remote health monitoring interventions based on individual health data.

13.7.2 Health and Wellness Programs

Health and wellness programs in the metaverse provide individuals with immersive platforms for virtual fitness classes, mental health support groups and personalized wellness activities. In the metaverse, these programs utilize their interactive features to promote holistic well-being by gamifying wellness activities and incorporating social aspects that motivate people to lead healthier lives.

13.7.3 Virtual Fitness and Wellness

The integration of the metaverse in fitness and wellness is a great chance to help people adopt positive lifestyles that seek prevention more than treatments. Physical activity and general well-being are among the various ways through which individuals can be engaged within this world of reality. The interactive characteristic of these environments in the metaverse enhances consistency in exercise and physical fitness because they are game based [34]. It encourages individuals' participation in exercising by gamifying it, leading to avoidance of sedentary lifestyle–related health threats. The ability of metaverse to host virtual support groups and deliver wellness programs has huge consequences for community development as well as mental health. Virtual wellness programs facilitate exchange of experiences, advice, resources, etc., among participants, thus enhancing their overall mental health status. Integration of virtual fitness and wellness into the metaverse addresses different dimensions of good health while encouraging physical activities as a form of preventive care.

13.7.4 Gamification of Health

Incorporating gaming principles into the metaverse presents a new way to engage with users' health as players interact with each other using avatars. When rewards, challenges or competitions are included in games, they become gamified experiences which motivate users toward better lifestyle choices. Research shows how effective gamification is in changing healthcare environment and behavior, especially on matters concerning patient's health [35]. In order to encourage healthy behaviors such as frequent physical exercise or adherence to medication regimens within the metaverse, gamification can be implemented, for instance, through VR fitness games. This approach helps avoid a sedentary lifestyle, hence improving their overall well-being by making exercise more interesting. Furthermore, this could be a way of incorporating gamification into the metaverse for the sake of improving patient adherence to treatment. Gamified mobile applications in healthcare are highly beneficial [36]. The inclusion of gaming elements in virtual health platforms spurs people's motivation and dedication to their given therapies. The possibility for personalizing and executing efficient methods of enhancing health based on individual choices through adopting custom game experiences in the metaverse is available. The emergence of the metaverse brings with it an exciting opportunity to turn routine daily health activities into pleasurable and enduring habits by employing the use of gamified mobile health apps.

13.7.5 Data Visualization and Analysis

Unlike the common data visualization and analysis techniques used in healthcare, an immersive and detailed representation of information can be experienced in the metaverse environment. These dynamic visualization techniques enhance the understanding of health data and are helpful for quick decision-making by healthcare professionals. Representation of intricate health data in three-dimensional (3D) space within the metaverse is a drastic shift from conventional methods of medical data representation. Complex datasets like 3D medical imaging or genomics are conventionally challenging to analyze in healthcare settings. Health professionals are now able to use the metaverse virtual environment to view health data in 3D, which allows for more immersive and intuitive ways of analyzing it. Studies have shown that VR-based 3D visualization of medical imaging is a useful tool for spatial representation, resulting in better diagnostics [37, 38]. In the metaverse, health data are represented on the fly, allowing deep analyses and discussions among various teams that result into better patient care decisions. The adoption of 3D visualizations while using medical imagery has enhanced the learning experience and improved memory retention [39]. Thus, the convergence between the representation of health data on metaverse platforms is aimed at assisting physicians' analytical skills and definitely has impacts on every level of medical education.

13.7.6 Population Health Management

A novel approach in healthcare is the use of various population health management applications available in the metaverse. There are extensive collections of

AI-based tools to analyze population health records and understand differences among each record pertaining to individual's well-being. With this tool, clinicians as well as public health officials may gain insight into community wellness, predict spread of diseases, identify root causes behind poor health status and plan presentable interventions accordingly. Metaverse technologies advocate for public health analytics in terms of their ability to work with diverse datasets and enhance the decision-making process that is necessary for planning public health activities [40, 41]. Metaverse applications in population health management help to generate and implement evidence-based solutions. Real-time visualization and analytics of data by public health experts can enable monitoring of the effectiveness of interventions, for tracking outcomes that have been achieved as well as for modifying strategies where necessary. Dynamic and interactive modulation of public health measures during a crisis were shown by [42] in their research work. The use of metaverse technologies in population health management enhances the efficacy of public health initiatives, thereby empowering decision-makers to formulate better interventions for their communities. Figure 13.1 presents an overview of the possible advantages and discrepancies of metaverse applications in the electronic governance of the healthcare industry.

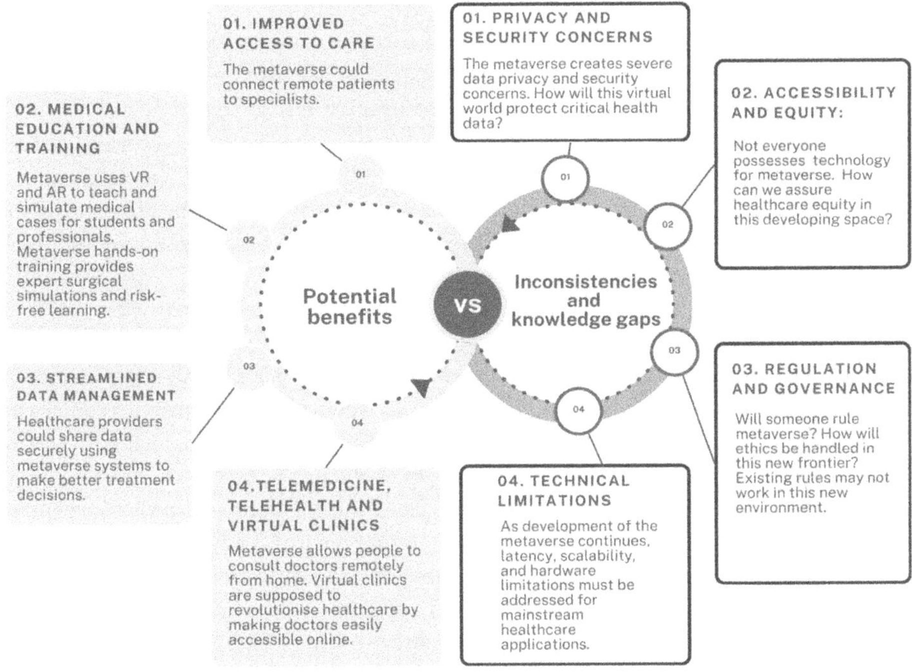

Figure 13.1   Potential benefits and inconsistencies of metaverse applications in the healthcare sector.

13.7.7 Assistive Technologies for Metaverse Implementation in Healthcare Governance

Recent updates in other advanced technologies, such as blockchain, brain–computer interfaces and spatial audio technology have played an important role in implementing a metaverse within the healthcare industry. Within the metaverse, cloud computing is instrumental for propelling healthcare into the future through provision of scalable, adaptable and available storage and processing systems for huge volumes of data. In virtual medical environments, cloud computing facilitates seamless fusion of patient records, image tests and real-time monitoring systems which avails critical information to health providers even if they may not be physically present. Also, platforms based on clouds enhance healthcare collaboration among multidisciplinary teams as it allows instantaneous distribution of information. Healthcare on the web using the cloud and edge computing could thus obliterate past limitations that were hindrances to personalized immersive virtual worlds with resilient clinical encounters.

Immutable ledgers created with blockchain technology can retain patients' details securely, hence privacy and trustworthiness are guaranteed. Smart contracts integrated into these networks, however, simplify interactions between insurance firms and medics. There is no barrier from paperwork or miscommunication with regard to billing; likewise, appointments are scheduled accordingly using this means as well. Blockchain has created a basis for a more inclusive virtual healthcare environment. It is essential in helping patients because decentralized identity systems can verify who they are across different channels so that their private data cannot be exposed to hackers. These models prioritize transparency around patient data while incentivizing sharing participation in clinical trials that cultivate an innovation ecosystem within the metaverse. Blockchain technology also speeds up drug production, and distribution of drugs has been used before by some big pharmaceuticals companies.

Pharmaceuticals seems like it could be one of those industries where we find numerous applications of blockchain technologies essentially being put to practice. Furthermore, developments in haptic feedback devices, 3D scanners and cameras, motion capture and spatial audio technology as well as brain–computer interfaces also contribute heavily to implementation of a metaverse within healthcare. The virtual world may be approached with the help of the haptic feedback devices which give feeling just like that of touch. Haptic feedback mechanisms provide realistic digital experiences by conveying textures, temperatures and resistance through gloves, suits and controllers. The digital twins of real-world objects and settings of the metaverse are created using 3D scanners and cameras. It makes possible the virtualization of physical things found in our surroundings, including items, people, places etc. By following every movement made by the user, avatars can accurately reproduce real-world actions into virtual ones by way of motion capture technology. This is crucial if experiences need to be interactive or captivating. Virtual spaces can become more realistic representations of the real thing through spatial audio technology, where direction, distance and environment are some factors considered, thus making it more immersive. Brain–computer interfaces, known as emerging technologies, have potential to allow users control over virtual environments through their brain signals. Through this specific emerging innovation for persons who unable to move, together with push wheelchairs, could increase interaction levels. Brain–computer interfaces are the new technological device that enables individuals to operate their brain signals virtually controlling the environments while using them. For example, this feature might improve communication for individuals who have epilepsy, autism, cerebral palsy or difficulty in speaking or moving due to neurological issues. In addition, AI technologies can be used for personalizing user experiences on dynamic content creation, intelligent virtual assistants and nonplayer characters (NPCs) inside the metaverse.

13.8 Regulatory Compliance and Privacy

The metaverse is a blending of opportunities and challenges in e-governance of healthcare, which has to be carefully examined for its ethical, privacy and accessibility considerations to fully realize its potential benefits. Therefore, the critical criteria which need to be considered while overseeing metaverse healthcare projects are as follows.

13.8.1 Digital Health Records (DHR) and Interoperability Standards

The DHRs of individuals within the metaverse should be created, kept, shared and protected with the help of e-governance. E-governance must have interoperability standards and regulations so that there can be a smooth flow of information among different virtual healthcare platforms in the metaverse. The metaverse comprises many virtual worlds and health apps that require interoperable protocols to facilitate cooperation among them and securely share health data. Different aspects of e-governance exist for ensuring effective governance, confidentiality, security, integration of DHRs, standardization and interoperability into the metaverse.

Standardizing and interoperating are vital in the metaverse because it allows easy collaboration on the various devices across platforms. E-governance legislation should specify the framework, storage and transfer of health data in the metaverse. In order to ensure uniformity and reliability on a virtual healthcare platform (VHP), Health Information Exchange (HIE) regulations should be put in place by authorities governing exchange of medical data between different providers' information systems. Standardization implies creating standardized frameworks as well as data formats for health information processing. Through such approaches toward a standardized format, VHPs can uniformly comprehend and analyze health data, thereby enabling ease sharing of information during transactional processes.

Governments would prefer that there exist a standard understanding of clinical terms in various virtual healthcare systems through standard definitions or interpretations given for items (e.g., lack of ambiguity). By having e-governance frameworks, one can determine who owns what particular health data in virtual healthcare, whether it is doctors, patients or other stakeholders. Regulations would help streamline the transfer of DHRs between different virtual healthcare platforms, thereby ensuring correct sharing, understanding and utilization of health information across numerous virtual healthcare settings. Accordingly, governments would set guidelines governing application programming interfaces (APIs) for applications in their digital health systems to guarantee adherence to one common set of standards for data transmission within the metaverse. Thus, their use supports interoperable apps and systems creation across the global data, which involves creating uniform data formats and frameworks for health information. VHPs can consistently comprehend and analyze health data, facilitating smooth information exchange.

To protect DHRs in the healthcare metaverse, e-governance standards should be put in place. Policy development should therefore include encryption standards, access controls and secure data transfer protocols [43]. Biometrics, multifactor authentication and other reliable methods of identity verification are some of the secure identity verification techniques that can be implemented by e-governance strategies for authenticating plus authorizing DHR users in the metaverse. Identity and Access Management (IAM) protocols forming part of interoperability standards need to include standardized authentication techniques. In virtual platforms, these protocols ensure similar ways for validating user information, thus improving security. Healthcare professionals and patients must establish and improve standard authentication methods on various virtual platforms to authenticate use by them.

There are a few key areas to consider when implementing e-governance into the metaverse so that DHRs can be properly integrated and operated within regulated compliance and ethical boundaries. Government should also develop DHR policies for audit and regulatory purposes for the protection of patients' rights under health and data protection laws. The change of virtual healthcare platforms within the digital world requires long-term storage policies and guidelines for DHR due to rapid advancement of technology in the area. To cope with rapid technological developments, the e-governance framework should remain flexible to incorporate technological change. In this regard, it is important to industry players to update these standards. It is equally important to adhere to the ethical norms governing the use of health data in cases of misuse or illegal dissemination of health data. Therefore, regulatory measures are required to ensure adherence as well as penalties for non-compliance. Virtual healthcare platforms can be certified or verified to comply with interoperability standards by regulatory entities, thereby enhancing trust in system stability and compatibility.

13.8.2 Regulatory Compliance in the Metaverse Healthcare

Healthcare metaverse regulatory compliance is essential for privacy, data protection and medical practice standards. Metaverse platforms must follow data minimization and right-to-erasure regulations set by governments. User consent to health data collection, processing, sharing and revocation will be more accessible with e-governance frameworks [44], suggesting precise consent forms, granular consent options and revocation procedures. Governments will set security and encryption standards to protect health data during transmission and storage. Encrypting the metaverse will prevent unauthorized access.

Continuous compliance checks and standardized protocols will enable seamless data exchange between virtual healthcare platforms. Practitioner ethics and virtual provider licensing will be regulated in telemedicine. E-governance frameworks will audit data ownership and health record portability, and unethical providers may be penalized. For the protection of health data and virtual healthcare services, the healthcare metaverse needs highly efficient judicial, ethical and technical regulatory frameworks.

13.8.3 Virtual Health Consultations

Governments regulate virtual health consultations in the metaverse to ensure implementation of stipulated standards and ethical guidelines, through licensing and credentialing processes. This will help to maintain standards of professionalism and build trust in distance healthcare. We need to give necessary priority to quality health services, since it is crucial factor of user satisfaction. Virtual healthcare interactions should follow codes of conduct and ethical standards for protection of data and privacy of the patients as well as professional conduct of the medical professionals. Government standardization mechanisms with deterrents such as fines and other punishments for defaulters could be helpful in effective implementation these mechanisms. The regulations of privacy should also specify encryption and access controls to protect patient data during virtual consultations. Telemedicine platforms should refer cases beyond their capabilities to the most competent specialists. Disparities among communities need to be addressed, especially among marginalized communities which lack digital literacy for taking care of their well-being. Telemedicine insurance systems could be of assistance in this regard. While promoting metaverse cybermedicine service entities and patient rights, governments need to regulate user experience, safety, interoperability and reliability in virtual healthcare environments when promoting metaverse cybermedicine service entities and patient rights.

13.8.4 Telemedicine Regulations

It is necessary to incorporate proper definitions of virtual medical services and guidelines for remote diagnostics to secure telehealth platforms. It is equally important to regulate medical services both in the metaverse and the physical world. Governments must determine which medical conditions and treatments suit metaverse remote consultations, considering virtual healthcare technologies and the need for in-person care. Clearly defined telemedicine services allow healthcare providers and patients to reap the benefits of telehealth without compromising safety or quality [45].

In addition, the healthcare metaverse-assisted e-governance includes remote diagnostics guidelines and tool use regulations to ensure accuracy, reliability and medical standards. Governments must have approval procedures for telehealth platforms and diagnostic tools to promote innovation and patient well-being. Telehealth platforms must also be secured by e-governance protocols for data protection, encryption and secure communication channels to protect patient data and confidentiality in metaverse virtual medical interactions.

13.8.5 Security and Authentication

Highly efficient e-governance implementation is needed to protect health data and authenticate virtual healthcare services in the healthcare metaverse. Governments must be keen in setting metaverse cybersecurity standards, emphasizing advanced encryption algorithms to protect health data during transmission and storage. Regulatory bodies can maintain trust in the virtual healthcare ecosystem by enforcing encryption standards to protect patient data from cyberattacks [46].

Multifactor authentication (MFA) is essential to metaverse security in e-governance. If the government mandates MFA, healthcare providers and patients must use multiple methods to verify their identities on virtual healthcare platforms. This extra security improves verification and reduces unauthorized access. The standardization of the MFA requirements would be essential for interoperability in e-governance frameworks, ensuring consistency and reliability across virtual healthcare services. Governments must require regular security audits, vulnerability assessments and quick breach response for strengthening the healthcare metaverse's resilience and trustworthiness [47].

13.8.6 Public Health Initiatives

Vaccination campaigns, disease monitoring as well as health education are some of the metaverse public health initiatives that e-governance could support. In the healthcare metaverse, e-governance for public health initiatives employs technology in expanding and enhancing critical health programs. Virtual vaccination campaigns are organized by governments to facilitate inclusive participation from various populations. Similarly, e-governance enables users to schedule appointments, access vaccine safety and efficacy information or even simulate vaccinations at virtual vaccination clinics for educational purposes. The use of the metaverse to promote widespread vaccination helps in achieving herd immunity against communicable diseases [48].

Public health driven by e-governance requires metaverse disease monitoring. Meanwhile, governments do this through data analytics and surveillance,

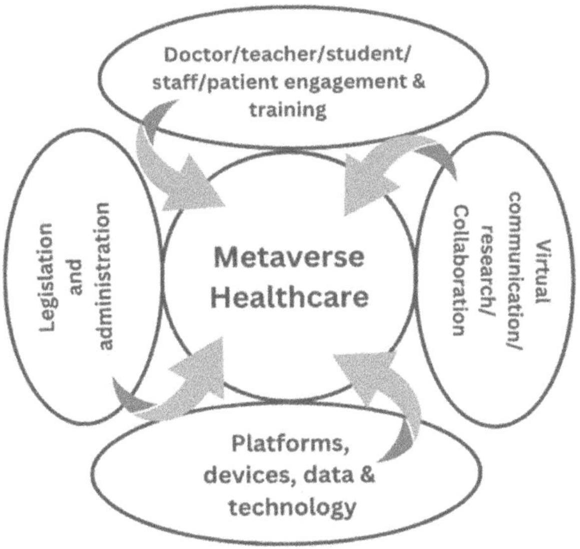

Figure 13.2 Ecosystem of healthcare in the metaverse.

including real-time analysis of virtual health records, analysis of user interactions and patterns of outbreak identification using AI algorithms. It is not difficult for regulatory bodies to react quickly to new threats regarding public health issues, efficiently allocate resources and prevent illness in a virtual population thanks to advanced systems for monitoring diseases.

Additionally, there is need for metaverse e-governance in relation to health education programs. Governments establish and maintain virtual platforms on which information about prevention of disease spread, healthy living tips as well as management of illnesses can be widely disseminated. These programs may include immersive educational experiences, interactive simulations and healthcare professional virtual seminars. Governments empower users to make informed health decisions using the metaverse for health education, improving virtual public health. Developing a healthcare metaverse and e-governance measures requires technological advances, societal acceptance and changing regulatory frameworks. These ideas are speculative based on healthcare technology directions. The main pillars of metaverse application of the healthcare ecosystem are given in Figure 13.2.

13.9 Challenges, Potential and Future Research Scope of Metaverse-Supported Healthcare Governance

It is indeed such a complex landscape that challenges and potential of the metaverse present in the e-governance of healthcare. This is because not all people have access to metaverse technologies, as they are not accessible universally due to a lack of infrastructure or devices, mostly in underserved and remote areas. For full metaverse-supported health governance to be achieved, this digital divide must be addressed. Additionally, there are insurmountable levels of difficulties surrounding data security and privacy. Trust can only be preserved if robust cybersecurity measures and compliance with data protection regulations are implemented, as these platforms hold sensitive health information. The way different healthcare stakeholders within the metaverse ecosystem can collaborate effectively and optimize efficiency requires interoperability standardization of various technologies [49].

The metaverse, on the other hand, holds great potential for the growth of e-governance in the healthcare sector. It could be used, for instance, to come up with immersive and interconnecting bespoke health services, which then shall redefine both involvement and compliance of therapeutic approaches as prescribed to the patient. Simulations and exercises have been considered very important means for skills development and professional enhancement of the health workforce. The simulations also help provide some ideas for possibly better planning of effective public health campaigns and care for prevention. Essentially, it needs to focus on modern technologies for meeting emerging individual and community needs. In addition, advanced data analytics, machine learning and AI are believed to completely change how health research takes place. Researchers will study big datasets of patients in such a way that they will be able to come up with personal treatment plans and even predict diseases' trends. Additionally, genomics and precision medicine breakthroughs occurring in the world today mean that we are now able to approach personalized therapies as we start from the very cause of diseases. However, with continued advancement of technology at an increasingly faster pace; telemedicine wearable technologies remote monitoring systems will change patient–provider relations, thus bringing access closer to home, enabling proactive management.

Effective regulation and surveillance aimed at the healthcare ecosystem and virtual services necessitate a comprehensive e-governance system. Table 13.2 provides an overview of various healthcare domains in the metaverse and the supportive e-governance frameworks and highlights assistive technologies associated with them. Therefore, we can see that one of those areas where metaverse-supported e-governance might act as a game changer for medical research, policy formulation processes or service delivery modes. Thus, this approach can be envisaged as leading toward a more agile, effective and patient-centered healthcare environment. The future research landscape on e-governance in healthcare using metaverses is intricate and complex, providing a wide range of opportunities for investigation as well as innovation. This opens up the possibility for scholars to investigate how accessibility and inclusiveness could be improved in healthcare provision as metaverse technology advances. However, to make this possibility a reality, we need to develop innovative applications that are revolutionary in nature. Therefore, it is necessary to investigate how edge computing or AI among other cutting-edge technologies can be incorporated into metaverse design for supporting better real-time

Table 13.2 The Primary Healthcare Sectors in the Metaverse and the Supporting Pillars of e-Governance

Major Healthcare Areas in the Metaverse	*The Supporting Pillars of e-Governance*	*Assistive Technologies*
1. Medical education and training 2. Remote patient monitoring 3. Telemedicine and telehealth 4. Therapeutic interventions 5. Collaborative research and development 6. Telemedicine and telehealth 7. Health and wellness programs 8. Data visualization and analysis 9. Population health management	1. DHR and interoperability standards 2. Regulatory compliance in metaverse healthcare 3. Virtual health consultations regulations 4. Telemedicine regulations 5. Security and authentication 6. Public health initiatives	1. VR 2. AR 3. Blockchain 4. Edge technology 5. AI 6. Data mining

data analytics and decision-making processes. Introduction of these revolutionary technologies has the potential to completely change the manner in which patient care is offered. The rapid ongoing research, policy formulation as well as service provision related to the metaverse are triggering a paradigm shift in healthcare ecosystems. This transition should involve several stakeholders such as researchers, clinicians, policy makers and technical experts for creating a more holistic approach to address issues related to healthcare. To address the disparities in healthcare with respect to the increasing population, policy makers need to consider more data-driven approach by incorporating evidence-based practices as well as patients' perspectives while formulating policies targeting prevention care. The field is moving from provider-centric systems of delivery toward patient-centric models focused on disease prevention, early detection and overall well-being. The appropriate strategic integration of these innovations could enhance better efficiency, accessibility and equity for different populations worldwide.

We need to also consider the social and ethical issues associated with the governance of healthcare through the metaverse platform for critical examination. Digital equity, user privacy and data security along with other factors need further attention. The research on scalability and interoperability of metaverse platforms should be considered in different contexts or locations within the health sector for developing standard global e-governance frameworks. The future research should also take up the task of perfecting immersive educational training programs within the metaverse applicable to long-term health outcomes and public health strategies evaluations. Hence, taken together the emergence of the research landscape within this area, an unprecedented opportunity is available for overcoming existing impasses and finding new ways that may eventually revolutionize the e-governance paradigm for companies involved in the medical industry.

13.10 Conclusion

A paradigm shift is happening now within the healthcare sector as it increasingly adopts innovative, streamlined, interactive and other forms of governance in healthcare that are transforming the entire industry. Through VR and AR platforms, remote access to complicated medical data interpretation and analysis has become a reality, thus making healthcare more affordable while saving time with high operational efficiency. This immersive 3D experience enhances not only the quality of healthcare but also revolutionizes transfer of health information, training and education, telemedicine consultations, virtual diagnostics, remote monitoring and so forth. In addition, assurance of privacy and security in patient record keeping and data transfer can be assured by combining virtual data with cutting-edge data management technologies such as blockchain. The inclusion of the metaverse in health systems could attract extensive involvement of the public in preventive healthcare. Various technologies have recently been introduced in the metaverse that support e-governance for dynamic, efficient and customer-oriented services. These systems incorporating VR and AR have the potential to develop platforms for immersive healthcare engagement, training and collaboration apart from providing facilities for doctors to virtually participate in conferences or undergo virtual training remotely, irrespective of their geographical locations. Furthermore, the metaverse component of e-governance of healthcare simplifies administrative tasks leading to increased efficiency and transparency besides various other benefits. It also helps to speed up the decision-making process and eliminates bureaucracy through waning administrative burdens. The inclusion of smart contracts supported by blockchain technology can enhance data integrity and security for enabling safe sharing across different medical domains. It can also enhance coordination between people within the healthcare system, which in turn enhances the efficiency of service delivery. Many technologies of the metaverse healthcare system have the capability to support personalized, interactive and secured patient care for a more immersive experience. This chapter presents an overview of potential medical situations that may arise in relation to healthcare governance facilitated by the metaverse. It discusses the opportunities and challenges associated with these scenarios. The ongoing research in e-governance in healthcare services, policy making and virtual technology developments is revolutionizing healthcare in the metaverse to an ever-dynamic and efficient patient-centered system.

References

1. Jones, Ted, Todd Moore, and James Choo. "The impact of virtual reality on chronic pain." PLoS One 11.12 (2016): e0167523.
2. Nica, Elvira. "Virtual healthcare technologies and consultation systems, smart operating rooms, and remote sensing data fusion algorithms in the medical metaverse." American Journal of Medical Research 9.2 (2022): 105–120.
3. Lewis, Kadriye O., Vitaliy Popov, and Syeda Sadia Fatima. "From static web to metaverse: Reinventing medical education in the post-pandemic era." Annals of Medicine 56.1 (2024): 2305694.
4. Salvetti, Fernando, Roxane Gardner, Rebecca D. Minehart, and Barbara Bertagni. "Enhanced reality for healthcare simulation." In Recent Advances in Technologies for Inclusive Well-Being: Virtual Patients, Gamification and Simulation (2021): 103–140. Springer.
5. Liu, Justina Yat Wa, et al. "The effects of immersive virtual reality applications on enhancing the learning outcomes of undergraduate health care students: Systematic review with meta-synthesis." Journal of Medical Internet Research 25 (2023): e39989.
6. Bashir, Ali Kashif, et al. "Federated learning for the healthcare metaverse: Concepts, applications, challenges, and future directions." IEEE Internet of Things Journal 10.24 (2023): 21873–21891.
7. Veras, Mirella, et al. "A framework for equitable virtual rehabilitation in the metaverse era: Challenges and opportunities." Frontiers in Rehabilitation Sciences 4 (2023): 1241020.
8. Bansal, Gaurang, et al. "Healthcare in metaverse: A survey on current metaverse applications in healthcare." IEEE Access 10 (2022): 119914–119946.
9. Rachmad, Yoesoep Edhie. "MediVerse: Challenges and development of digital health transformation towards metaverse in medicine." Journal of Engineering, Electrical and Informatics 2.2 (2022): 72–90.
10. Damaševičius, Robertas, and Olusola O. Abayomi-Alli. "The future of telemedicine: Emerging technologies, challenges, and opportunities." Metaverse Applications for Intelligent Healthcare (2024): 306–338.
11. Steinhubl, R. Steven, Dawit Feye, Adam C Levine, Chad Conkright, Stephan W Wegerich, and Gary Conkright. "Validation of a portable, deployable system for continuous vital sign monitoring using a multiparametric wearable sensor and personalised analytics in an emergency medical centre." BMJ Innovations 1.3 (2015): 165–171.
12. Topol, Eric J. "High-performance medicine: The convergence of human and artificial intelligence." Nature Medicine 25.1 (2019): 44–56.
13. Patel, Shyamal, Hyung Park, Paolo Bonato, Leighton Chan, and Mary Rodgers. "A review of wearable sensors and systems with application in rehabilitation." Journal of NeuroEngineering and Rehabilitation 12.1 (2015): 1–17.
14. Golinelli, Davide, Erik Boetto, Gherardo Carullo, Andrea Giovanni Nuzzolese, Maria Paola Landini, and Maria Pia Fantini. "Adoption of digital technologies in health care during the COVID-19 pandemic: Systematic review of early scientific literature." Journal of Medical Internet Research 22.11 (2020): e22280.
15. https://www.eosurgical.com/blogs/news/how-will-surgeons-operate-in-the-metaverse (as accessed on March 9, 2024)

16. https://www.vph-institute.org/news/surgery-meets-the-metaverse.html (as accessed on March 9, 2024)

17. Bashshur, Rashid L., Gary W Shannon, Noura Bashshur, and Peter M Yellowlees. "The empirical evidence for telemedicine interventions in mental disorders." Telemedicine and e-Health 22.2 (2016): 87–113.

18. Khairat, Saif, et al. "A mixed-methods evaluation framework for electronic health records usability studies." Journal of Biomedical Informatics 94 (2019): 103175.

19. Antypas, Konstantinos, and Silje C. Wangberg. "An Internet- and mobile-based tailored intervention to enhance maintenance of physical activity after cardiac rehabilitation: Short-term results of a randomized controlled trial." Journal of Medical Internet Research 14.6 (2012): e171.

20. Chaudhry, Sarwat I., Jennifer A. Mattera, Jeptha P. Curtis, John A. Spertus, Jeph Herrin, Zhenqiu Lin, Christopher O. Phillips, Beth V. Hodshon, Lawton S. Cooper, and Harlan M. Krumholz. "Telemonitoring in patients with heart failure." New England Journal of Medicine 363.24 (2016): 2301–2309.

21. Ali, Sikandar, et al. "Metaverse in healthcare integrated with explainable AI and blockchain: Enabling immersiveness, ensuring trust, and providing patient data security." Sensors 23.2 (2023): 565.

22. Epstein, Ronald M., Kevin Fiscella, Cara S. Lesser, and Kurt C. Stange. "Why the nation needs a policy push on patient-centered health care." Health Affairs 34.3 (2015): 376–380.

23. Papadopoulos, Theofilos, et al. "Interactions in augmented and mixed reality: An overview." Applied Sciences 11.18 (2021): 8752.

24. Botella, Cristina, Javier Fernández-Álvarez, Verónica Guillén, Azucena García-Palacios, and Rosa Baños. "Recent progress in virtual reality exposure therapy for phobias: A systematic review." Current Psychiatry Reports 19 (2017): 1–13.

25. Riva, Giuseppe, Rosa M. Baños, Cristina Botella, Fabrizia Mantovani, and Andrea Gaggioli. "Ransforming experience: The potential of augmented reality and virtual reality for enhancing personal and clinical change." Frontiers in Psychiatry 7 (2016): 164.

26. Laver, K. E., S. George, S. Thomas, J. E. Deutsch, and M. Crotty. "Virtual reality for stroke rehabilitation." The Cochrane Database of Systematic Reviews 11.11 (2017): CD008349.

27. Murala, Dileep Kumar, Sandeep Kumar Panda, and Sujata Priyambada Dash. "MedMetaverse: Medical care of chronic disease patients and managing data using artificial intelligence, blockchain, and wearable devices state-of-the-art methodology." IEEE Access 11 (2023): 138954–138985.

28. Barnes, Robert. "Healthcare diagnosis and treatment in the metaverse: Remote sensing algorithms, networked wearable devices, and virtual patient data." American Journal of Medical Research 9.2 (2022): 41–56.

29. Perkins, James. "Immersive metaverse experiences in decentralized 3D virtual clinical spaces: Artificial intelligence-driven diagnostic algorithms, wearable internet of medical things sensor devices, and healthcare modeling and simulation tools." American Journal of Medical Research 9.2 (2022): 89–104.

30. Aashima, Mehak Nanda, and Rajesh Sharma. "A review of patient satisfaction and experience with telemedicine: A virtual solution during and beyond COVID-19 pandemic." Telemedicine and e-Health 27.12 (2021): 1325–1331.

31. Burton, Lindsay, et al. "Empowering patients through virtual care delivery: Qualitative study with micropractice clinic patients and health care providers." JMIR Formative Research 6.4 (2022): e32528.

32. Daye, Dania, et al. "Point-of-care virtual radiology consultations in primary care: A feasibility study of a new model for patient-centered care in radiology." Journal of the American College of Radiology 18.9 (2021): 1239–1245.

33. Privorotskiy, Ann, et al. "Augmented reality in anesthesia, pain medicine and critical care: A narrative review." Journal of Clinical Monitoring and Computing 36.1 (2022): 33–39.

34. Liu, Zhen, et al. "Virtual reality aided therapy towards health 4.0: A two-decade bibliometric analysis." International Journal of Environmental Research and Public Health 19.3 (2022): 1525.

35. Johnson, Daniel, et al. "Gamification for health and wellbeing: A systematic review of the literature." Internet Interventions 6 (2016): 89–106.

36. Altuwayrib, Saleh A., Khin Than Win, and Mark Freeman. "Gamified Medication Adherence Applications for Chronic Health Conditions: Scoping Review." International Conference on Persuasive Technology. Cham: Springer Nature Switzerland, 2023.

37. Pfandler, Michael, et al. "Virtual reality-based simulators for spine surgery: A systematic review." The Spine Journal 17.9 (2017): 1352–1363.

38. Pires, Filipi, Carlos Costa, and Paulo Dias. "On the use of virtual reality for medical imaging visualization." Journal of Digital Imaging 34 (2021): 1034–1048.

39. Smith, Kathryn L., Yang Wang, and Luana Colloca. "Impact of virtual reality technology on pain and anxiety in pediatric burn patients: A systematic review and meta-analysis." Frontiers in Virtual Reality 2 (2022): 751735.

40. Zhang, Haolan, et al. "A survey on big data technologies and their applications to the metaverse: Past, current and future." Mathematics 11.1 (2022): 96.

41. Muthumeenakshi, R., S. Balasubramaniam, Charanjeet Singh, Pallavi V. Sapkale, and Moresh M. C. Mukhedkar. "An efficient and secure authentication approach in VANET using location and signature-based services." Ad Hoc & Sensor Wireless Networks 53 (2022): 59–84.

42. Yang, Yin, et al. "Smart health: Intelligent healthcare systems in the metaverse, artificial intelligence, and data science era." Journal of Organizational and End User Computing (JOEUC) 34.1 (2022): 1–14.

43. Ullah, Hidayat, et al. "Exploring the potential of metaverse technology in healthcare: Applications, challenges, and future directions." IEEE Access (2023): 69686–69707.

44. Gollagi, Shantappa G., and S. Balasubramaniam. "Hybrid model with optimization tactics for software defect prediction." International Journal of Modeling, Simulation, and Scientific Computing 14.02 (2023): 2350031.

45. Kostick-Quenet, Kristin, and Vasiliki Rahimzadeh. "Ethical hazards of health data governance in the metaverse." Nature Machine Intelligence 5.5 (2023): 480–482.

46. Mohammadzadeh, Zahra, Shokri, M., Saeidnia, H.R., Kozak, M., Marengo, A., Lund, B.D., Ausloos, M., and Ghiasi, N. "Principles of digital professionalism for the metaverse in healthcare." BMC Medical Informatics and Decision Making 24.1 (2024): 201.

47. Balasubramaniam, S, and K. S. Kumar. "Fractional feedback political optimizer with prioritization-based charge scheduling in cloud-assisted electric vehicular network." Ad Hoc & Sensor Wireless Networks 52.3-4 (2022): 173–198.

48. Tan, Ting Fang, et al. "Metaverse and virtual health care in ophthalmology: Opportunities and challenges." The Asia-Pacific Journal 11.3 (2022): 237–246.

49. Ali, Saba Ghazanfar, et al. "A systematic review: Virtual-reality-based techniques for human exercises and health improvement." Frontiers in Public Health 11 (2023): 1143947.

Chapter 14

Issues, Challenges, and Research Direction in Integrating Metaverse and Healthcare Industry

Naresh Kumar Kar, Manoj Kumar Pandey,
Jyoti Upadhyay, Priyanka Gupta, and Celestine Iwendi

14.1 Introduction

The healthcare sector is of paramount significance to both the community and the whole country. The healthcare industry has raised an important concern for everyone, importantly since the COVID-19 pandemic. Artificial intelligence (AI), augmented reality (AR) and virtual reality (VR) have improved the way of diagnosis in healthcare industry as it can provide added technologies for diagnosis of various diseases [1]. The healthcare industry has recently done lots of improvement in various directions like various wearable devices, IoT devices, machine learning, blockchain (BC), VR, etc. VR and AR are combined in the metaverse, an online realm or technology connected via a network [2]. The metaverse is a cutting-edge technology that integrates virtual, mixed, and augmented reality applications. It is frequently described as an Internet of the future. The hospital industry is growing very fast, and along with that the technologies are also developing day by day. The researchers have done so much work in this area, and this area is continuously growing. The involvement of the metaverse in diagnosis has proved a remarkable achievement in this area. In the healthcare industry, wearable devices and

DOI: 10.1201/9781003491668-14

monitoring systems have also added an extra advantage, as they can be used to store the medical data related to a patient and can be processed later on for identifying the types of disease and types of treatment that must be given to patients [3]. Chronic disease is common and increasing nowadays, and it can also be treated very efficiently using emerging technological advancements such as the Internet of Things (IoT), blockchain, VR, etc. Heart diseases, cancer, cerebrovascular disease, hypertension, chronic respiratory disease, and joint disease are types of chronic disease. AI-based medical applications are a category of applications that enhance their performance through the utilization of training data. Consequently, data pertaining to a specific ailment are gathered utilizing innovative technologies and subsequently processed to achieve the intended outcomes. The security and integration of these collected data are also important concerns that must be taken care of very carefully. Healthcare data are rapidly growing, and integrating the metaverse with healthcare can be an important direction for diagnosing various diseases [4].

The incorporation of the metaverse into the healthcare field marks a step toward an era of patient care, medical research, and health-focused engagements. This innovative integration entails blending VR and AR technologies within healthcare, leading to an impact on how professionals provide services and how individuals engage with their own health. The immersive environments of the metaverse offer an approach to education allowing students and healthcare practitioners to practice complex surgeries explore anatomical structures and engage in realistic patient interactions for skill enhancement in a safe digital setting [5]. Moreover, patient care reaches heights with clinics and telehealth platforms in the metaverse, offering accessible and personalized healthcare solutions that break down geographical barriers for inclusive care.

Additionally the metaverse accelerates research by promoting collaboration and data sharing through virtual labs and simulations to fast-track innovative treatments development. Well-being is redefined as people can partake in fitness sessions, mental health support communities, and preventive health activities to encourage a proactive approach to self-care. Nevertheless, merging these aspects requires an examination of privacy and security concerns to guarantee that the metaverse contributes positively to healthcare. This involves harmonizing progress with the values of patient-focused care and medical ethics. As the metaverse becomes an integral part of the healthcare landscape, the industry stands on the precipice of a paradigm shift, where the boundaries between physical and digital realms blur to forge a more interconnected, accessible, and innovative healthcare ecosystem.

This chapter deals with the various aspects related to integrating healthcare with the metaverse, and also discusses challenges, issues, and research directions. The introduction is covered in the Section 14.1, review of literature is covered in the Section 14.2, various issues and challenges are covered in the Section 14.3, and Section 14.4 covers future research directions and the conclusion.

14.1.1 Introduction to the Metaverse

The metaverse was introduced in the year 1992 by the science fiction writer Neal Stephenson in his *Snow Crash* novel and has since been established as a buzzword, even luring the corporate world to get interested in it, like the developers and engineers did [6].

The metaverse represents a highly futuristic conception that our physical and virtual worlds will be smoothly and loosely integrated into shared digital space, rich and immersive for everything from work and play to everything in between. The metaverse is a virtual world where human avatars interact with computer-generated environments, products, and other human avatars. With the advancing of technology, growing VR and AR, while being infused in our lives with digital experiences, have largely increased the popularity of the notion of the metaverse over the years.

The metaverse users typically navigate through a persistent, immersive, and interconnected digital space. A key element of a metaverse includes 3D graphics, AI, blockchain, and other emerging technologies such as 5G, computer vision, and robotics. The various companies in the tech industry are exploring the development of metaverse platforms to create more immersive and interconnected digital experiences.

It is clear from the literature that the idea of utilizing metaverse technology continues to evolve and most of the people have identical ideas. The metaverse has generated important interest and discussion among technologists, developers, and the general public. Furthermore, it is widely thought that the metaverse comprises a complex system of virtual world, where individuals can be busy with avatars to generate a deeply immersive meet. Digital twin technology could be utilized to create a reflective image of the real world, and AR can create an immersive experience. Furthermore, Facebook has changed its name to Meta, as the metaverse has lots of potential in the future. The metaverse is used in many fields, like healthcare [7, 8], education [9], the tourism industry [10], agriculture [11], social networking, entertainment, and gaming [12, 13]. Figure 14.1 shows the metaverse core technologies.

14.1.2 Metaverse Importance for Healthcare Industry

A vast array of cutting-edge technologies is combined in the metaverse, which is the result of numerous technical advancements. More specifically, the idea of the metaverse is not new. With the addition of blockchain, cloud computing, digital twins, AI, extended reality (XR), and other new technologies, it is more akin to the resurrection of a timeless idea and its concretization. Numerous professionals, academic institutions, and associated businesses have provided definitions of the metaverse from various research vantage points since 2021, when the metaverse first appeared.

Ownership, storage, and use of data might all alter under this new paradigm. Possibilities for delivering services across national borders and assisting with tailored and predictive treatment arise [14].

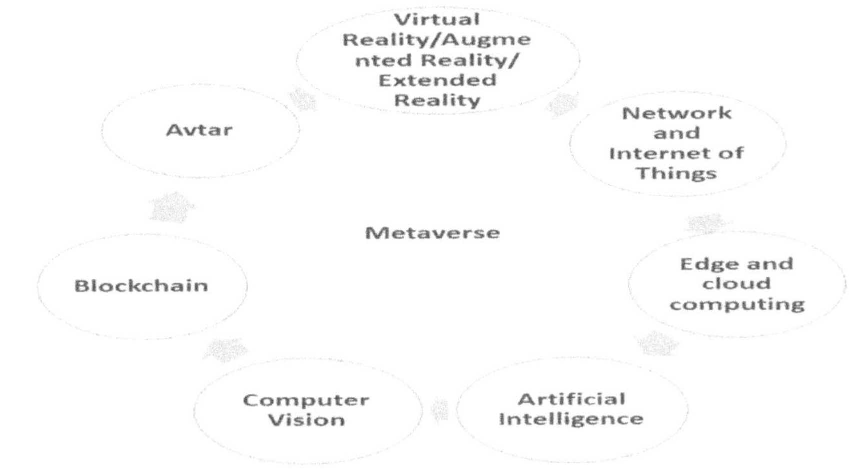

Figure 14.1   Metaverse core technologies.

Imagine a world in which individuals receive individualized treatment regimens that are customized based on specific health data, and patients may easily access healthcare services across virtual boundaries. Patients can choose remote medical care in virtual worlds through the use of the metaverse, and this may include virtual consultations with specialists doctors from anywhere in the world utilizing wearable devices based remote vital signal monitoring [15, 16]. Patients having mobility difficulties, and those living in distant places now have better access to healthcare facilities utilizing the metaverse.

The metaverse could be better utilized by medical practitioners receiving immersive medical education and training. VR simulations can offer practical exposure in patient care, surgery, and emergency response situations. This will improve healthcare providers abilities and expertise in a secure setting [17]. The metaverse gives us ability to communicate with others to consult one another in a virtual environment. In terms of education, it can facilitate students and teacher cooperation in a fully immersive three-dimensional environment that can simulate a real classroom [18]. Virtual three-dimensional structures may be visualized thanks to metaverse technology, which also makes it easier to collaborate and engage in small groups. It also enhances the mentor relationships with students and also offers self-directed learning and look after the growth of the healthcare industries. [18]. The metaverse has quickly become an essential part of healthcare, accelerating digital transformation and extending its application in medical education and surgery.

The metaverse has made it easier to analyze and visualize complicated medical data, and now healthcare professionals are getting better access to the patient conditions and treatment planning by using virtual environments to analyze medical imaging data, such as MRIs and CT scan data in three-dimensional spaces. The imagining of anatomical organizations and comprehension of sophisticated relationships between the organs and systems are made possible through a three-dimensional model of the human body. Medical practitioners can investigate diseases as well as the various organs' structures, functioning, and interconnections. This will contribute to information acquisition and enhance therapeutic and diagnostic abilities of the doctor. Medical professionals can now view the blood flow through vessels in real time with a blood flow visualization device [19].

Applications for AR and VR in the metaverse can provide immersive fitness experiences, such as interactive workout regimens, virtual training courses, and individualized training plans. These encounters can increase the appeal and accessibility of exercise, encouraging people to stick to a regular fitness schedule. A twin epicyclic geared motor actuator that may provide torque feedback is used by the metaverse device. Utilizing hysteretic damping in the virtual environment, it created torque profiles that mimic real-world interactions [20]. The manufactured gadget also includes an anatomical digital twin model in MR format, and thermographic and electromyogram sensors are used to evaluate the device's functionality. It assessed the wearable's haptic quality and adaptability as an immersive metaverse tool and carried out support vector machine-based motion feature categorization analysis [20]. Different sorts of technology have been employed to address a variety of diseases in both profitable and research applications. The most popular has been the usage of smartphones, tablets, and e-Health apps. These are either used to passively gather data from the mobile device (for example, GPS position, daily steps) or involve daily surveys that the user must complete regarding their emotional state. People with responsiveness deficit and hyperactivity disorder (ADHD) or autism spectrum disorder (ASD) have benefited from gesture recognition technology, such as Leap Motion, to enhance their cognitive and motor abilities.

With the use of immersive experiences, interactive technologies, and virtual settings, the metaverse provides a plethora of creative applications that assist people in reaching their well-being objectives.

14.2 Various Core Technologies of Metaverse Used in the Healthcare

Large-scale data integration with intelligent machines is made possible by this revolution, which allows for human-free autonomous decision-making. The Internet of Health Things links wearables and medical equipment to provide real-time monitoring. Healthcare systems that combine digital and physical components are known as medical cyber-physical systems. The privacy and security of the health data are two of the primary concerns for any metaverse-enabled system, and the health cloud is a repository used for safely storing and analyzing medical data, and extracting useful data from the database is known as big data analytics. These extracted useful data are fed into the machine learning algorithms to further improve the planning and diagnosis process of patients. In order to provide security to the records, blockchain is a technique that can provide a transparent and safe medical records repository [21].

VR and AR platforms are utilized in the metaverse virtual environment to establish a dynamic and integrated virtual healthcare ecosystem. With utilization of virtual clinical labs and home consultations with medical professionals, patients in the metaverse can get the care they need. Metaverse technologies are used by medical professionals to be updated on the newest medical developments, conduct surgical simulations, and receive enhanced training. Furthermore, these involvements offer innovative ways for patient treatment, including the utilization of VR treatment, which has demonstrated efficacy in addressing anxiety disorders. Additionally, researchers from all around the world can collaborate on drug development, medical investigations, and creative healthcare solutions thanks to the metaverse in healthcare, which makes it easier for researchers to do joint study in virtual labs.

A computer-generated recreation of reality is called VR, a term used to designate immersive multimedia or computer-based simulated reality that gives users an extremely amazing experience [22]. Unlike traditional media, VR is based on a three-dimensional framework and controlled by specialized technology such as tracked controllers, room-scale sensors, and VR goggles. The major tech companies such as Google, Apple, HTC, Sony, and Meta (formerly Facebook) are working on VR gear like haptic gloves, visual trackers, 3D mice, and omnidirectional treadmills for motion controllers. These gadgets are offering incredible features to the customers. For instance, the Oculus Quest 2 is a VR platform that includes built-in CPUs. Numerous nations, including the USA, Japan, China, South Korea, and Taiwan, are concentrating on the VR sector as a crucial technological avenue with the potential to strengthen their economies overall [23].

By adding digital components to the physical environment, AR enhances it. AR, in contrast to VR, superimposes digital data on the real world rather than creating a fully digital environment. Heads-up displays, smart glasses, and smartphones are some examples of gadgets that help do this. Holographic displays and real-time information are two examples of what AR may offer [24]. To put it another way, AR is the process of adding digital elements to the real environment by superimposing digital images over it. One of the best demonstrations of AR is Pokémon Go, which allows us to superimpose digital figures over the actual world with the use of our cell phones. Similar to this, we employ a variety of filters on Snapchat for our social media posts to enhance our appearances, such as bunny ears, various makeup styles, etc.

Digital and physical elements are combined in mixed reality (MR) to create an environment where information and digital objects coexist with the actual world. Microsoft's HoloLens is an excellent illustration of MR technology. While interacting with digital holograms, users can maintain awareness of their physical environment [25].

14.3 Applications of Metaverse Technologies in Healthcare

The metaverse in healthcare provides an optimistic environment and enables surgeons to learn and practice complex surgeries with exceptional accuracy. Augmented reality also aids in navigating intricate anatomical structures by preventing damage to surrounding tissues. The following are a few examples of metaverse uses for medical care [26]:

i. **Virtual Consultations Using the Metaverse:** By facilitating virtual consultations, follow-ups, and appointments between medical professionals and patients, the metaverse platforms enhanced accessibility to healthcare services.

ii. **Medical Training and Simulation for Better Exposure:** Healthcare workers can improve their virtual learning experiences by using metaverse environments for realistic medical instruction, surgical operations, and simulations.

iii. **Patient Education and Engagement for Their Own Care:** Metaverse technology can help patients become more health-literate and involved in their own care by developing instructional contents for the patients.

iv. **Enabling of Remote Monitoring and Telehealth:** The utilization of the metaverse enables remote monitoring for the patient in real time from a distance.

v. **Satisfying interventions:** Metaverse techniques have the prospect of enhancing satisfying interventions like immersive experiences for pain management or VR treatments for mental health issues.

vi. **Collaborative research and conferences:** Metaverse platforms permit researchers and medical professionals to work together on projects and participate in virtual conferences.

vii. **Enabling Health Data Visualization:** The metaverse technologies can facilitate the study and interpretation of medical information by enabling the visualization of complex health data in three-dimensional areas.

viii. **Rehabilitation and Physical Therapy:** VR enables patients to engage themselves into interactive and engaging rehabilitation programs.

ix. **Enhancement of Health and Wellness:** Applications of the metaverse can support wellness programs, treatment plan adherence, and healthy behavior of the patients.

x. **Healthcare facility design and planning:** The inclusion of the metaverse technology can offer designing and planning of healthcare facilities in a virtual environment. It also helps architects and healthcare planners to optimize workflows and a layout prior to actual operations.

These applications showcase the potential of metaverse technologies to enhance various aspects of healthcare, making it more accessible, engaging, and efficient. Figure 14.2 shows the applications of metaverse technologies in healthcare.

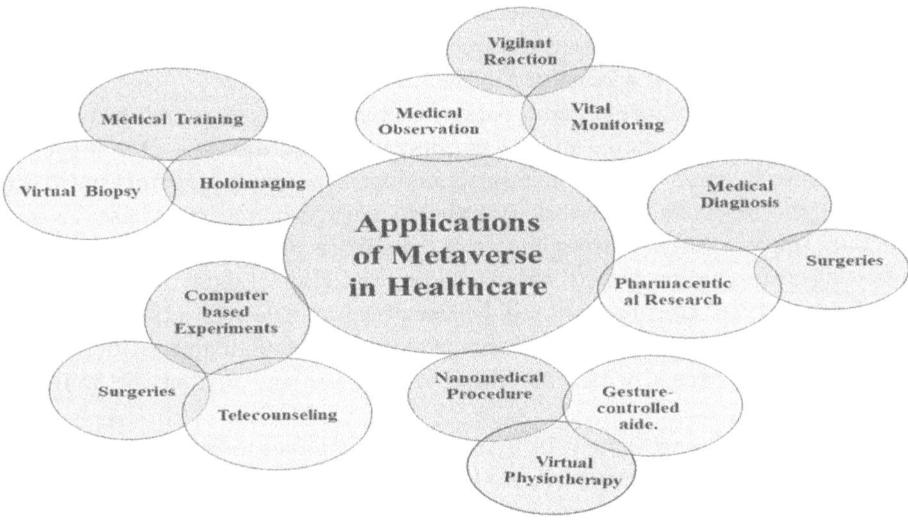

Figure 14.2   Applications of metaverse technologies in healthcare.

14.4 Review of Literature

Recent years have seen the appearance of numerous surveys on utilizing the meta-verse in various medical sectors, as the metaverse's popularity in the healthcare industry has been growing quickly. The word "metaverse" describes a new form of Internet that uses VR, headgear, blockchain technology, and avatars to merge the real and simulated worlds. The metaverse is not merely a place to retreat from the busy outside world and enjoy a sedentary existence; it is a place in which individu-als will spend a significant amount of their time consuming services and amenities. Thanks to modern technologies that enable us to participate in this online com-munity at any time and from any location, we may now interact with the metaverse. These include handsets and smart watches, the latter of which may monitor physi-cal activity, offer home or nursing care, and help patients manage their chronic illnesses on their own.

The first attempt to provide a thorough assessment that looks at the most recent metaverse advancements in the healthcare sector was made by Bansal et al. [27]. The survey covered seven fields: telemedicine, medical education, mental wellness, health, fitness, animal care, and medicines. They went over metaverse applications and had in-depth discussions on the technological problems and potential fixes in each area to aid in the creation of a long-lasting, self-sufficient, and future-proof medical healthcare system solution. Finally, they emphasized the difficulties that need to be resolved before the healthcare sector can completely adopt the metaverse. They constituted a noteworthy endeavor to provide an all-encompassing perspec-tive on metaverse inside the healthcare sector. The values that can be brought by the metaverse to the healthcare business today were represented in their paper. Based on their findings, they put forth research problems that must be addressed before metaverse technology is widely used in the healthcare sector.

Murala et al. [28] suggested a patient-centered technology architecture that uses wearables, blockchain, and AI to control chronic diseases. Our suggested architecture is reliant on the metaverse setting. Patients and doctors must register on the blockchain network in order to engage in the metaverse. Avatars will accompany guests throughout the experience after they arrive. A complete log of text, photographs, videos, audio, and clinical data collected during physician–patient consultations will be assembled, transferred to the blockchain, and preserved forever. These details are examined by explainable artificial intelligence (XAI) systems, which use them to diagnose and predict the course of diseases.

The ongoing improvement in living standards places an increasing demand on healthcare and medical services. Even though the current medical pattern has somewhat improved, there are still significant problems, including a lack of medical resources, ineffective medical care, and low levels of medical technology. Medical facilities can be upgraded by using the metaverse as a novel mechanism to solve these issues in the traditional healthcare sector. In general, the metaverse is a dynamic feedback mechanism that makes it easier for the virtual and real worlds to cooperate and coexist. Yang et al. [29] tries to stimulate more study in this area by summarizing the present state of research on several healthcare application scenarios for the metaverse, highlighting its obstacles and future prospects.

Lee et al. [30] presented a metaverse sentiment mapping system that could offer objects in the metaverse additional face expression detecting skills. They identified facial expressions using emotions filtering and a deep learning algorithm using webcam-captured expressions. To establish a mechanism for item alteration within the metaverse, the cleaned emotions data were subsequently transmitted via an IoT portal and the metaverse connecting component. This allows users to use metaverse items to communicate their feelings to other users, which may promote emotional communication inside the metaverse. The authors proposed the utilization of an Artificial Intelligence of Things device for emotion detection, which employs a deep learning model to identify facial expressions. This device would be integrated into their methodology for mapping emotion data into the metaverse.

Seven distinct emotional states can be identified in webcam-captured human expressions by utilizing the convolutional neural network (CNN) for model development for facial expression identification like anger, annoyance, fear, pleased, neutral, sad, and startled. A face expression identification algorithm that filters emotions is developed, allowing users to choose which feelings to include into the metaverse and avoiding misunderstandings. The clarified feelings are denoted as blocks in the metaverse, allowing consumers to exchange reactions with other users and establish reaction-based services.

The metaverse is a cutting-edge technology that can help with a number of healthcare-related concerns, such as mental health, connection with friends and family, virtual physical wellness, and health access without regard to location. The application of the metaverse and its potential applications in the healthcare sector were examined and compiled by Athar et al. [31]. They go into further detail on the primary difficulties that could arise in the future when utilizing metaverse technology. Here is a summary of their research: (i) How the metaverse can improve education, healthcare collaboration, monetization, fitness, and medical performance and results. (ii) The impact of a metaverse employing AR and VR in the medical field and the prospect of the metaverse in healthcare through the use of AI and other smart technologies. (iii) Using the metaverse to improve telesurgery, telemedicine, and individualized care results. (iv) A brief review of the potential applications and difficulties of a metaverse in the medical field.

Laws, data security, and interoperability are a few of the challenges the metaverse healthcare industry will confront. New protocols, standards, and infrastructure will be needed to overcome the variety of problems that the healthcare sector faces as the metaverse becomes more integrated into the system. Bhatia and Joshi [5] conducted research of these issues. The necessity to combine training with cutting-edge technologies has grown due to technological improvements. This will allow professionals with more training to give patients a more rehabilitative environment. This study looks at how the metaverse can help with the aforementioned problems.

The safety of digital patient health information is a major concern with metaverse installations. A number of components of the suggested procedure for implementing the embedded Esantem smart health system under the metaverse were investigated by Dilibal and Tur [32], including the potential for enhanced human–computer interaction, handling of clinical information from wearable biomedical devices and its safety in a digital setting, and the methods by which traditional healthcare could be adapted for use in the metaverse. In preparation for future study directions, the main obstacles to the progress of the metaverse in healthcare industries also revealed in this work, along with potential solutions like blockchain technology for patient data security. This study focuses on the challenges encountered inside the metaverse of the Esantem smart health system that includes various wearable biomedical devices, including the Mobile XMI gadgets, to perform real-time medical examinations. Moreover, the intricate technological parts of the Esantem smart medical system serve to schematically unveil the tailored interfaces between patients and physicians.

The world has become accustomed to the metaverse and its revolutionary potential. It's expected to transform gaming, social interactions with friends, shopping, and other activities. The medical care industry's fortunes could be altered by metaverse. Pandey et al. [33] looked into every possible use for this breakthrough. It can be applied to outdated therapeutic and educational facilities; some of these benefits are listed below. They continued to highlight the healthcare industry as the worthiest sector throughout this report. The medical care industry's fortunes could be altered by the metaverse and the benefits are as follows.

The IoT, AR, VR, AI, and other technologies are all included in the metaverse. It is now feasible to concentrate on health condition of patient in a more accurate, efficient, and focused way because to the convergence of healthcare and metaverse technology. Scholars are attempting to expedite the use of the metaverse for clinical diagnostics as well as patient diagnosis by utilizing the many imaging technologies available there. Making a diagnosis no longer requires a doctor to be present in person. Much work is being done to enhance the metaverse environment so that patients can be diagnosed in a very precise and efficient way. The study of Mahdi et al. [34] concentrated on the ways in which the metaverse has simplified the healthcare sector and the range of services it provides. In an attempt to improve the healthcare field in the metaverse, the proposed work of Mahdi et al. [34] provided a comprehensive analysis of diagnostic and clinical advancements made in the metaverse. The work concentrated on the state-of-the-art advancements that will revolutionize the metaverse healthcare sector.

The healthcare sector has been investigating ways to improve patient satisfaction and expand access to treatment. It is uncertain whether patient data will continue to be treated with the utmost confidentiality in a field where it is vital. Mejia and Rawat [35] investigated various application of the metaverse in the healthcare as well as the state, difficulties, and viewpoint of relevant practices and technology. More precisely, they addressed the difficulties in protecting patient privacy in a healthcare metaverse and the experience of practicing outpatient telemedicine with body sensor networks.

The current state of metaverse innovation and quantum computing in the healthcare and pharmaceutical industries were outlined by Bajkoti et al. [36], who also counted the many applications and use cases. This paper investigates how quantum computing might help with genetics and clinical research, diagnostics, and image restoration, while the metaverse can offer telemedicine, continuous monitoring, and readiness. They looked at the difficulties and barriers these inventions face as well as the potential long-term benefits of using them in healthcare. Their research indicates that the pharmaceutical and healthcare sectors could undergo a significant transformation in the future due to advancements in quantum computing and the metaverse, which could provide affordable, customized, and high-quality healthcare to individuals worldwide.

The healthcare industry has made extensive use of the metaverse and its enabling technologies. Prakash et al. [37] examined these uses and looked into potential security risks. Three metaverse components — blockchain, avatars, and XR — were determined to be crucial for the design of future healthcare systems through the literature analysis. Metaverse-based healthcare solutions will take on diverse dimensions depending on how these components are combined in different degrees. They also examined the dangers connected to these elements alone and in combination.

The entire risk assessment was predicated on an analysis of vulnerabilities, the body of current research, the pattern of cyberattacks in the medical business, and emerging cyberattacks. Using the vulnerabilities found on the Common Vulnerabilities and Exposures (CVE) website, an analysis of the hazards related to the metaverse, healthcare, and their integration was carried out.

Studies indicate that by 2027, the medical domain's metaverse revenue is predicted to reach $640 billion. Various industries, including finance, manufacturing, media, entertainment, and others, are utilizing healthcare tools to incorporate cutting-edge technology into their respective sectors. The current status of metaverse technology in digital healthcare and its applications in the metaverse were covered by Mozumder et al. [38]. Additionally, the difficulties the metaverse poses for the healthcare sector were covered. They talked about the potential effects of the metaverse on healthcare delivery and its future in that regard. Finally, they presented a paradigm for metaverse healthcare based on XAI, BC, and immersive technology, which has the potential to enhance patient outcomes and revolutionize the healthcare sector [39].

Individuals have the ability to engage with their virtual representations in an environment facilitated by advanced technologies known as the metaverse, which combines the physical and digital realms. The prospect of the medical metaverse and the possible applications of these technologies in digital medicine were the main topics of Elkafrawy et al.'s [40] study. This study uses qualitative methods to analyze and assess previous books and webpages. In the healthcare sector, the metaverse has the potential to replicate visual signals, including eye contact, gestures, and facial expressions, which are the main methods of communication. The metaverse technique can be perceived as a means to enrich the efficiency of the medical structure by facilitating worldwide education, standard training, treatment, and creation of worldwide research data. Given the significant amount of time that young people spent in front of their displays, it is possible for them to begin training and acquiring new skills in the metaverse [41].

Jeljeli et al. [42] studied the idea of decision-making in medical care and treatment in the United Arab Emirates (UAE). In order to collect information from doctors employed by various healthcare institutions in the three UAE cities, the researchers utilized a cross-sectional methodology. Data analysis using structural equation modeling reveals that the virtual models and reported outcomes of metaverse technology that are used for medical usage are mostly determined by relatedness and autonomy. The perceived benefit and virtual simulation also have a role in physicians' intentions to use metaverse technology in healthcare in the UAE. Overall, the findings demonstrated the metaverse's critical role in medical operations and diagnosis, supporting the self-determination theory and the study's underlying assumptions. The studies suggest that the medicine and diagnosis sectors in the UAE have undergone a metaverse revolution, resulting in enhanced precision and effectiveness in healthcare. The study's weaknesses are also addressed within this particular setting.

14.5 Issues and Challenges of Metaverse Technologies in Healthcare

Integrating metaverse technologies with the healthcare industry presents several challenges and issues that are discussed in the literature. While the metaverse has the potential to revolutionize healthcare, there are various concerns that need to be addressed. While the metaverse has the prospect to transform healthcare delivery, the following issues are commonly discussed in the context of this integration. Here are some of the issues and challenges identified in the literature, as shown in Figure 14.3.

14.5.1 Data Security and Privacy

Concerns regarding data security and privacy are raised by the storage and management of sensitive health data within the metaverse [41]. One of the biggest challenges is preventing unauthorized access to patient information and making sure that healthcare data regulations are followed. Widespread adoption depends on addressing privacy issues and ensuring strong data security safeguards. Immersion healthcare data creation and interchange occur within the metaverse. It is crucial to guarantee strong encryption, access controls, and adherence to data protection regulations.

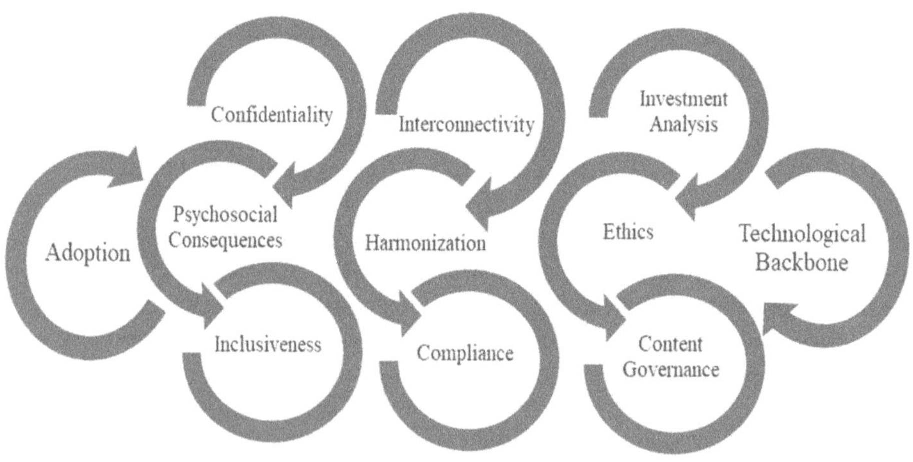

Figure 14.3 Issues and challenges in integrating the metaverse with healthcare technologies.

14.5.2 Interoperability and Standards for Standard Communication

Interoperability is a big challenge while integrating the metaverse into the existing medical environment. A healthcare ecosystem highly depends on attaining good communication and data exchange between various platforms and technologies. However, the standards and technologies used by healthcare frequently change [42].

14.5.3 Regulatory Compliance and Legal Frameworks

Respecting the patient privacy, data security, and other legal mandates is essential for the ethical application of metaverse technology in healthcare. The Health Insurance Portability and Accountability Act (HIPAA) and other healthcare regulations must be modified in order to accommodate a virtual healthcare system. A clear legal framework is necessary to manage liability, accountability, and ethical issues in an efficient manner.

14.5.4 Ethical Dilemmas in Virtual Healthcare System

The literature discussed the moral results of employing metaverse technologies in healthcare. The involvement of the metaverse raises the ethical questions about informed permission. A careful balance between innovation and ethical considerations is necessary to maintain trust in virtual healthcare [43].

14.5.5 Digital Divide and Accessibility

The literature shows that how critical it is to close the digital divide in order to guarantee that everyone has the access to healthcare solutions facilitated by the metaverse. The objective of the metaverse is to ensure universal access to virtual healthcare system.

14.5.6 Technical Infrastructure and Connectivity

The technical challenges like bandwidth constraints and network latency could prevent metaverse technology from being widely used in healthcare. It might be difficult to guarantee dependable hardware, minimal latency, and high-speed Internet connectivity for the infrastructure [44].

14.5.7 User Training and Acceptance

Integrating the metaverse technologies into healthcare requires healthcare professionals and patients to adapt to new workflows and interfaces. Healthcare workers ranging from physicians to administrative assistants need specific training to use metaverse technology with the efficiency.

14.5.8 Financial Investments and Return on Investment

The investments in terms of money are necessary for the implementation of metaverse technology in the healthcare industry and achieving the return on investment. The long-term financial viability and return on investment must be carefully evaluated. For virtual healthcare to be widely adopted, it must first be determined whether it is economically feasible or not.

14.5.9 Content Regulation and Quality Assurance

Ensuring patient safety in the metaverse requires good quality and accuracy of healthcare material. For patient safety, it is critical to guarantee that the dependability and correctness of health information in the virtual system.

14.5.10 Cultural Sensitivity and Diversity

The literature investigates how incorporating metaverse technologies into healthcare might have an impact on society and culture. Healthcare may be observed in a different way in different cultures, so the metaverse should take cultural sensitivity into attention.

14.5.11 Social and Psychological Impact

It is very important to carefully measure how immersive technologies affect patients and healthcare. It is critical to comprehend how interactions with virtual healthcare may impact mental health and well-being in order to minimize any unfavorable effects.

14.6 Future Research Directions and Conclusion

AI, VR, and AR are some of the key metaverse technologies utilized in medical systems. In order to improve patient outcomes and healthcare services, these technologies are incorporated into the metaverse environment. VR and AR offer immersive experiences for telemedicine, medical education, and training, while AI is used to evaluate medical data and develop customized treatment regimens. Wearable technology allows for remote patient monitoring via the IoT, gathering real-time data for therapeutic purposes. The amalgamation of these technologies within the metaverse setting offers novel prospects for the healthcare sector. These encompass augmenting healthcare accessibility, establishing transparent and safe healthcare data ecosystems via blockchain, and elevating the caliber of care via digital anti-aging

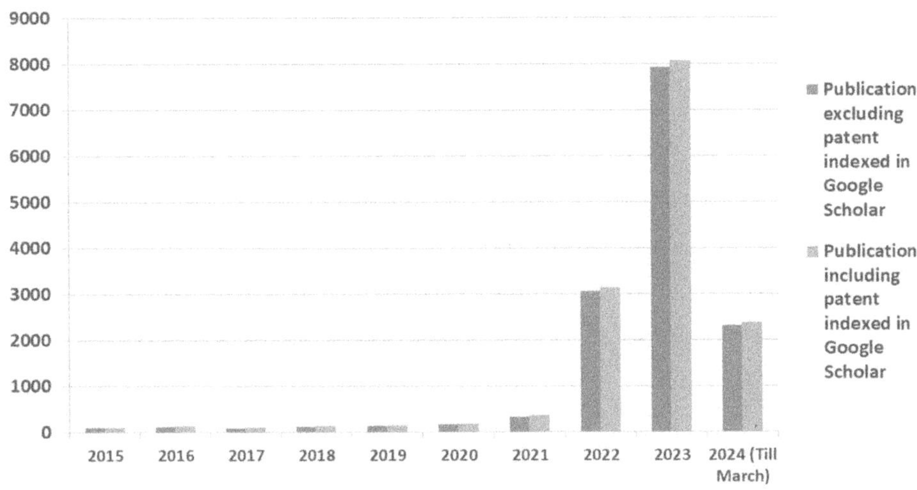

Figure 14.4   Number of publications in the year 2015 to March 2024 indexed in Google Scholar.

healthcare. These technological breakthroughs possess the capacity to revolutionize the healthcare sector and enhance care for patients on a global scale.

Looking at the literature, we find that the number of publications in the field of "Metaverse in healthcare" is consistently growing with the year. Figure 14.4 shows the number of publications related to the metaverse in the healthcare industry indexed in Google Scholar from 2015 to March 2024, and it shows that the number of publications is consistently increasing with every year. Likewise, Figure 14.5 shows the number of publications related to "metaverse in healthcare" in the ACM Digital Library for last five years, and it is shows that the number of publications in the year 2020 is 1,963, for 2021 the number of publications is 2,384, for 2022 the number is 2,699, for 2023 the number 3,750, for 2024 (until March) the number of publications is 921.

Future research directions include the following points on which future researchers can work: (i) Good and adaptive algorithms must be developed to tackle security and privacy issues. (ii) Good regulatory compliance and legal frameworks must be developed for applying the metaverse in the healthcare industry with ease. (iii) VR and AR tools need to be cheaper and flexible in order to achieve wide access for the healthcare industry. (iv) Work must be done to bridge the gap that separates the digitally included from the digitally excluded. (v) Technical infrastructure and connectivity must be enhanced by incorporating latest technologies, such as 5G connectivity and other fast networks connectivity. (vi) Increasing the users training so that the technologies can be used efficiently and its worldwide reach can be promoted, and also to broaden acceptance of these technologies. (vii) The social and psychological impact of adapting these technologies must be reviewed for better adaptability and productivity.

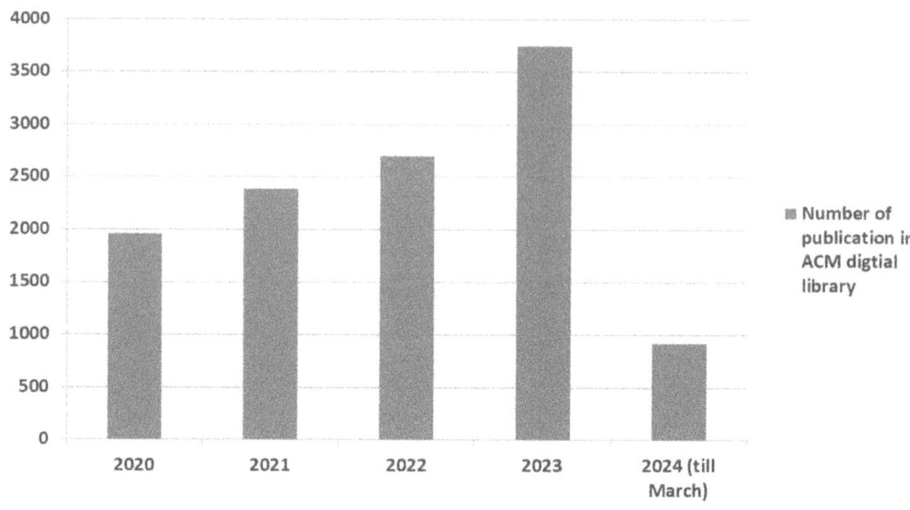

Figure 14.5   Number of publications in the year 2020 to March 2024 in the ACM Digital Library.

The integration of the metaverse has revolutionized the healthcare industry, but lots of improvement in this field is needed to make it more reachable to the general people worldwide. Winning peoples' confidence is also a one of the challenges of this field, so future research must work in this direction.

References

1. Ali, M., Naeem, F., Kaddoum, G., & Hossain, E. (2023). Metaverse communications, networking, security, and applications: Research issues, state-of-the-art, and future directions. IEEE Communications Surveys & Tutorials, 26(2), 1238–1278.
2. Aljanabi, M., & Mohammed, S. Y. (2023). Metaverse: Open possibilities. Iraqi Journal for Computer Science and Mathematics, 4(3), 79–86.
3. Bashir, A. K., Victor, N., Bhattacharya, S., Huynh-The, T., Chengoden, R., Yenduri, G., & Liyanage, M. (2023). Federated learning for the healthcare metaverse: Concepts, applications, challenges, and future directions. IEEE Internet of Things Journal, 10(24), 21873–21891.
4. Dwivedi, Y. K., Hughes, L., Baabdullah, A. M., Ribeiro-Navarrete, S., Giannakis, M., Al-Debei, M. M., & Wamba, S. F. (2022). Metaverse beyond the hype: Multidisciplinary perspectives on emerging challenges, opportunities, and agenda for research, practice and policy. International Journal of Information Management, 66, 102542.
5. Bhatia, B., & Joshi, S. (2023). Applications of Metaverse in the Healthcare Industry. In 2023 International Conference on Innovative Data Communication Technologies and Application (ICIDCA) (pp. 344–350). IEEE.

6. Joshua, J. (2017). Information bodies: Computational anxiety in Neal Stephenson's snow crash. Interdisciplinary Literary Studies, 19(1), 17–47.

7. Thomason, J. (2022). Metaverse, token economies, and non-communicable diseases. Global Health Journal, 6(3), 164–167.

8. Yang, D., Zhou, J., Chen, R., Song, Y., Song, Z., Zhang, X., & Bai, C. (2022). Expert consensus on the metaverse in medicine. Clinical eHealth, 5, 1–9.

9. Hwang, G. J., & Chien, S. Y. (2022). Definition, roles, and potential research issues of the metaverse in education: An artificial intelligence perspective. Computers and Education: Artificial Intelligence, 3, 100082.

10. Gursoy, D., Malodia, S., & Dhir, A. (2022). The metaverse in the hospitality and tourism industry: An overview of current trends and future research directions. Journal of Hospitality Marketing & Management, 31(5), 527–534.

11. Khansulivong, C., Wicha, S., & Temdee, P. (2022, January). Adaptive of New Technology for Agriculture Online Learning by Metaverse: A Case Study in Faculty of Agriculture, National University of Laos. In 2022 Joint International Conference on Digital Arts, Media and Technology with ECTI Northern Section Conference on Electrical, Electronics, Computer and Telecommunications Engineering (ECTI DAMT & NCON) (pp. 428–432). IEEE.

12. Shin, D. (2022). The actualization of meta affordances: Conceptualizing affordance actualization in the metaverse games. Computers in Human Behavior, 133, 107292.

13. Jungherr, A., & Schlarb, D. B. (2022). The extended reach of game engine companies: How companies like epic games and unity technologies provide platforms for extended reality applications and the metaverse. Social Media+ Society, 8(2), 20563051221107641.

14. Bailey, R., & Parsheera, S. (2021). Data localization in India: Paradigms and processes. CSI Transactions on ICT, 9(3), 137–150.

15. Abdel-Rahman, O. (2021). Patient-related barriers to some virtual healthcare services among cancer patients in the USA: A population-based study. Journal of Comparative Effectiveness Research, 10(2), 119–126.

16. Upadhyay, N., Kamble, A., & Navare, A. (2023). Virtual Healthcare in the new normal: Indian healthcare consumers adoption of electronic government telemedicine service. Government Information Quarterly, 40(2), 101800.

17. Ahuja, A. S., Polascik, B. W., Doddapaneni, D., Byrnes, E. S., & Sridhar, J. (2023). The digital metaverse: Applications in artificial intelligence, medical education, and integrative health. Integrative Medicine Research, 12(1), 100917.

18. Qu, Q., Hatami, M., Xu, R., Nagothu, D., Chen, Y., Li, X., & Chen, G. (2024). The microverse: A task-oriented edge-scale metaverse. Future Internet, 16(2), 60.

19. Daineko, Y., Ipalakova, M., Tsoy, D., Alipova, B., Kozhakhmetov, A., & Mustafina, A. (2024). Towards metahospital: Augmented and virtual reality in medicine. Procedia Computer Science, 231, 373–378.

20. Ha, M., Lee, J., Cho, Y., Lee, M., Baek, H., Lee, J., & Lee, W. G. (2024). A hybrid upper-arm-geared exoskeleton with anatomical digital twin for tangible metaverse feedback and communication. Advanced Materials Technologies, 9(2), 2301404.

21. Pons, P., Navas-Medrano, S., & Soler-Dominguez, J. L. (2022). Extended reality for mental health: Current trends and future challenges. Frontiers in Computer Science, 4, 1034307, 1–9. doi: 10.3389/fcomp.2022.1034307.

22. Mäkinen, H., Haavisto, E., Havola, S., & Koivisto, J. M. (2022). User experiences of virtual reality technologies for healthcare in learning: An integrative review. Behaviour & Information Technology, 41(1), 1–17.
23. Zhao, H., Zhao, Q. H., & Ślusarczyk, B. (2019). Sustainability and digitalization of corporate management based on augmented/virtual reality tools usage: China and other world IT companies' experience. Sustainability, 11(17), 4717.
24. Fida, B., Cutolo, F., di Franco, G., Ferrari, M., & Ferrari, V. (2018). Augmented reality in open surgery. Updates in Surgery, 70(3), 389–400.
25. Doolani, S., Wessels, C., Kanal, V., Sevastopoulos, C., Jaiswal, A., Nambiappan, H., & Makedon, F. (2020). A review of extended reality (XR) technologies for manufacturing training. Technologies, 8(4), 77.
26. Mehta, S., & Sharma, D. (2023). Wearable technology in healthcare engineering. In Emerging Nanotechnologies for Medical Applications (pp. 227–248). Elsevier.
27. Bansal, G., Rajgopal, K., Chamola, V., Xiong, Z., & Niyato, D. (2022). Healthcare in metaverse: A survey on current metaverse applications in healthcare. IEEE Access, 10, 119914–119946.
28. Murala, D. K., Panda, S. K., & Dash, S. P. (2023). MedMetaverse: Medical care of chronic disease patients and managing data using artificial intelligence, blockchain, and wearable devices state-of-the-art methodology. IEEE Access. 11, 138954–138985. doi: 10.1109/ACCESS.2023.3340791.
29. Yang, Y., Zhou, Z., Li, X., Xue, X., Hung, P. C., & Yangui, S. (2023). Metaverse for healthcare: Technologies, challenges, and vision. International Journal of Crowd Science, 7(4), 190–199.
30. Lee, H. M., Ham, S. M., Moon, H., Kwon, H. M., Rho, J. H., & Seo, J. (2023, June). A Metaverse Emotion Mapping System with an AIoT Facial Expression Recognition Device. In 2023 IEEE International Conference on Metaverse Computing, Networking and Applications (MetaCom) (pp. 704–707). IEEE.
31. Athar, A., Ali, S. M., Mozumder, M. A. I., Ali, S., & Kim, H. C. (2023, February). Applications and Possible Challenges of Healthcare Metaverse. In 2023 25th International Conference on Advanced Communication Technology (ICACT) (pp. 328–332). IEEE.
32. Dilibal, C., & Tur, Y. (2022, October). Implementation of Developed Esantem Smart Healthcare System in Metaverse. In 2022 International Symposium on Multidisciplinary Studies and Innovative Technologies (ISMSIT) (pp. 1027–1031). IEEE.
33. Pandey, A., Chirputkar, A., & Ashok, P. (2023, March). Metaverse: An Innovative Model for Healthcare Domain. In 2023 International Conference on Innovative Data Communication Technologies and Application (ICIDCA) (pp. 334–337). IEEE.
34. Mahdi, H. F., Sharma, B., Sille, R., & Choudhury, T. (2023, June). Metaverse and Healthcare: An Empirical Investigation. In 2023 5th International Congress on Human-Computer Interaction, Optimization and Robotic Applications (HORA) (pp. 1–6). IEEE.
35. Mejia, J. M. R., & Rawat, D. B. (2022, July). Recent Advances in a Medical Domain Metaverse: Status, Challenges, and Perspective. In 2022 Thirteenth International Conference on Ubiquitous and Future Networks (ICUFN) (pp. 357–362). IEEE.
36. Bajkoti, A. S., Tiwari, S., Ranjan, T., Bisht, R. S., & Mittal, A. (2023, August). Role of Quantum Computing and Metaverse in the Field of Healthcare and Medicine. In 2023 5th International Conference on Inventive Research in Computing Applications (ICIRCA) (pp. 306–311). IEEE.

37. Prakash, R., Nayar, G. R., & Thomas, T. (2023, November). Security Risk Assessment of Metaverse Based Healthcare Systems Based on Common Vulnerabilities and Exposures (CVE). In 2023 IEEE International Conference on Recent Advances in Systems Science and Engineering (RASSE) (pp. 1–10). IEEE.

38. Mozumder, M. A. I., Sumon, R. I., Uddin, S. M. I., Athar, A., & Kim, H. C. (2023, June). The Metaverse for Intelligent Healthcare Using XAI, Blockchain, and Immersive Technology. In 2023 IEEE International Conference on Metaverse Computing, Networking and Applications (MetaCom) (pp. 612–616). IEEE.

39. Balasubramaniam, S, Nelson, S. G., Arishma, M., & Rajan, A. S. (2024). Machine learning based disease and pest detection in agricultural crops. EAI Endorsed Transactions on Internet of Things, 10, 1–8.

40. Elkafrawy, P., Abbas, H., AlFarra, J., Alam, L., & Junaid, M. (2023, January). The Redefinition of mHealth Applications in the Metaverse. In 2023 20th Learning and Technology Conference (L&T) (pp. 14–19). IEEE.

41. Gollagi, S. G., & Balasubramaniam, S (2023). Hybrid model with optimization tactics for software defect prediction. International Journal of Modeling, Simulation, and Scientific Computing, 14(02), 2350031.

42. Jeljeli, R., Farhi, F., Shawabkeh, F., Al Marei, A. A., Mohammed, M. M., & Setoutah, S. (2023, June). The Role of Self-Determination Theory in Adopting Metaverse for Healthcare and Diagnostics among Healthcare Professionals. In 2023 International Conference on Multimedia Computing, Networking and Applications (MCNA) (pp. 95–102). IEEE.

43. Balasubramaniam, S, Syed, M. H., More, N. S., & Polepally, V. (2023). Deep learning-based power prediction aware charge scheduling approach in cloud based electric vehicular network. Engineering Applications of Artificial Intelligence, 121, 105869.

44. Turab, M., & Jamil, S. (2023). A comprehensive survey of digital twins in healthcare in the era of metaverse. BioMedInformatics, 3(3), 563–584.

Chapter 15

Monitoring the Virtual Realm: Ethical Dilemmas and Connotations in the Metaverse–Artificial Intelligence Connection

Meera Mathew

15.1 Introduction: Digital Landscape Evolution

Artificial intelligence (AI) has been applied in every aspect of life that currently every other entrepreneurial sector looks to for innovations. With its quick progress, a new age has begun. Because of the metaverse's seemingly limitless potential and objectives, it is currently all the rage in the digital world. From one-to-one, to one-to-many, and many-to-many communication landscapes, we have now moved to augmented realities. Users will be able to engage in interactive experiences through the metaverse that have the possibility of helping augment actual events with computer-generated perception data. The technology of augmented reality also uses supplementary tools, like smart glasses, and add-on applications and programs for displaying digital information on actual things and surroundings.

Since the metaverse can incorporate many different types of intellectual property, investors in it must prioritize intellectual property issues. For instance, in terms of copyrights – contrary to popular belief, there are a number of augmented reality–related characteristics that can be protected by copyright, such as the

DOI: 10.1201/9781003491668-15

maps — although many individuals assume they are exempt from copyright laws, this isn't always the case. Many nations have adopted the position that "multiple features of maps to be legally protected" when making decisions concerning law. Likewise, there is no consensus on the most efficient approach to deal with the options, organization, and representation of data in archives. The same concerns exist over branding, particularly with regard to names or symbols that are deployed to provide immersive experiences and may be protected as trademarks. This could involve utilizing a certain domain name [1].

The metaverse has emerged as the cutting edge of technical and digital discoveries and attracts a lot of investors. It's a setting where the digital and real worlds interact and may significantly affect basic aspects of day-to-day existence. Using virtual reality (VR) headsets, augmented reality (AR) glasses, smartphone applications, and other technology, individuals may interact, work, and have fun in what is essentially an eternally linked world of virtual communities. It also encompasses other facets of your virtual existence, such social networking and e-commerce. The metaverse develops into a very big, extremely open, dynamically optimized system as application situations get more advanced [2]. Progress in cutting-edge technologies in various areas — biotechnology, automation, and computational intelligence — have shown immense promise for long-term prosperity. AI and data pooling are two examples of digital technologies that are being used today to detect and diagnose problems in the environment, health, and agriculture as well as to carry out routine chores like paying bills and managing traffic. Businesses and governments alike are becoming more equipped to collect and utilize data for economic and nonfinancial gains. People's lives have already been impacted by AI-based apps in manners which are frequently not completely understood or appreciated. Until now, the private sector has been a major force behind this subtly spreading AI technology, with a primary concentration on merchandise for consumers. It is incorrect to think of the digital transformation as existing independently.

Algorithms that operate on inadequately varied data have the potential to reproduce and sometimes intensify institutional and interpersonal prejudices. Insufficient diversity within the IT industry may result in an inadequate approach to addressing this topic. But because this innovation has so much potential and significance, its creation and utilization should not be restricted; at the same time, policymakers at all levels must pay attention given to the technology's emerging scope and repercussions [3]. Human rights can be upheld and exercised through their usage, but they can also be violated, as in the case of tracking our whereabouts, purchases, interactions, and behaviors. Ultimately, judges and regulatory bodies will need to determine the jurisdiction or country's laws related to a brand's metaverse procedures, specifically those happening on platforms positioned outside the United States. It's worth remarking that the metaverse and Web 3.0 are still in embryonic stages. Illustrations have been described of nonfungible token (NFT) auctions instigating a surplus on bitcoin platforms, consequential in substantial business fees or failed acquisitions. Brands cannot depend on evolving technologies to be immaculate; hence they must be organized for impending encounters and ensuing public dealings ramifications.

In making an allowance for the metaverse as a place for promotional goings-on, brands, advertisers, and marketers must take into consideration basic legal reflections. As the metaverse progresses, social media influencers are projected to shift into this digital galaxy, in concert with their listeners. Looking forward, expansions in computer-generated imaginings and VR could blur the lines amid virtual influencers and real individuals, raising apprehensions, predominantly regarding children's safety, as children may struggle to discern virtual entities from honest individuals.

15.2 Metaverse: Functioning and Challenges

The concept of metaverses has been much deliberated in both science narrative and gaming spheres. However, scholarly consideration devoted explicitly to the metaverse in jurisprudence has been somewhat lacking. In May 2021, it was noted that legal attention to the metaverse is still in its beginning. Thus, researchers often use the notion of "virtual worlds," which has received sizable academic responsiveness, to deduce potential legal issues that may arise in the metaverse [4]. In addition, there is a huge literature on the legal and regulatory phases of AI, principally robotics, drones, and autonomous vehicles. Metaverse epitomizes a cutting-edge expansion that could develop the manner people absorb in virtual backgrounds for exertion, edification, and social interface.

The term "metaverse" was coined by author Neal Stephenson in his novel *Snow Crash* (1992) and was introduced in science fiction works such as *Ready Player One*. Hints of conceivable future reiterations of the metaverse can be initiated in occurrences such as "Striking Vipers" from *Black Mirror*, season five. In that episode, people are familiarize with approaches in a VR martial arts video game that necessitates a neural linking among the player's brain and the VR maneuver. This raises thought-provoking interrogations about the thinkable allocation of emotions established in the metaverse to real-life contacts as represented in the episode. Currently, there is no collectively agreed-upon definition of what constitutes a metaverse. Nonetheless, for a metaverse to fully transpire, various auxiliary infrastructures, comprising 5G networks, VR technologies, holographic presentations, and radical graphic and data processing proficiencies, would need to be advanced and integrated simultaneously. Some scholars, such as Ball, have attempted to delineate key features of a metaverse [5]. These include its aptitude to facilitate both the physical and virtual worlds, enable a fully functioning economy, and provide incomparable interoperability that tolerates users to transfer their avatars and assets impeccably between different parts of the metaverse, notwithstanding who accomplishes those features. Importantly, the metaverse is labeled as an "embodied Internet" pigeonholed by devolved governance concerning numerous stakeholders rather than being measured by a single being. The metaverse embodies a leeway of the cyber-physical social scheme that joins physical systems, human society, and cyber systems through complex relations. The enlargement of the metaverse is assumed to go through four general stages [6]:

- **Preliminary Phase:** This segment is categorized by the procedure of VR equipment, which sanctions users to submerge themselves in the pictorial and acoustic understandings of the metaversion. In a chapter led primarily by gaming companies, blockchain knowledge, cryptocurrencies, and non-fungible tokens (NFTs) are evolving, building it so that it is easier to own an exceptional digital asset.
- **Boosted Sensory Immersion:** The following stage concentrates on increasing sensory immersion through the incorporation of measure and touch-enhancing hardware, such as haptic suits. These improvements empower users to pretend movement within the virtual situation, increasing the inclusive familiarity.
- **Advanced Virtual Reality:** At this juncture, advanced VR technologies target to pretend real practices by diffusing evidence straight to the brain via neural signals. Claims include administration in quantifiable backgrounds and neural data assortment to recognize behavioral answers in a virtual situation.
- **Final integration:** The ultimate step is the uninterrupted amalgamation of the virtual and physical worlds over advanced neurotechnology. At this point, the modification between the metaverse and physical reality converts to undetectable mode, marking a central milestone in industrial growth. While the metaverse has mammoth prospects, its unfettered nature forms the menace of criminal sign and exploitation. Threats from the virtual world can have a logical bearing on physical arrangement, personal well-being, and collective safety.

Privacy and data protection are the main areas that need special attention, and these shortcomings need special care because the users are diverse and any new subtypes of data could be created. With users voluntarily providing data without informed consent of the data being taken other than for a special purpose, what ramifications these data collections would have are not sorted. Some researchers, especially in the area of psychology, show that digital innovations have the latent ability to upgrade different cognitive and cerebral processes, including the process of communication, and it can affect natural intellect abilities, including facial sensitivity response and deliberation as well as functional and locomotive abilities [7]. Children ordinarily become significantly uneasy when they experience neurodevelopmental disorders. There are various concerns regarding the ethical use of biometric data, as especially while in usage these can go as recording and thus unexpected user behaviors such as voices, movement of hands, behavior, etc., can be absorbed.

Resolving safety problems and confirming moral behavior take precedence over the unparalleled prospects for revolution and engagement that the metaverse offers. The metaverse is an online community virtual environment that can be visited on several devices wherein the one who wants to use different avatars can make use of such options. International associations, philosophical norms, and operational rules are necessary to guarantee user rights and social comfort while fully realizing the promise of the metaverse. And in such instances, how to hold individual metaverse operators rightfully accountable would also be a concern because of the anonymity that avatars afford. Apart from these assurances, there exist noteworthy administrative and sociotechnical obstacles.

This collaboration can transpire through VR, amplified authenticity, or a mishmash of both, such as with VR glasses. A characteristic representative of the metaverse is its self-determining economy, which holds noticeable value and is interrelated with the everyday economy. While several of its subservices were formerly offered on separate podiums, the amalgamation of these services within the metaverse epitomizes a momentous encroachment. The thematic foundations and constructed milieus within changed divisions of the metaverse are dogged by their separate providers, with high-tech enactments fluctuating accordingly. Presently, the metaverse finds submission in gaming and social media daises, but its impending future encompasses "virtual conferences, live-streamed procedures like shows and fashion demonstrations, digital libraries, and the revolution of e-commerce through simulated shopping" familiarities [8]. Moreover, organizations are discovering different submissions, such as developing virtual atmospheres for healthcare, including virtual therapy and remote surgeries, as well as augmenting online education and public services like virtual conferences. Interconnectivity and interoperability across altered territories of the metaverse are simplified by NFTs. These tokens allow for the tokenization of goods within one area of the metaverse, empowering their virtual procurement and ensuing use in other metaverse provinces.

For instance, tokenized clothing from a luxury brand can be established in different virtual environments. The presence of metaverses contributes to uncountable legal considerations. Due to the incorporation of numerous technologies and dependence on servers, hosting, software, peripherals (for instance, VR eyeglasses and haptic gloves), content conception, and blockchains to attain and register tokenized assets, a large quantity of legal issues arise. These embrace copyrights, data security, civil law, trademarks, NFTs, cybersecurity, intellectual property rights, advertising regulations, and compliance with emerging regulatory frameworks such as the European Union (EU) AI regulation. In addition, as metaverses progress, it is expected to affect the nature of work and the perception of the workplace, which requires consideration of labor legislation and labor regulations. The development of the metaverse is currently in its infancy, but its potential impact on human existence is enormous. According to one perspective, the metaverse is a parallel universe that exists alongside the physical world, where individuals reside as avatars and VR acts as one of many access portals. This insight suggests profound repercussions for business, offering openings for transformations in marketing, tourism, leisure, hospitality, management, health, education, and social connectivity [9]. For those who choose to participate in the metaverse, the continuous amalgamation of the corporal and virtual worlds offers a rich array of experiences and interactions, intensifying the territory of possibility far beyond contemporary understanding. Platform providers strive to allow users and organizations to customize their own virtual domains, but ethical, safety, regulatory, and security issues abound. Unwanted behaviors such as harassment, sexualization of communication, and exploitation of data have already increased on current metaversal platforms, as well as unfettered gambling. Worryingly, research conducted by the Center to Combat Digital Hate (CCDH) shows an alarming number of abuses in metaversal environments, including bullying, exposure to open content, racism, threats, and solicitation of minors.

With the dawn of AR knowhow, inserting digital simulation models into real-world environments has become progressively common. For illustration, builders can view on land and envision the buildings they want to figure nearby. Using headsets, the whole team of designers, structural architects, and site supervisors can engross themselves in the building's cybernetic milieu and make real-time variations, such as accumulating or eradicating fundamentals, to witness the deduction of these variations on the arrangement and its conformation along with the visions nearby. We could go from having physical events to virtual ones in the future, making it possible for people to attend meetings, seminars, and concerts. People from all over the world will be able to participate in events as a result, increasing their inclusivity and accessibility. This new presentation of AR technology not only expands the productivity and precision of the edifice progression but also encourages joint policymaking among project participants. In tallying, the condensed landscape of the metaverse, without fundamental specialists and lacking boundaries, epitomizes a paradigm shift in the administration of digital spaces. As this multipart setting continues to progress, it is central to be preemptive and practical in vindicating risks, and confirming that the potential upshots of the metaverse are effusively comprehended. Regardless of many possible drawbacks, the metaverse will undoubtedly expand and adapt in the next years. However, the legal system needs to be strong with the advancement of VR and other technologies; there needs to be a distinction between actual and virtual worlds.

15.3 Legal Issues Pertaining to the Metaverse

The lines separating reality from imagination might become increasingly hazy in the dynamic environment that is produced by VR and metaverses. This phenomenon calls into question the boundaries of what is morally and legally permissible behavior, particularly with reference to the idea of consensual action. Avatars and virtual worlds, which serve as people's extensions or even take on their personalities, are significant elements of this terrain. Conduct that is inappropriate in these digital environments has substantial consequences that might have a significant psychological impact. Resolving these complex difficulties requires sensitivity and care because virtual connections are ever-changing and may impact people's personal welfare [10].

Using avatars to engage in immersive meetings and conversations in 3D environments, the metaverse is an online environment that bypasses geographical barriers. Workflows are believed to be streamlined and productivity increased by the metaverse by giving employees access to real-time information and direction. To boost their efficiency in performing repair tasks, technicians can read instructions and diagrams overlapping their particular field viewpoint when wearing AR glasses. By noticing their designs in three dimensions using AR, artists, technologists, and constructors can improve their understanding of physical connections to arrive at more intelligent decisions concerning design. AR apps can translate spoken language in real time for people with hearing losses or give visually challenged users with subtitles of visual features. The EU hopes to establish Web 4.0 and digital spaces that align with the principles of the EU, guarantee safeguarding human rights protection, and simultaneously support the growth of creative European businesses through the implementation of both the Digital Services Law and Digital Markets Law. This collaborative efforts within various states of EU may be able to ease user privacy concerns, promote market regulation, and decrease the impact of inadvertent monopolies in conjunction with less focused advertising [11]. Limiting access to unlawful information and reducing the amount of time data are retained for targeted marketing are two examples of these integration-facilitating regulations. The draft EU AI regulation, in a similar vein, aims to fortify users' resistance to marketing ploys, data exploitation, and practices of excessive data retention by introducing new categories and requirements for "high-risk" AI applications. The document also addresses steps to stop or restrict AI systems that target vulnerable groups, use manipulative "sub-subjective techniques," facilitate social assessment processes on behalf of government agencies, or use "real-time" biometric remote identification systems in areas that are open to the public — areas where there are exclusions for police enforcement [12].

While these initiatives have tangible implications, incorporating Extended Reality (XR) regulations into the metaversion, including data aggregation and biometric methods such as eye movement tent data, is essential to create a strong regulatory foundation for the future. Meanwhile, in 2022, Japan announced the creation of its own Web 3.0 Policy Office under the auspices of the Ministry of Economy, Trade, and Industry, tasked with overseeing all activities related to emerging social technologies, including blockchain, NFTs, and the metaverse. Therefore, under the Cybersecurity Bill, the United Kingdom (UK) indicated that it intends to regulate the metaverse actions of businesses and people that fall within its purview. On the other hand, the US does not have any customary rules that are unique to the meta-verse or the Web 3.0 architecture; instead, it keeps counting on current legislation to manage the metaverse, including issues of consumer protection and intellectual property rights. Online limits and constraints expose users to a greater number of actual consequences. These effects span a broad spectrum of illicit activity, includ-ing the theft of cryptocurrencies, the unlawful selling of NFTs, white-collar crime, and money laundering. Challenges exist over fiscal avoidance and fraud along-side other sexual offences, such as trafficking in youngsters. Future occurrences that might arise in the metaverse are depicted as possible dangers on the shadowy hand. Furthermore, the conferring of legal force on these online environments is a major source of worry. For human users, an avatar acts as a representation that can either extend their real identity or embody an entirely separate virtual persona [13]. Central to the appeal of virtual environments is the veil of anonymity offered by avatars, giving users a platform to experiment without fear of social judgment. Without the legality of AI or virtual avatars, rights, duties, freedom, and privileges cannot be decided. The lack of clarity arises from legal considerations, including but not limited to the following inquiries:

- How should jurisdictions address situations where avatars commit acts that are considered illegal in a particular country?
- What mechanisms should be employed to handle property interests and transactions within virtual worlds?
- How would intellectual property rights, such as copyright law, operate within virtual spaces, and how should copyrightable creations be managed from the perspectives of both game developers and players?
- What methods can be utilized to track behavioral responses, particularly concerning privacy and ethical concerns, and especially in scenarios involv-ing children or minors engaging in virtual gaming environments?

Additionally, there exists widespread skepticism regarding the accuracy of machine learning (ML) systems. However, in the absence of ethical guidelines and deployment regulations, there is a foreseeable risk of exploitative ML implementa-tions, incentivizing user spending and compromising data privacy by corporations. Many studies have highlighted that companies like Meta (and indeed various other tech firms) have obtained numerous patents related to the utilization of technol-ogy for tracking biometric data, such as eye movements. However, there remains a significant gap in discussing the intended use or purpose limitation of such tech-nologies and the ethical guidelines adopted or to be adopted for such purposes. Consequently, it becomes imperative to assess how the Indian legal framework is equipped to address the challenges posed by the metaverse and whether the cur-rent legal regime is adequate to regulate and prevent illegal activities in virtual environments.

15.4 Legal Implications of Metaverse in India and Evaluation on Current Existing Legal Framework

In India, cybercrimes fall within the purview of the Information Technology Act, 2000 (IT Act) and the Indian Penal Code, 1860. The proposed criminal laws have undergone few changes in line with the IT Act but not in consonance with global standards dealing with the metaverse. The legislative framework concerning cyber activities in India surpasses that of many other nations with comparable user bases. Consequently, the country is well positioned to develop and institute foundational regulations and ethical standards for the metaverse. Certain transgressions necessitate the corporeal presence of individuals. For instance, the act of homicide cannot transpire unless an individual is physically terminated. Similarly, transgressions such as battery, acid assault, culpable manslaughter, and abduction, among others, denote offenses that rely on the physical embodiment of the perpetrator. In these instances, the human physique constitutes the principal objective. Consequently, it appears implausible for such offenses to occur within the metaverse, as users do not transport their physical form into this virtual realm [14].

Conversely, there exist offenses that do not mandate the physical proximity of individuals. For instance, the act of demeaning a woman's modesty can transpire within the metaverse if a male avatar undertakes actions (such as gesturing) in the presence of a female avatar that evoke adverse sensations in the actual woman operating the avatar, thus constituting an affront to her modesty. Similarly, transgressions such as inciting religious animosity, cyberstalking, and making criminal threats, among others, do not hinge on the physical existence of the victim. In such cases, the primary target is the human psyche. Consequently, these offenses can be perpetrated within the metaverse, as users bring their cognitive faculties into this virtual environment.

To do this, one first step is to examine current laws, including the IT Act and the Indian Penal Code, to see how well they apply to or may be modified for the metaverse. For example, the IT Act is being broadened to include cybersquatting and phishing, among other types of theft. Those illegal acts can also be carried out in the metaverse and deal with crimes like theft of identification, rug pulling, and other misdeeds involving the theft of virtual avatars and other online assets that are used fraudulently for negotiations or to manipulate pricing. The use of existing laws has caused dispute because of the special characteristics of the metaverse. Antitrust has encountered issues of existence ever since the creation of the virtual world. The Competition Act of 2002 preserves antitrust rules by classifying any agreement, coalition, or plot as impeding trade. It also forbids arbitrary limitations. Thus, such measures can be taken if many applications are competing in an industry and one illegally controls the market or poses a danger to becoming a monopoly. The majority of anticompetitive behaviors that occur in the real world may also occur in the metaverse in some capacity, but because of the fundamental characteristics of the metaverse and the blockchain, these behaviors are invisible and unpunishable, allowing businesses to engage in them without consequence. Private distributed ledgers can be used by unfair organizations to exchange commercially sensitive information, such pricing knowledge, among themselves. Those who have been approved by the blockchain's owner are able to access these blockchains. Although officials cannot access these messages and cannot, therefore, punish such actions, they may still seek access to such material by using applicable legislation. In contrast, in the current situation, it is simple for authorities to visit firms' locations in order to obtain proof of such violations. Because digital goods are so easily copied, the metaverse may potentially see a rise in claims of trademark theft. Businesses are currently concerned about registrations for their physical products being applied to their digital equivalents. Blockchain technology presents a possible solution for businesses, even if there is now a void in government regulation that can provide remedies for virtual intellectual property rights (IPR) infractions. Once data are added to the blockchain technology, that data cannot be removed or altered without the use of an agreement system, making the data an inviolable and unchangeable archive of the information.

When a business's virtual products or services are not located on a single metaverse platform, this form of technology can be applied. With the use of this technology, IPR associated with products and services are both protected and integrated. Enclosed are summaries of the key materials, their ownership background, and the extent of the applicable rights. These details can determine the approved and prohibited uses of the product. Furthermore, this information is associated with the product throughout the duration of its digital existence, even when it switches across platforms. This is allegedly a successful strategy for safeguarding the proprietary rights of an organization [15]. As was already noted, the fact that not one user may alter data on a blockchain without the consent of other users greatly improves security. Disguise is a key component of blockchain technology. A false identity, or the inability to determine a user's true identity in the physical world regardless of whether their online identity is publicly accessible, is another crucial feature of blockchain computing. Nevertheless, this raises some very particular and specific problems, even in light of the potential benefits of blockchain technology. For instance, if one virtual avatar abuses another, will the harasser be held accountable for their deeds? The enforcement of laws could become troublesome since there would be no comprehension of or implementation of regulations in such worlds, leaving police unable to hold anybody accountable for their actions in the metaverse. Since it is anticipated that users of the virtual world will come from a wide range of backgrounds, countries, and places, the topic of whose legal system will govern the digital sphere and metaverse surroundings arises. A number of government organizations are gravely concerned about the increased uncertainty surrounding competence in a virtual world without borders. There is still a lot of ambiguity around this issue, and the authorities have not provided a clear statement. Developing and combining laws is the only practical answer. The regulations must adapt to the world's shifting conditions by adding several clauses to address emerging issues and offer answers.

Furthermore, India recently enacted the Digital Personal Data Protection Act (DPDPA), 2023 although it is yet to be implemented. Presuming that the extraterritorial jurisdiction of the DPDPA encompasses the metaverse, the existing deficiency in the regulation's oversight regarding the transmission, evolution, and propagation of private data within an immersive environment would subvert the objectives of the regulation. One of the technical attributes inherent to the metaverse is the principle of interoperability, facilitating the seamless interaction and exchange of data among various devices, platforms, and environments. The primary objective behind linking these diverse elements is to furnish the end user with an immersive virtual experience within the metaverse. Upon accessing a specific metaverse platform, the end user gains the ability to partake in assorted virtual activities, establish connections with external devices, platforms, and environments, and engage with fellow end users through the utilization of an avatar. From our perspective, the avatar assumes the role of the "central figure" and consequently, "the primary focus" within the metaverse, serving as the virtual conduit bridging the end user with this digital immersive realm.

Initially, it appears that the DPDP Act establishes a reciprocal relationship with the broader information technology regulations set forth by the Government of India. The aspect of information acquisition reflects an interaction with the IT Act and the Information Technology (Intermediary Guidelines and Digital Media Ethics Code) Rules, 2021, granting the central government the authority to seek information from the Data Protection Board ("Board"), trustees or intermediaries. However, the lack of specifics suggests an examination of the extent, intention, and protections associated with this information retrieval, necessitating adherence to the legal principles outlined in the *ratio decidendi* of Justice K.S. Puttaswamy & Anr. vs. Union of India & Ors AIR 2017 SC 4161 [*Puttaswamy* judgment]. Additionally, there is indication of integration between the DPDPA and the Information Technology (Procedure and Safeguards for Blocking for Access of Information by Public) Rules, 2009, merging concerns of data protection with the regulation of access to computer resources. This arrangement seems to empower the government, following due process and ensuring the right to be heard, to instruct agencies or intermediaries to restrict information access, safeguarding public interests. Such a combination of mechanisms provides a strong tool to mitigate the risks of noncompliance, but a comprehensive plan is necessary for its operational implementation.

With the entry into force of the DPDPA in 2023, India has taken a significant step toward improving data protection and privacy. Under its jurisdiction, DPDPA, approved by the Government of India in August 2023 after years of reflection and consultation with stakeholders, establishes a principled framework for data protection compliance. Although DPDPA implementation and enforcement has been delayed until 2024, stakeholders are actively preparing for the new regulatory environment. Under the DPDPA, the duty to comply with the data rests with data controllers. These commitments cover various aspects such as consent and notification requirements, personal data security measures, restrictions on cross-border data transfers, data breach notification protocols, basic data rights, and complaints-handling mechanisms. The Data Protection Board of India has been designated as the regulatory authority responsible for monitoring compliance with the DPDPA.

Penalties for noncompliance with the DPDPA are significant, ranging from 500 million to 2.5 billion. In addition, the central government is expected to introduce rules that clarify compliance aspects such as notification requirements, consent management, data breach procedures, exceptions to data processing, and complaint-handling mechanisms. The general population can shortly remark on the afore-mentioned rules, and the DPDPA will probably go into effect in June 2024 or later. The Information Technology Act of 2000 and the accompanying Information Technology (Reasonable Security Practices and Procedures and Sensitive Personal Data or Information) Guidelines of 2011 will serve as the present foundation for confidentiality of data until the DPDPA takes effect. Furthermore, newer revisions to the IT Act's penalty clauses have increased the severity of fines for infractions, highlighting how crucial data safety and compliance are in the digital era. Similarly, in the metaverse, images that violate the rules may be subject to sanctions without necessarily implicating the specific user, especially when neither the user nor the creator of the avatar is directly at fault. The application of sanctions to individuals or organizations that violate established standards. The metaverse predominantly functions as a user-centric platform, whether through human-controlled avatars, company-created avatars for character merchandising, or ML-based avatars enhancing platform interactions. Regulation of the metaverse necessitates adherence to three principles: transparent governance, emphasis on human rights, and public accountability decentralized from any singular nation. So the question of whether the DPDPA is enough to regulate the metaverse, as it would have many more vertical and horizontal sectoral ramifications. Upon the notification of the provisions outlined in the DPDPA, it is anticipated that the existing Information Technology (Reasonable Security Practices and Procedures and Sensitive Personal Data or Information) Rules of 2011 will be superseded. As of the present moment, the government has not officially disclosed the timeline for the enforcement of the DPDPA. However, based on publicly available information, it is inferred that the DPDPA may be formally notified during the initial quarter of 2024. It is pertinent to acknowledge that the government reserves the prerogative to specify distinct dates for the notification of individual provisions, thereby necessitating corresponding compliance measures.

15.5 Conclusion

AI presents the opportunity for a fully automated governance framework for the metaverse. However, outcomes of AI governance algorithms may exhibit bias and inequity as they derive from collective Internet usage and social interactions. A potential remedy involves developing a multilayered governance model – data governance and algorithmic accountability form the initial layer of protection, ethical criteria and norms guide decision-making and data processing at the second layer, while the final social and legal layer addresses regulatory responsibilities allocation [16]. Nevertheless, collaborative efforts are imperative for developing a governance framework for the metaverse to prevent regulatory authority from consolidating within any single nation. To achieve this, a fully free association beyond current international entities can be formed, or a metaverse supervisory element can be established inside the United States [17]. A few things to consider as legislators explore metaverse-explicit regulations at the national or international levels are as follows:

- **Giving representations specific legal personality:** In the metaverse, customers are very important. Assigning distinct legal personas to characters helps shield customers from impersonators concealing their true selves beneath obscure or artificially intelligent characters. Talks about endowing AI with blessed autonomy are ongoing, and similar attributions may extend to symbols, preventing them from taking the place of customer actions [18].
- **Providing representations with capabilities comparable to organizational aspects:** In the real world, enlisting organizations value regular treatment from their financiers or shareholders. Similarly, representations in the metaverse, as inhumane extensions of human action, may benefit from expanded capabilities akin to those of businesses. Using symbols as business elements in the metaverse would improve responsibility for both intelligent machines and client-driven systems. By promoting competent behavior, the combination would create an additional trustworthy and accountable online setting.
- **Information security and assurance:** Difficulties concerning information protection and licensed innovation freedoms in the metaverse equal contemporary issues. Existing licensed innovation and buyer assurance regulations wrestle with these worries. In any case, current information security guidelines, including India's Computerized Individual Information Assurance Act [19], deficiently address the broadness of biometric information collectible in the metaverse. Clashes every now and again emerge in both the physical and virtual domains, originating from contrasts in culture, religion, governmental issues, and different minority gatherings. The virtual world, specifically, worsens these struggles because of its absence of actual obstructions and requirements, prompting issues such as digital harassing via web-based entertainment stages and enormous-scope savagery in web-based gaming conditions. Clients of current web-based stages have the choice to withdraw from such bad encounters by framing more modest virtual networks with similar people. Be that as it may, this getaway course isn't promptly accessible in the metaverse, a total virtual universe where beginning once more is testing. This can be accomplished by laying out a metaverse oversight substance inside the unified countries or making a totally free association of past

existing worldwide bodies. As state-run administrations think about metaverse-explicit guidelines at public or worldwide levels, a few contemplations merit consideration [20].

- **Allowing avatars unmistakable legitimate personhood:** Clients hold principal significance in the metaverse. Doling out discrete lawful personalities to symbols can shield clients against others covering their characters behind symbol obscurity or man-made intelligence-empowered symbols. Conversations encompassing blessing independence to AI are progressing, and comparative attributions might reach out to symbols, safeguarding them from becoming substitutes for client activities [21].

- **Blessing avatars with privileges similar to corporate elements:** In the actual domain, enrolled organizations appreciate unmistakable treatment from their partners or owners. Also, symbols in the metaverse, as nonhuman augmentations of human action, may profit from stretched out privileges similar to those of companies. Engaging avatars to work as corporate substances would upgrade responsibility, whether client- or AI-driven, empowering dependable ways of behaving inside the metaverse interface [22].

- **Information security and assurance:** In the metaverse, there arise challenges with data security and authorized innovation rights at par with other contemporary problems. These concerns are wrestled with by current buyer guarantee and licensed creativity policies. However, existing security of information laws, such as the Indian IT laws, inadequately tackle the extent to which biometric data are recoverable in the metaverse. In terms of economics, AR has proven quite useful in a number of industries, including advertising, instruction, and wellness. This could not only sustain itself commercially but also be of great use to the metaverse. However, in the virtual world, any sort of disagreements arising between avatars can worsen by the absence of physical boundaries and constraints [23]. Violent behavior in multiplayer gaming contexts and online harassment via social media sites are two prominent instances of these issues. Contemporary Internet users have the option to avoid these regrettable encounters by forming smaller virtual communities with others who share their interests. Conflicts frequently arise from differences in society, faith, legislation, and various minority categories in both the real and digital worlds.

Because avatar actions can be newly generated not exactly as neuro-related characters, understanding the situation is indispensable to recognizing malevolent intent. Furthermore, there are many different avatar actions, which make it challenging to establish precise guidelines for what defines malicious behavior. Researchers have proposed a multifactor approach to accurately identify malicious behavior, taking into account objects, social interactions, objects' body language, and facial expressions. Protecting individual avatars from harassment and stalking might not be enough to stop these types of behaviors because malevolent avatars can still cause harm in public virtual spaces. While there's a chance that the current types of cybercrime could worsen, there's also a chance that a completely new kind of crime will manifest [24].

Stalkering, assault, abuse, child exploitation, copyright violations, and financial fraud, including Ponzi schemes and other schemes, are all considered potential crimes in the metaverse. As previously mentioned, it is difficult to assess such possible criminality using Lau's theory. Is the nature of these crimes truly new, or do they mimic real-world crimes but function as distinct entities that allow criminological principles to be applied? The latter seems more straightforward, allowing law enforcement agencies to carry out their duties in accordance with established protocols. But there could be dangers if this viewpoint is strictly adhered to without taking into account other points of view. The metaverse is still in its early stages of development, and the future is still unknown. As such, it is essential to keep an open mind. A more practical option would be to give users the power to teleport or vanish quickly in order to avoid malevolent avatars. To prevent malevolent avatars from gradually identifying trends, customers can further enhance their confidentiality and safety by creating numerous avatars and selecting them at random.

Avatars are utilized in the metaverse for interactions, and users control them. Techniques for encrypting messages can help ensure confidentiality and information secrecy when communicating. Because communications are secured with a unique key that can only be decrypted by the person who intended to receive it, adversaries are unable to access content without consent. However, the deployment of robust means of encryption and the preservation of keys to encryption secrecy are necessary for optimal communication transmit cybersecurity.

Conventional encryption methods do a good job of protecting audiovisual material, but they additionally have the potential to render it even harder for consumers to view the content visually, making surfing more challenging. Thumbnail-preserving encryption balances anonymity and graphic availability by revealing coarser visual characteristics while concealing finer details. This method enhances users' overall metaverse experience by enabling them to see encrypted images and videos while preserving some level of visual coherence. Although there are still gaps in the laws pertaining to involuntary actions or spontaneous motions in the metaverse, static biometrics are typically protected under existing information security regulations as sensitive or personal data. In the IoT, it is challenging to defend people's rights because data processing and collection are private activities [25].

Since it is difficult for law enforcement to get and validate information, stakeholders must establish their roles, responsibilities, and access conditions. The proper tools and training are also necessary for handling the complexities of digital forensics in order to preserve an effective legal and enforcement system. Data security problems may persist or intensify in the metaverse if proper regulations are not in place, as targeted marketing and prodding might become more prevalent due to its all-encompassing nature and possibly cause challenges with personal targeting. Given the global scope of the metaverse, further international collaboration on privacy legislation may be essential. Legal problems in metaverses are similar to those in other online markets; they include small-time fraud, con artists, and minors making unauthorized transactions. The metaverse networks have substantial pressure to implement restrictions when current laws are insufficient to prevent these damages exclusively in the appearance of aggressive antipathy.

In the metaverse, contractual liberty is essential, and there is a tendency toward lessening government intervention in private management through leading supplier self-management. In the metaverse, control can take numerous shapes and originate from a variety of places, including laws of territorial governments, provider regulations, and standards set by communities. Internal and outside disagreements are possible; however, what really counts is how restrictions affect users who are dealing with many limitations at once. As such, it is imperative to tackle the conflicts resulting from various regulatory origins in the metaverse and offer perspectives pertinent to various governing frameworks. The agreements and conditions of service that regulate the majority of the metaverse community usually serve as the primary source of restrictions on a service provider's flexibility. Companies are bound by these conditions constitutionally and not only for their own advantage, thus they must abide by them. Nonetheless, a lot of terms of service have provisions that give suppliers a lot of leeway and significantly favor them. The provisions granting total discretion should be interpreted cautiously in a metaverse wherein adherence to the rule of law is essential to avoiding arbitrary authority.

There are two main issues with contract law in the metaverse. In the beginning, there's the matter of the contracts that users and platform providers such as "Activision Blizzard" or "Linden Labs" have. Defined clauses to safeguard user rights are absent from these agreements, which can be found in "Terms of Services" or "End User Licencing Agreements." Decisions by the courts that preserve customer satisfaction and consumers' legal rights intensify the scenario and bring about unequal treatment. Furthermore, because of the many ways that people and companies connect (C2C, C2B, or B2B), binding contracts among those who use platforms create ambiguity. Because of the complexity present in real-world situations, the implementation of laws like those pertaining to consumer protection can be ambiguous. The introduction of smart contracts also poses challenges to the protection of human rights in virtual environments since data collection and processing are private.

Parties must be explicit about their responsibilities and need for access, given the difficulties law enforcement has in collecting and verifying data. The proper tools and expertise are also necessary to properly handle the complexities of electronic forensics in order to build a solid legal and enforcement framework. Without enough laws, worries about confidentiality of information can continue or potentially grow severe in the metaverse, where completely targeted advertising and manipulation might intensify, possibly leading to problems related to private targeting. The metaverse's worldwide reach suggests that further international cooperation on privacy laws may be necessary. Legal problems in simulated universes are comparable to those in other online marketplaces; they involve instances of fraud, purchases made by minors without authorization, and small-scale businesses fraud. Because of the fierce competition they face, the platforms that make up the metaverse have a strong incentive to impose limits when the regulations in place are ineffective to prevent these abuses.

The introduction of electronic agreements in the metaverse will not help. Users will not read the agreements and by default they tick to terms and conditions. Smart contracts might help in e-commerce dealings in terms of efficiency and achieving rapid results, but how far it will address the legal issues that could arise in future is the question. Because virtual property is intangible and sovereignty issues make it difficult to enforce intellectual property rights, the law of properties finds it difficult to handle the question of digital ownership. Plus, significant obstacles can also be found in the areas of supervision, taxation, data protection, and electronic safety. There are limitations on legislation governing the use of cash and payment methods in the parallel universe.

Regulations on cryptocurrencies, which are controlled by laws relating to money and central banks, hinder attempts by central banks to ensure price stability. Nevertheless, it's important to understand that metaverse control may come with costs. Given the nascent stage of the metaverse, the risk of stifling innovation through premature regulation, and the lack of obvious serious market failures requiring public intervention, the commission's call for evidence may be seen as premature or as prematurely prioritizing regulatory measures over fundamental market dynamics. Prior to technology consuming humankind, people should consider potential future scenarios and create the necessary legal frameworks.

References

1. Kahambing, J. G. (2024) Fourfolded objects, or toward a philosophy of object-oriented curation, *The Museum Journal*, 67(2), 28–34.
2. McStay, A. (2023) The metaverse: Surveillant physics, virtual realist governance, and the missing commons, *Philosophy and Technology*, 36(1), 1–26.
3. Smart, P. (2022) Minds in the metaverse: Extended cognition meets mixed reality, *Philosophy and Technology*, 35, 1–29.
4. Turner, C. (2023) The metaverse: Virtual metaphysics, virtual governance, and virtual abundance, *Philosophy and Technology*, 36(4), 1–8.
5. Avci, E. A. (2023) Research on the ontology of virtual actions (Sanal Eylemlerin Ontolojisi Üzerine Bir Araştırma), *Journal of Academic Social Science*, 11(145), 280–293.
6. Beck, D., Morgado, L. and O'Shea, P. (2023) Educational practices and strategies with immersive learning environments: Mapping of reviews for using the metaverse, *IEEE Transactions on Learning Technologies*, 45–55.
7. Alfaisal, R., Hashim, H. and Azizan, U. H. (2022) Metaverse system adoption in education: A systematic literature review, *Journal of Computers in Education*, 13(5), 1–45.
8. Almarzouqi, A., Aburayya, A. and Salloum, S. A. (2022) Prediction of user's intention to use metaverse system in medical education: A hybrid SEM-ML learning approach, *IEEE Access*, 10(1), 43421–43434.

9. Alam, A., and Mohanty, A. (2022). Metaverse and Posthuman Animated Avatars for Teaching-Learning Process: Interperception in Virtual Universe for Educational Transformation. In: Panda, M., *et al.* Innovations in Intelligent Computing and Communication. ICIICC 2022. Communications in Computer and Information Science, vol 1737. Springer, Cham. https://doi.org/10.1007/978-3-031-23233-6_4

10. Ahmad, P., Asif, J. A. Alam, M. K. and Slots J. (2020) A bibliometric analysis of periodontology 2000, *Periodontology 2000*, 82(1), 286–224.

11. Barahona, M. (2016) Challenges and accomplishments of ELT at primary level in Chile: Towards the aspiration of becoming a bilingual country, *Education Policy Analysis Archives*, 24(82), 54–67.

12. Bhavana, S. and Vijayalakshmi, V. (2022) AI-based metaverse technologies advancement impact on higher education learners, *WSEAS Transactions on Systems*, 178–184.

13. Cheong, Y. and Lee, Y. (2022) A case study on elementary convergence education using metaverse platform, *Korean Association for Learner-Centered Curriculum and Instruction*, 22(16), 561–580.

14. Zhao, T. (2022) If the metaverse becomes an ontological event, *Journal of Human Cognition*, 6(1), 3–17.

15. Fakhri, M., Silvianita, A. and Yulias, D. (2021) Assessing quality of work life toward junior high school teacher during pandemic Covid-19, *Journal of Management Information & Decision Sciences*, 24(6), 1–8.

16. Beovich, B., Olaussen, A. and Williams, B. (2021) A bibliometric analysis of paramedicine publications using the Scopus database: 2010–2019, *International Emergency Nursing*, 59–101.

17. Daz, T. B., Karagölge, Z. and Ceyhun, İ. (2020) Üstün Yetenekli Öğrencilerin Kimya Dersine Yönelik Görüşlerinin İncelenmesi: Erzurum Bilsem Örneği, *Atatürk Üniversitesi Kazım Karabekir Eğitim Fakültesi Dergisi*, 41, 159–179.

18. Muthumeenakshi, R., Singh, C., Sapkale, P. V., and Mukhedkar, M. M. (2022). An Efficient and Secure Authentication Approach in VANET using Location and Signature-Based Services. *Adhoc & Sensor Wireless Networks, 53.*

19. Aribowo, E. K. (2019) Analisis bibliometrik berkala ilmiah names: Journal of Onomastics dan peluang riset onomastik di Indonesia, *Aksara*, 31(1), 85.

20. Aksnes D. W. and Sivertsen, G. (2019) A criteria-based assessment of the artificial intelligence and algorithms, *Journal of Data and Information Science*, 4(1), 1–21.

21. Boulton, C. A., Kent, C. and Williams, H. T. (2018) Virtual learning environment engagement and learning outcomes at a "bricks-and-mortar" university, *Computers & Education*, 126, 129–142.

22. Gaviria-Marin, M., Merigo, J. M. and Popa, S. (2018) Twenty years of the journal of knowledge management: A bibliometric analysis, *Journal of Knowledge Management*, 22(8), 1655–1687.

23. Calongne, C., Sheehy, P. and Stricker, A. (2013) Gemeinschaft Identity in a Gesellschaft Metaverse, in *The Immersive Internet*, R. Teigland and D. Power, (Eds.) Palgrave Macmillan UK, 180–191.

24. Yardley I. (2024) The identity of one: Conservation of the circle, https://medium.com/the-circular-theory/the-identity-of-one-a6f37686cece (last accessed on 15 April, 2024)

25. Kadry, S., Dhanaraj, R. K. and Manthiramoorthy, C. (2024) Res-Unet based blood vessel segmentation and cardio vascular disease prediction using chronological chef-based optimization algorithm based deep residual network from retinal fundus images, *Multimedia Tools and Applications*, 1–30.

Index

W